MW00736843

Blood Management:
Options for Better Patient Care

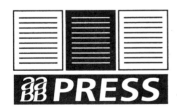

PRESS

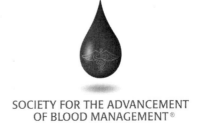

SOCIETY FOR THE ADVANCEMENT
OF BLOOD MANAGEMENT®

Other related publications available from the AABB:

Standards for Perioperative Autologous Blood Collection and Administration, 3rd Edition
Edited by Sarah J. Ilstrup, MD

Perioperative Blood Management: A Physician's Handbook, 1st Edition
Edited by Jonathan H. Waters, MD, and Jerome L. Gottschall, MD

The Transfusion Committee: Putting Patient Safety First
Edited by Sunita Saxena, MD, and Ira A. Shulman, MD

To purchase books or to inquire about other book services, including chapter reprints and large-quantity sales, please contact our sales department:
- 866.222.2498 (within the United States)
- +1 301.215.6499 (outside the United States)
- +1 301.951.7150 (fax)
- www.aabb.org>Bookstore

AABB customer service representatives are available by telephone from 8:30 am to 5:00 pm ET, Monday through Friday, excluding holidays.

Blood Management:
Options for Better Patient Care

Editor

Jonathan H. Waters, MD
Magee-Womens Hospital
University of Pittsburgh Medical Center
Pittsburgh, Pennsylvaniaa

AABB Press
Bethesda, Maryland
2008

AABB
8101 Glenbrook Road
Bethesda, Maryland 20814-2749

ISBN NO. 978-1-56395-253-1
Printed in the United States

Library of Congress Cataloging-in-Publication Data

Blood management : options for better patient care / editor, Jonathan H. Waters.
    p. ; cm.
Includes bibliographical references and index.
ISBN 978-1-56395-253-1
1. Blood--Transfusion. 2. Blood banks. I. Waters, Jonathan H.
[DNLM: 1. Blood Transfusion. 2. Blood Banks--organization & administration.
3. Perioperative Care. WB 356 B6539 2008]

RM171.B588 2008
362.17'84--dc22

2008008088

Contributors

Egle Bavry, MD
Cleveland Clinic
Cleveland, Ohio

Antonio Cassara, MD
Children's Hospital of Pittsburgh
University of Pittsburgh
Medical Center
Pittsburgh, Pennsylvania

Davy H. Cheng, MD, MSc, FRCP(C)
University of Western Ontario
London, Ontario, Canada

Ann Craig, MBChB
University of Western Ontario
London, Ontario, Canada

Robert Dyga, RN, CCP
BioTronics
University of Pittsburgh
Medical Center
Pittsburgh, Pennsylvania

Patricia A. Ford, MD
Joan Karnell Cancer Center
Philadelphia, Pennsylvania

T. Clark Gamblin, MD
UPMC Liver Cancer Center
University of Pittsburgh
Pittsburgh, Pennsylvania

David A. Geller, MD
UPMC Liver Cancer Center
University of Pittsburgh
Pittsburgh, Pennsylvania

Lawrence Tim Goodnough, MD
Stanford University
Stanford, California

Timothy J. Hannon, MD
St. Vincent Hospital and
Healthcare Center
Indianapolis, Indiana

Felicia A. Ivascu, MD
William Beaumont Hospital
Royal Oak, Michigan

Vivek Maheshwari, MD
UPMC Liver Cancer Center
University of Pittsburgh
Pittsburgh, Pennsylvania

Gregory A. Nuttall, MD
Mayo College of Medicine
Rochester, Minnesota

William C. Oliver, MD
Mayo College of Medicine
Rochester, Minnesota

Sherri Ozawa, RN
Englewood Hospital and
Medical Center
Englewood, New Jersey

Antonio Pepe, MD
University of Miami
Miami, Florida

Fiona E. Ralley, BSc, MBChB, FRCA
University of Western Ontario
London, Ontario, Canada

Gary D. Reeder, CP
Hema Rx Corporation
Broomfield, Colorado

Tanuja Rijhwani, MBBS, MPH
Englewood Hospital and
Medical Center
Englewood, New Jersey

Paula Santrach, MD
The Mayo Clinic
Rochester, Minnesota

Carl I. Schulman, MD, MSPH
University of Miami
Miami, Florida

Aryeh Shander, MD, FCCM, FCCP
Englewood Hospital and
Medical Center
Englewood, New Jersey

Doreen E. Soliman, MD
Children's Hospital of Pittsburgh
University of Pittsburgh
Medical Center
Pittsburgh, Pennsylvania

Judith A. Sullivan, MS, MT(ASCP)SBB, CQA(ASQ)
AABB
Bethesda, Maryland

Dale F. Szpisjak, MD, MPH
Uniformed Services University
of the Health Sciences
Bethesda, Maryland

Elora Thorpe, RN, BSN
St. Luke's Hospital of Kansas City
Kansas City, Missouri

Minh-Ha Tran, DO
University of Pittsburgh
Pittsburgh, Pennsylvania

Jo Valenti, RN
Kennedy Health System
Stratford, New Jersey

Janet F. R. Waters, MD, MBA
John P. Martha Neuroscience
and Pain Institute
Johnstown, Pennsylvania

Jonathan H. Waters, MD
Magee-Womens Hospital
University of Pittsburgh
Medical Center
Pittsburgh, Pennsylvania

Mark H. Yazer, MD, FRCP(C)
The Institute for Transfusion Medicine
University of Pittsburgh
Pittsburgh, Pennsylvania

Table of Contents

*Lawrence Tim Goodnough, MD; Minh-Ha Tran, DO;
   and Mark H. Yazer, MD, FRCP(C)*

Patricia A. Ford, MD

Mark H. Yazer, MD, FRCP(C)

Preface

THIS BOOK REPRESENTS A COLLECTIVE EF-
fort of many authors to give the reader a theoretical
and technical understanding of blood management
practices. Blood management encompasses a wide
variety of strategies intended to optimize patient outcome, including efforts to reduce or avoid allogeneic transfusion
as well as to administer allogeneic components and products
most appropriately.

Many of the techniques espoused in this text are not new; yet
many of the strategies have not gained widespread usage. The
reason for this is threefold. First, little information is available to
describe how to perform these techniques. Second, because
generally no quality measures have been used with the techniques, adverse patient outcomes have resulted. Finally, many of
the techniques are minimally effective as stand-alone strategies.

Perhaps the best "mission statement" for this body of work
could be summed up as the following: to emphasize that optimal patient care should involve a combination of blood management strategies rather than just one or two. When multiple
strategies are combined, a dramatic synergy can be obtained,
often producing surprisingly good patient outcomes. In this author's experience using combined blood management strategies,
patients have tolerated 15- to 20-L blood losses without the
need for allogeneic blood components.

This textbook was written in conjunction with a handbook using a large proportion of the same base material. In keeping with a handbook format, the editors of *Perioperative Blood Management: A Physician's Handbook*, 1st edition, condensed many chapters written for this textbook into a more concise, easily accessible resource. Thus, readers of the handbook may find much of the material familiar, including some passages that have been left unchanged. Still, large portions of this book, including many whole chapters—on topics such as program development, cancer, and quality systems, to name a few—are completely new. The expansion of the chapter on blood management in pediatric surgery is particularly significant as it is an area with very little available in the literature. As a whole, this much fuller text is intended to give the interested reader a broader understanding of the concepts and techniques that represent the practice of blood management.

The book is intended to be a reference for surgeons, anesthesiologists, perfusionists, transfusion specialists, clinicians, nurses, and other members of the health-care team who provide care to patients undergoing surgery. It reflects a joint effort by AABB and the Society for the Advancement of Blood Management (SABM). Both organizations have identified the need for a variety of resources to educate health-care providers about the application of these techniques; this book is one tool. The latest advances in blood management may be followed by taking advantage of the offerings from AABB or SABM through their Web sites, annual meetings, and other educational resources.

It has been a rewarding experience to participate in the alliance between AABB and SABM to inform practitioners and help to enrich their expertise in this fascinating area of patient care. Special thanks are due to Laurie Munk and Jay Pennington at AABB for their relentless assistance in producing this valuable resource.

Jonathan H. Waters, MD
Editor

About the Editor

Jonathan H. Waters, MD, is Chief of Anesthesia Services at Magee-Womens Hospital, part of the University of Pittsburgh Medical Center. In addition, he is Medical Director of the Perioperative Blood Management Program of the University of Pittsburgh Health System. Before arriving at Magee in 2004, he was Head of OB/Gyn Anesthesia as well as Director of the Autotransfusion Service at the Cleveland Clinic Foundation. During his tenure at the Clinic, he developed the first AABB-accredited blood management program.

Dr. Waters received an undergraduate degree in physics at Missouri University of Science and Technology (formerly the University of Missouri-Rolla) before attending medical school at George Washington University and completing a residency at New York University Medical Center. His areas of expertise include transfusion management, fluid resuscitation, and acid-base theory. He has been honored to present his research at the New York Academy of Medicine, the Hong Kong Academy of Medicine, and the Mexican College of Anesthesiologists. He has also been invited as a visiting professor at numerous academic institutions, including Duke University and Sloan-Kettering Cancer Institute.

In addition to conducting research, Dr. Waters maintains active roles in many professional societies. In September 2007, he began a two-year term as President of the Society for the Advancement of Blood Management. He has served on the editorial board of the journal *TRANSFUSION* and is a member of the AABB Clinical Transfusion Medicine Committee as well as the Transfusion Committee for the American Society of Anesthesiologists. As a main program coordinator for the Perioperative Blood Management Track of AABB's annual Spring Conference, he has assisted in organizing and executing this educational activity since its first program in 2003.

In: Waters JH, ed.
Blood Management: Options for Better Patient Care
Bethesda, MD: AABB Press, 2008

1

Why Blood Management?

JONATHAN H. WATERS, MD, AND
MARK H. YAZER, MD, FRCP(C)

MULTIPLE THERAPIES CAN BE USED TO REDUCE the use of allogeneic blood. This chapter provides an overview of such therapies. Beforehand, the risks associated with allogeneic transfusion will be discussed to give some understanding of why it is important to incorporate blood management practices. In addition to those risks, an important factor driving the increased use of perioperative blood management strategies is the cost of allogeneic

Jonathan H. Waters, MD, Chief and Visiting Associate Professor, Department of Anesthesiology, Magee-Womens Hospital, University of Pittsburgh Medical Center, Pittsburgh, Pennsylvania, and Mark H. Yazer, MD, FRCP(C), Medical Director, RBC Serology Reference Laboratory, The Institute for Transfusion Medicine, and Assistant Professor, Department of Pathology, University of Pittsburgh, Pittsburgh, Pennsylvania blood. The number of allogeneic Red Blood Cell (RBC) units transfused in the United States has risen from 11,804,000 in 1999 to 13,720,000 in 2004—an increase of 16%.[1] The estimated cost of those transfusions was in excess of $2 billion.[2] That cost does not take into account the complications associated with RBC transfusions.[3] According to a study by Vamvakas and Caven,[4] length of hospital stay is increased by 1.3% per RBC unit transfused, and hospital charges are increased by 2.0%. Likewise, Blumberg and colleagues[5] have shown a linear increase in length of stay with every unit of blood transfused. Thus, the $2-billion price tag does not truly represent the cost of allogeneic transfusions.

Risks of Allogeneic Blood Transfusion

Infectious Complications

Before considering the techniques of blood management, readers should understand the risks of allogeneic blood transfusion and should compare them with the risks of autologous blood transfusion (see Table 1-1). The risk of infectious complications is foremost in the minds of most people when they consider allogeneic transfusion. Modern donor screening and testing techniques have markedly reduced the risk of disease transmission; however, that risk is raised considerably when multiple units are transfused. For instance, the risk of having an infectious complication of any type, including human immunodeficiency virus (HIV), hepatitis C, and human T-cell lymphotropic virus (HTLV), is approximately 1:30,000 following transfusion of a single unit of blood.[6] But the patient receiving 10 units has an exposure risk close to 1:3000. Certainly, the risk of more common reactions is even more enhanced when multiple units are transfused. The current risk of receiving an HCV- or HIV-positive unit of blood that has undergone nucleic acid testing is approximately 1:1.9 million and 1:2.1 million, respectively.[7] Dis-

Table 1-1. Risks of Allogeneic vs Autologous Blood

Risks	Allogeneic Blood	PAD	Autologous Blood	
			Normovolemic Hemodilution	Blood Recovery
Viral exposure	+	–	–	–
Bacterial contamination	+	+	–	+
Immunomodulation	+	–	–	–
Reduced 2,3-DPG effects	+	+	–	–
Citrate exposure	+	+	+	–
Hyperkalemia	+	+	–	–
Mistransfusion (ABO incompatible transfusion)	+	+	–	–
Volume overload	+	+	Less likely	Less likely

"+" indicates a positive risk; "–" indicates no risk. PAD = preoperative autologous donation; DPG = diphosphoglycerate.

cussions that follow show that patients who require massive transfusion benefit most from blood recovery techniques.

Immunomodulation

The risk of immunosuppression following allogeneic blood transfusion is mentioned less often but can be of greater importance to short-term patient outcome than will be the risks of viral transmission.[8] The possibility that the transfusion of allogeneic blood might cause an immunosuppressive effect was first noticed in kidney transplant patients more than 30 years ago; transplant patients had a better outcome with their graft when they were transfused with allogeneic blood.[9] The apparent immunosuppression induced by blood transfusion is known as transfusion-related immunosuppression (TRIM) and is thought to be caused by the passenger lymphocytes in blood products. A recent study of a large number of renal allograft patients who were randomly assigned to receive or not to receive transfusions before transplantation once again demonstrated the apparent TRIM effect; those patients who were transfused before transplantation had significantly better 1- and 5-year graft survival rates.[10] Thus, the TRIM effect is beneficial for some patients.

Conversely, TRIM might worsen the condition of other patients. It is possible that the TRIM effect might cause enough immunosuppression to allow for increased cancer growth and to cause posttransfusion infections (ie, infections not borne in the component itself). A recent review by Blajchman[11] has highlighted the controversies in those areas. Blajchman combined the results of 87 observational and three randomized control trials (RCTs) of patients with various types of cancer and demonstrated that most studies indicated that allogeneic transfusion has a "significant adverse effect" on the survival of those patients. Causing an adverse effect was not an absolute trend, however. For most of the cancer types reviewed, at least one study each showed that allogeneic transfusion did not have an adverse effect on outcome. For patients with cervical and breast cancer, more studies suggested that allogeneic transfusion did not have a significant adverse effect on survival than those suggesting that TRIM was detrimental.[11]

The literature is equally divided when it comes to assessing the role of TRIM in causing postallogeneic transfusion infections. Blajchman reviewed eight RCTs that have been conducted to investigate whether TRIM is involved in causing perioperative infections in transfused patients. Although those studies could not be combined into a meta-analysis, the results were evenly split as to whether or not TRIM was associated with perioperative infections. Perhaps the TRIM effect is small and thus would require a high enrollment of patients for it to be demonstrated.[11]

Some controversy clearly exists regarding the extent of immunosuppressive effects; nevertheless, a sizeable body of literature seems to support the TRIM effect of allogeneic blood transfusion. Given that the mechanism of TRIM is currently thought to be related to white cells (or their breakdown products) that are present in blood components, a number of investigators have suggested that leukocyte reduction may ameliorate the risk of immunomodulation.[12-14] Currently, most countries of the industrialized world, with the exception of the United States and South Africa, use prestorage leukocyte-reduced blood products.[15] Mixed results have been published about whether such manipulation removes all of the TRIM effect.[16,17] A recently published Canadian study highlights the uncertainty of TRIM amelioration by leukocyte reduction.[18]

The charts of several thousand transfused patients who had cardiac surgery or hip fracture repair or who had spent time in an intensive care unit (ICU) were divided into two groups: those transfused before the nationwide implementation of universal leukocyte reduction (mid-1999) and those transfused after that implementation. The primary outcomes included suspected or confirmed infection and in-hospital mortality, while the secondary outcomes included various organ failures, antibiotic use, transfusion reactions, and fever. The group that was transfused with leukocyte-reduced blood suffered significantly less in-hospital mortality (p = 0.04), less antibiotic use, and fewer fevers (both p <0.01). The rates of infection were not significantly different between the two groups.[18] In any case, using autologous blood or blood from a perioperative blood recovery process would avoid the TRIM effect by giving patients their own white cells back.

Storage Lesion

Blood storage brings not only risks of immunomodulation and viral exposure but also alteration of the blood. The term "storage lesion" describes a number of metabolic and biochemical changes that occur in stored red cells. The most significant of the storage injuries is the decreased level of 2,3-diphosphoglycerate (2,3-DPG) in the stored cells. Decreased levels of 2,3-DPG shift the oxyhemoglobin dissociation curve to the left, making it more difficult for oxygen to be released from hemoglobin at the tissue level. In effect, the hemoglobin has higher affinity for the oxygen that it carries, thus rendering it less able to release the oxygen when it arrives in the tissue microvasculature. Restoration of normal levels of 2,3-DPG can take up to a day to occur following the reinfusion of stored blood; the time it takes for restoration means that the oxygen delivery of transfused blood is somewhat reduced compared to in-vivo blood. The clinical significance of this left shift has not been determined.

In a rat model of hemorrhagic shock, red cells stored for 28 days in citrate-phosphate-dextrose (CPD), SAGM, or citrate-phosphate-dextrose-adenine-1 (CPDA-1) were unable to raise the intestinal pO_2, thereby suggesting an important physiological consequence of the reduced levels of 2,3-DPG in stored blood. Only fresh red cells achieved that goal. Other metabolic parameters, including intestinal oxygen consumption and mesenteric venous pO_2, were improved following the transfusion of most varieties of fresh and stored red cells. Curiously, CPD-stored cells were an exception.[19]

Another study looking at changes in systemic oxygen uptake in rats transfused with 28-day-old CPDA-1 rat blood also demonstrated a failure to improve tissue oxygenation,[20] while a study of euvolemic, anemic patients in the ICU who were randomly assigned to receive either fresh (5 days old) or stored (20 days old) leukocyte-reduced RBC units failed to show any clinically significant differences between the two groups in terms of gastric tonometry or global indices of tissue oxygenation.[21] Thus, the clinical consequences of the transfusion of stored RBC units with reduced levels of 2,3-DPG remain uncertain. The use of perioperatively recovered blood would avoid the storage lesion; however, preoperatively donated and stored autologous blood would be affected.

Additionally, during storage the red cell undergoes a reduction in intracellular adenosine triphosphate (ATP), sialic acid, and nitric oxide, which results in a change in the red cell shape and deformability.[22-24] That conformational change may impair the red cell's ability to traverse through the smallest vessels (eg, capillaries) of the microcirculation. Some emerging evidence suggests that such conformational changes may impair tissue oxygen concentration.[25] This storage defect applies to both allogeneic and stored autologous blood but does not apply to intraoperatively recovered blood.

Storage of blood can also lead to electrolyte abnormalities. Increases in patient potassium concentrations can occur from lysis of red cells as they age during storage.[26] Although the amount of potassium per milliliter in a 42-day-old unit of RBCs preserved with additive solution (AS) can appear staggering, the relatively minute plasma volume of the unit renders the total amount of potassium very small. For example, the potassium concentration at the outdate of an AS-preserved RBC unit can reach levels of upwards of 50 mEq/L. Because there are approximately only 30 mL of plasma in the entire unit, the overall amount of potassium in the unit is less than 2 mEq.[27] However, in spite of the small quantity of potassium in a typical AS RBC unit, life-threatening hyperkalemia can occur under circumstances of massive transfusion when the kidney's ability to remove the potassium is overwhelmed.

Another electrolyte abnormality stemming from transfusion is hypocalcemia; it can occur when the citrate anticoagulant in the transfused unit chelates the patient's autologous calcium. Normally, citrate is rapidly metabolized in the liver, and its use as a blood-bank anticoagulant is clinically benign under typical circumstances. However, at rapid transfusion rates or in patients who metabolize citrate slowly (such as small children and patients with hypothermia, hypotension, or liver dysfunction), hypocalcemia can occur. Hypocalcemia can lead to myocardial and clotting dysfunction. Again, by using preoperatively recovered and washed blood, those adverse metabolic reactions can be avoided.

Mistransfusion

Receiving a mistransfusion, that is, receiving ABO-incompatible RBCs, is a leading transfusion-related cause of death. Mistransfusions are entirely preventable and are largely caused by clerical errors in the procurement of the patient specimen, in patient identification, or during pretransfusion testing in the blood bank. Although autologous blood is required to be stored separately from allogeneic units, this practice is not a guarantee of safety. Clerical errors can still occur with autologous blood, thereby resulting in mistransfusions just as they do with allogeneic units. The risks of mistransfusion are virtually nonexistent with intraoperatively recovered blood and with acute normovolemic hemodilution, assuming that patients' blood is reinfused before they leave the operating room.

Circulatory Overload

In addition, volume overload reactions can occur with both autologous and allogeneic RBC transfusions. Those reactions, which are characterized by dyspnea, decreased oxygen saturation, and chest pain, are caused by the inability of the recipients' cardiovascular and respiratory systems to handle the increased intravascular volume associated with transfusion. In fact, it is likely that some autologous RBC units are "readministered" to the recipient simply because they are available and not necessarily for actual medical reasons. That practice might increase the incidence of volume overload reactions among autologous blood recipients. Such reactions are probably less common in patients receiving perioperatively recovered blood and acute normovolemic hemodilution because of the generally smaller volumes of product administered, the close scrutiny of the patient, the ability to regulate the patient's volume status quickly in the operating room, and the fluid losses sustained during the operation itself.

Other Adverse Effects

Other adverse effects of transfusion include acute and delayed hemolytic reactions, allergic and anaphylactic reactions, bacterial contamination of blood products leading to septicemia in the recipient, and transfusion-related acute lung injury (TRALI). Those adverse effects will be covered in other chapters throughout this book.

Finally, interest has arisen over the possibility of transmission of disease-producing genes through blood transfusion.[28] Studies concerning the risk of such transmission in humans are limited to an increased risk of non-Hodgkin's lymphoma in patients who have received a blood transfusion.[29] Nevertheless, it is interesting to speculate about the ramifications of such a finding, which provides another reason to avoid allogeneic blood.

Blood management can encompass both the medical and surgical patient. For the surgical patient, perioperative blood management covers the time from the patient's surgical booking, through the operation itself, and into the recovery process. At each step of the way, effective use of blood preservation and recovery techniques can preserve scarce blood components and recover many of the components that would otherwise be lost. For a medical patient, areas for conservation are not as well defined. Therefore, this book will focus on the perioperative management of the surgical patient.

Overview of Blood Management Strategies

Blood management strategies should be addressed during the entire perioperative course. Different phases of a patient's operative course will mandate different approaches to blood management (see Table 1-2). This section uses a chronological approach to discuss various blood management strategies.

Table 1-2. Components of a Perioperative Blood Management Program

Blood management should be addressed over the entire perioperative course. Components for each stage of the perioperative period are outlined below:

Preoperative Period
1. Erythropoietin
2. Iron, folate, B_{12} supplements
3. Avoidance of anticoagulant medications
    a. NSAIDs
    b. Herbal supplements
    c. Antiplatelet drugs
    d. Heparin/warfarin

Intraoperative Period
1. Red cell avoidance
    a. Normovolemic hemodilution
    b. Preoperative autologous donation
    c. Blood recovery
2. Coagulation system avoidance
    a. Component sequestration
    b. Normovolemic hemodilution
3. Adjuncts
    a. Point-of-care testing
    b. Microsampling
    c. Drug therapy: desmopressin, aprotinin, ε-aminocaproic acid, recombinant Factor VIIa
    d. Deliberate hypotension
    e. Maintenance of normothermia
    f. Avoidance of normal saline
    g. Appropriate positioning

Postoperative Period
1. Recovered blood from wound drainage (washed or unwashed)
2. Erythropoietin
3. Hyperbaric oxygen therapy

NSAIDs = nonsteroidal anti-inflammatory drugs.

Preoperative Strategies

In the preoperative period, attention should be paid to the pro-spective surgical patient's hematocrit. A database review was conducted by the Cleveland Clinic Foundation of all patients who received transfusions during the perioperative period. Of 3079 patients who had received 1 to 2 units of blood during their surgery, the median preoperative hemoglobin was 12.1 g/dL for females and 13.2 g/dL for males. Those figures show that a large number of patients presented to the operating room with anemia and that the use of 1 to 2 units of blood may have been avoided by optimizing the patient's preoperative hemat-ocrit. Optimization of the hematocrit can take place through the use of iron, vitamins, erythropoietin, and androgens. Another is-sue that should be addressed is the patient's use of prescription and over-the-counter medications that impair coagulation, in-cluding herbal supplements, aspirin, and numerous new anti-platelet drugs.

Intraoperative Strategies

Patients who wish to avoid RBC transfusion during the course of a surgical operation have a number of alternative strategies to consider: preoperative autologous donation, normovolemic hemodilution, blood recovery, and component sequestration. There are also adjunctive strategies worthy of consideration.

Preoperative Autologous Donation

In the favored choice of many patients, preoperative autologous donation, patients donate their blood before a surgical proce-dure for their own subsequent use. The blood bank draws and stores the blood until the need arises for it, typically during sur-gery or in the postoperative period. However, more than 50% of those units are never used.[1,30] Thus, the cost of preoperative autologous donation, when compared to the health benefit gained, is high. It has been estimated to be as much as $23 million for every quality-adjusted year of life saved.[31] That cost, although it may be exaggerated, is but one of multiple disadvantages that exist.[32] Medical conditions such as anemia (hemoglobin <11 gm/dL), pregnancy, and indwelling intravenous lines may prevent preoperative donation. It has been suggested through mathematical modeling that, instead of preventing allogeneic transfusion, autologous RBC transfusions occur at an earlier time during a surgical procedure with significant blood loss.[33] Such action would seem to negate the purpose of donation. Autologous donation also requires advanced planning; mistransfusion, as detailed above, might occur; and bacterial contamination of the unit during processing is a possibility. In addition, storage causes some deterioration in the quality of the blood. For those reasons, preoperative autologous donation is now heavily discouraged as a blood management option.

Normovolemic Hemodilution

Normovolemic hemodilution is another technique designed to avoid allogeneic blood transfusion. The procedure entails drawing autologous blood and replacing it with intravenous fluids.[34,35] The replacement of blood with asanguinous colloid or crystalloid solutions maintains the normal circulating blood volume and oxygen delivery.[36] The primary goal of this technique is to create a relative anemia in the patient so that blood shed during the operative procedure effectively has a reduced number of red cells in it. Once the threat of blood loss is diminished, the harvested cells are returned to the patient. This technique minimizes the loss of crucial blood during the operative procedure.

The advantages to normovolemic hemodilution are as follows: 1) it may reduce the need for allogeneic blood during surgery, 2) no storage injury occurs to the blood, 3) the blood contains viable clotting factors, 4) minimal cost is incurred, and 5) the circuit used for this procedure can be kept in constant contact with the patient, thus making it a viable option for many patients who are members of the Jehovah's Witness denomination, as well as a way to prevent mistransfusion. The most significant disadvantage to normovolemic hemodilution is its ineffectiveness in preventing allogeneic transfusions. The estimated savings attributable to normovolemic hemodilution can amount to 100-200 mL, hardly enough to significantly reduce allogeneic exposure.[37]

Perioperative Blood Recovery

Blood recovery offers many advantages when compared to autologous preoperative donation and normovolemic hemodilution. A patient's entire blood volume can be processed before he or she needs allogeneic red cell supplementation if a focus is made to maximize the system's capture of red cells. For maximum efficiency, low suction pressures and washing of surgical sponges must be performed.[38]

Blood recovery is quite cost-effective. The cost of 1 unit of recovered blood is comparable to the cost of 1 unit of preoperatively donated blood; however, the blood recovery setup can be used to produce multiple subsequent units without significantly increasing the cost beyond the initial outlay. Subsequent recovery costs relate to the technologist's time in producing each unit. The cost of preoperative autologous donation increases linearly with each unit. With the blood recovery equipment, there are no limitations on the number of units that can be processed. In preoperative autologous donation, though, allogeneic avoidance is limited by the number of units that have been predonated.

Blood recovery also compares favorably in cost with allogeneic transfusions when larger volumes of blood loss are involved. As described, most costs of blood recovery relate to the setup cost, with a cost-neutral point being reached at approximately 2 units of recovered blood.

The major disadvantage to blood recovery is that it requires dedicated technical support. Without such dedication, inadequate washing and concentration of the blood can lead to anemia and disseminated intravascular coagulation. In an article on blood recovery, in an era that predated dedicated personnel, O'Hara and colleagues[39] from the Cleveland Clinic reported on a lack of red cell avoidance with the use of recovery techniques. They reported an average cell salvage unit hematocrit of 31%. Hematocrits of recovered blood should range between 50% and 70% depending on the method of processing and the machine used. Lower hematocrits in the recovered unit will hemodilute patients, thereby negating any positive benefit. A lack of both training and supervision of the personnel operating the equipment led to processing "on convenience." In other words, the blood was processed before enough red cells were collected so that the final product was predominantly normal saline rather than red cells.

Coagulation dysfunction following the administration of recovered blood has been attributed to activation of platelets and leukocytes during the centrifugation process.[40,41] In a study of the "salvaged blood syndrome" involving 36,000 cases, Tawes and Duvall[42] conclude that the problem occurs with inadequate bowl filling and inexperienced personnel. The experience of this chapter's authors supports that conclusion.

An Alternative to Transfusion of Clotting Factors and Platelets

Two interrelated methods for avoiding transfusion of plasma and platelets are available. Normovolemic hemodilution, which was discussed earlier, can be used to provide these blood components. If enough whole blood is removed, adequate plasma and platelets will be available to correct any perioperative coagulation dysfunction. The limitation to using normovolemic hemodilution for this purpose is that anemia can potentially limit the amount of whole blood that can be comfortably removed. Under this circumstance, component sequestration can be performed. In this technique, the whole blood that is removed is centrifuged into its components—plasma, red cells, and platelets. The red cells are given back in order to maintain an acceptable hemoglobin, whereas the plasma and platelets are kept for readministration at a later time.

Adjunctive Strategies

Many strategies can add to the efficacy of the previously discussed techniques. Primary to those adjunctive strategies is the use of point-of-care testing. Such testing allows the anesthesiologist or surgeon to make decisions based on quantitative data rather than on an estimate of the patient's need that is based on observing blood loss. Point-of-care testing allows microliter samples to be used to obtain hemoglobin, protime, and partial thromboplastin time, as well as to assess platelet number and function.

Other important strategies include microsampling and maintenance of patient temperature. Microsampling involves drawing the minimum amount of blood necessary to perform a chosen laboratory study. Maintenance of temperature is important to maintain functional platelets. Low patient temperature has also been implicated in leading to higher incidence of postoperative infection.

References

1. Whitaker BI, Sullivan M. The 2005 nationwide blood collection and utilization survey report, Bethesda, MD: AABB, 2006.
2. Wallace EL, Surgenor DM, Hao HS, et al. Collection and transfusion of blood and blood components in the United States. Transfusion 1995;35:802-12.
3. Lawrence VA, Birch S, Gafni A. The impact of new clinical guidelines on the North American blood economy. Transfus Med Rev 1994;8:232-41.
4. Vamvakas EC, Caven JH. Allogeneic blood transfusion, hospital charges, and length of hospitalization: A study of 487 consecutive patients undergoing colorectal cancer resection. Arch Pathol Lab Med 1998;12:145-51.
5. Blumberg N, Kirkley SA, Heal JM. A cost analysis of autologous and allogeneic transfusions in hip-replacement surgery. Am J Surg 1996;171:324-30.
6. Schreiber GB, Busch MP, Kleinman SH, Korelitz JJ. The risk of transfusion-transmitted viral infections: The Retrovirus Epidemiology Donor Study. N Engl J Med 1996;334:1685-90.
7. Dodd RY, Notari EP IV, Stramer SL. Current prevalence and incidence of infectious disease markers and estimated window-period risk in the American Red Cross blood donor population. Transfusion 2002;42:975-9.
8. Perkins H. Transfusion-induced immunologic unresponsiveness. Transfus Med Rev 1988;2:196-203.

9. Opelz G, Sengar DP, Mickey MR, Terasaki PI. Effect of blood transfusions on subsequent kidney transplants. Transplant Proc 1973;5:253-9.
10. Opelz G, Vanrenterghem Y, Kirste G, et al. Prospective evaluation of pretransplant blood transfusions in cadaver kidney recipients. Transplantation 1997; 63:964-7.
11. Blajchman MA. The clinical benefits of the leukoreduction of blood products. J Trauma 2006;60:S83-S90.
12. van de Watering LMG, Hermans J, Houbiers JGA, et al. Beneficial effects of leukocyte depletion of transfused blood on postoperative complications in patients undergoing cardiac surgery: A randomized clinical trial. Circulation 1998; 97:562-8.
13. Jensen LS, Kissmeyer-Nielsen P, Wolff B, Qvist N. Randomised comparison of leucocyte-depleted versus buffy-coat-poor blood transfusion and complications after colorectal surgery. Lancet 1996;348:841-5.
14. Vamvakas EC. Transfusion-associated cancer recurrence and postoperative infection: Meta-analysis of randomized, controlled clinical trials. Transfusion 1996; 36:175-86.
15. Blajchman MA. Transfusion-associated immunomodulation and universal white cell reduction: Are we putting the cart before the horse? Transfusion 1999;39: 665-70.
16. Blajchman MA. Allogeneic blood transfusions, immunomodulation, and postoperative bacterial infection: Do we have the answers yet? Transfusion 1997;37: 121-5.
17. Duffy G, Neal KR. Differences in post-operative infection rates between patients receiving autologous and allogeneic blood transfusion: A meta-analysis of published randomized and nonrandomized studies. Transfus Med 1996;6: 325-8.
18. Hebert PC, Fergusson D, Blajchman MA, et al. Clinical outcomes following institution of the Canadian universal leukoreduction program for red blood cell transfusions. JAMA 2003;289:1941-9.
19. van Bommel J, de Korte D, Lind A, et al. The effect of the transfusion of stored RBCs on intestinal microvascular oxygenation in the rat. Transfusion 2001; 41:1515-23.
20. Fitzgerald RD, Martin CM, Dietz GE, et al. Transfusing red blood cells stored in citrate phosphate dextrose adenine-1 for 28 days fails to improve tissue oxygenation in rats. Crit Care Med 1997;25:726-32.
21. Walsh TS, McArdle F, McLellan SA, et al. Does the storage time of transfused red blood cells influence regional or global indexes of tissue oxygenation in anemic critically ill patients? Crit Care Med 2004;32:364-71.
22. Stuart J, Nash GB. Red cell deformability and hematological disorders. Blood Rev 1990;4:141-7.
23. Greenwald TJ, Bryan DJ, Dumaswala VJ. Erythrocyte membrane vesiculation and changes in membrane composition during storage in citrate-phophate-dextrose-adenine 1. Vox Sang 1984;47:261-70.
24. Piagnerelli M, Boudjeltia KZ, Vanhaeverbeek M, Vincent JL. Red blood cell rheology in sepsis. Intensive Care Med 2003;29:1052-61.

25. Tsai AG, Cabrales P, Intaglietta M. Microvascular perfusion upon exchange transfusion with stored red blood cells in normovolemic anemic conditions. Transfusion 2004;44:1626-34.
26. Keidan I, Amir G, Mandel M, Mishali D. The metabolic effects of fresh versus old stored blood in the priming of cardiopulmonary bypass solution for pediatric patients. J Thorac Cardiovasc Surg 2004;127:949-52.
27. Brecher ME, ed. Technical manual. 15th ed. Bethesda, MD: AABB, 2005: 186-7.
28. Dzik WH, Okayama A. Can blood transfusion transmit disease-producing genes? Transfusion 1999;39:795-800.
29. Vamvakas EC. Allogeneic blood transfusion as a risk factor for the subsequent development of non-Hodgkin's lymphoma. Transfus Med Rev 2000;14:258-68.
30. Renner SW, Howanitz PJ, Bachner P. Preoperative autologous blood donation in 612 hospitals: A College of American Pathologists' Q-probes study of quality issues in transfusion practice. Arch Pathol Lab Med 1992;116:613-19.
31. Etchason J, Petz L, Keeler E, et al. The cost effectiveness of preoperative autologous blood donations. N Engl J Med 1995;332:719-24.
32. Blumberg N. Anesthesiology. New Engl J Med 1998;338:684-7.
33. Cohen JA, Brecher ME. Preoperative autologous blood donation: Benefit or detriment? A mathematical analysis. Transfusion 1995;35:640-4.
34. Ereth M, Oliver W, Santrach P. Subspecialty clinics: Perioperative interventions to decrease transfusion of allogenic blood products. Mayo Clinic Proc 1994; 69:575-86.
35. Olsfanger D, Fredman B, Goldstein B, et al. Acute normovolemic hemodilution decreases postoperative allogenic blood transfusion after total knee replacement. Br J Anaesth 1997;79:317-21.
36. D'Ambra M, Kaplan D. Alternatives to allogeneic blood use in surgery: Acute normovolemic hemodilution and preoperative autologous donation. Am J Surg 1995;170:49S-51S.
37. Goodnough LT, Grishaber JE, Monk TG, Catalona WJ. Acute preoperative hemodilution in patients undergoing radical prostatectomy: A case study analysis of efficacy. Anesth Analg 1994;78:932-7.
38. Ronai AK, Glass JJ, Shapiro AS. Improving autologous blood harvest: Recovery of red cells from sponges and suction. Anaesth Intensive Care 1987;15:421-4.
39. O'Hara PJ, Hertzer NR, Santilli PH, Beven EG. Intraoperative autotransfusion during abdominal aortic reconstruction. Am J Surg 1983;145:215-20.
40. McKie JS, Herzenberg JE. Coagulopathy complicating intraoperative blood salvage in a patient who had idiopathic scoliosis: A case report. J Bone Joint Surg 1997;79A:1391-4.
41. Bull BS, Bull MH. The salvaged blood syndrome: A sequel to mechanochemical activation of platelets and leukocytes? Blood Cells 1990;16:5-20.
42. Tawes RL, Duvall TB. Is the "Salvaged-cell syndrome" myth or reality? Am J Surg 1996;172:172-4.

In: Waters JH, ed.
Blood Management: Options for Better Patient Care
Bethesda, MD: AABB Press, 2008

2

Economics of
Blood Management

JANET F. R. WATERS, MD, MBA

 BLOOD MANAGEMENT IS BIG BUSINESS. DURing 2007, it is estimated that Americans paid 16.2% of their gross domestic income, or $2.272 trillion, on health care.[1] The cost of blood and blood products represents 1% of these health-care expenditures.[2] Cost-effective management of blood is of interest to patients, physicians, administrators, and insurers.

This chapter addresses cost considerations of the various modalities of blood management. It begins with an introduction to three types of cost studies that are often used by medical economists. This is followed by a survey of current cost data that covers several modalities of blood management, including the following:

Janet F. R. Waters, MD, MBA, General Neurologist, John P. Martha Neuroscience and Pain Institute, Johnstown, Pennsylvania

- Preoperative autologous donation (PAD).
- Bone marrow stimulation (erythropoietin).
- Blood recovery.
- Acute normovolemic hemodilution (ANH).
- Elevation of transfusion threshold.

Medical Economic Analysis

John Eisenberg provides a clear outline of medical economics in his JAMA article titled "Clinical Economics: A Guide to the Economic Analysis of Clinical Practices."[3] He describes three types of economic analyses: cost-identification, cost-effectiveness, and cost-benefit analyses.

Cost-Identification Analysis

A cost-identification study determines only the cost of a given treatment. It does not address the effectiveness of the treatment, nor does it give guidance as to the best treatment choice. It simply adds together all of the costs associated with providing a service or procedure. A well-done study will address direct and indirect costs, and it will include both fixed and variable components.

Direct costs are those that can be specifically traced to an activity, department, or product. Examples are the costs of labor, equipment, education, and supplies needed to provide a service. Direct costs may be fixed or variable. **Indirect costs** are those that cannot be traced to a process, department, or product. Examples in the hospital setting are electricity, heat, and security guards.

Fixed costs will remain the same regardless of the number of units or services provided, whereas **variable costs** will increase or decrease with production rates. For example, the cost of hiring three full-time technicians to provide blood recovery services is a fixed cost. The annual salary of these individuals will not change, assuming no overtime is needed. The disposables used during blood recovery are a variable cost. If only one patient per day receives blood recovery services, only one set of disposables is used. If five patients per day receive services, then five sets of disposables are used.

A cost-identification analysis will provide a compilation of indirect and direct fixed and variable costs to determine the cost of providing a service or procedure.

Cost-Effectiveness Analysis

Cost-effectiveness analysis measures both the cost and the outcome of a given treatment. Outcomes are reported in a unit of measurement such as years-of-life extension, years of continued productive employment, or quality-adjusted life years (QALYs). Measurement of QALYs gives an indication of how a given treatment will extend life and what the quality of those extended years will be. For example, a year of life with hemiparesis or pain might be equal to 0.5 years of healthy life.

Cost-effective analysis allows one to examine two or more treatment options that have differing costs and outcomes. It also allows one to consider an increase in use of resources if the increase will improve outcome. The results are generally presented as cost per unit of outcome.

Cost-Benefit Analysis

Cost-benefit analysis measures both cost and benefit by the same unit, often in dollars. Results are presented as ratios of benefit to cost or as net values of benefit minus cost. Eisenberg[3] describes an exemplary lead-screening study that includes cost-effective and cost-benefit components:

In the cost-effectiveness component of the study, free erythrocyte protoporphyrin screening was found to cost $2890 per case of learning disability prevented and $19,380 per case of mental retardation averted (cost per unit of outcome obtained).

The cost-benefit analysis demonstrated that in communities where the prevalence of lead poisoning is greater than 7%, free erythrocyte protoporphyrin screening also saves money for society. This suggests that at prevalence rates below 7% the cost will be greater than the benefit and that at prevalence rates above 7% the benefit (in terms of averted costs) will be greater than the cost.[3]

The value of any cost analysis is highly dependent on the perspective of the study. When assessing the costs described in each study, one must consider who is bearing these costs. Is it the patient, the hospital, the payor, or society as a whole? Because resources for medical care are limited, physicians must weigh and balance the use of additional resources to produce the best outcomes for the maximum number of patients. Economic analyses assist in that decision-making process.

Modalities of Blood Management

In the remainder of the chapter, the above principles will be applied in the review of current economic studies of blood management.

Preoperative Autologous Donation

Approximately 4% to 5% of blood that is collected is acquired through PAD.[4] The expense of PAD is higher than that of allogeneic blood. The additional costs of collection and storage combined with the frequent need to discard unused units bring the average cost of a PAD unit to a level that is 40% to 60% above the average cost of an allogeneic unit.[5]

In the 1980s, viral contamination of the US blood supply with human immunodeficiency virus (HIV) and non-A, non-B hepatitis led to widespread use of PAD. Legislative action in New Jersey[6] and California[7] mandated that this option be available and discussed with patients. The reduction in exposure to these infections was desirable from both a societal and economic perspective.

In subsequent decades, because the pretesting of blood has markedly reduced the presence of these viruses in the blood supply, the cost-effectiveness of PAD has been called into question. Currently, the rates of HIV contamination are estimated to have been reduced to 1 in 7,299,000 units. Hepatitis C is found in 1 in 3,636,000 units, and hepatitis B is found in 1 in 339,000 units.[8] Certainly, contracting these diseases can be devastating on an individual level. However, it must be considered that, from a broad financial perspective, the overall cost to the community of treating the few patients who become infected through allogeneic transfusion amounts to just a few dollars per unit transfused[9]—much lower than the cost of PAD per unit, not to mention the higher discard rate associated with PAD.

Bacterial contamination is a more common complication of transfusion, and it affects the PAD supply as well as the allogeneic supply. Bacteria can be introduced at the time of collection.[10] During storage, the bacteria level will increase, leading to catastrophic inoculation at the time of transfusion. Contamination with gram-negative organisms occurs in 1 unit per million of Red Blood Cells (RBCs).

Factors that favor a better outcome for autologous transfusion over allogeneic transfusion include the avoidance of transmission of infectious agents of diseases such as Chagas' disease and Creutzfeldt-Jakob disease, as well as other unknown agents that may make themselves evident at a future date. Again, because these diseases are relatively rare, the added cost of treating infected patients, when spread across all allogeneic units, is not significant,[4] especially when compared with the cost of PAD.

A number of studies have reported that allogeneic blood is associated with a higher rate of postoperative fever and infection.[11] Modulation of the immune system is felt to be responsible. This effect has been associated with a longer length of stay and higher costs of hospitalization.

One study[12] reviewed records of 487 patients undergoing colorectal cancer resection. The influence of allogeneic transfusion in explaining the variation in the observed length of stay was calculated after adjusting for the effects of 20 confounding factors that related to severity of illness, difficulty of operation, and risk of postoperative infection. The mean length of stay was 16.7 days in the transfused group, with hospital charges of $28,101, as compared with 10.3 days in the untransfused group at a cost of $15,978.

Another study[13] noted that the postoperative infection rate of patients undergoing hip replacement or spine surgery was 7 to 10 times higher in those who received allogeneic blood than in those who received no blood or PAD. The infection rate of the PAD group was the same as the infection rate of patients who received no transfusions at all. Allogeneic, but not autologous, blood transfusion was associated in a dose-dependent manner with longer hospital stays and higher charges. Total charges for patients receiving 1 to 3 units of autologous blood was $13,000, while patients receiving 2 to 3 units of allogeneic blood incurred hospital costs of $18,000.

At issue with the two studies is whether the need for allogeneic blood is a marker for more extensive disease, or whether allogeneic blood is in fact a causative agent in the extension of hospital stay and costs.

Another study has shown that the higher risks of infection associated with allogeneic blood transfusion are mitigated by leukocyte reduction.[14] Three groups of patients underwent colorectal surgery. Ninety-three patients received no transfusions and were hospitalized for 10 days at a cost of $7,030 per patient. Fifty-six patients received allogeneic blood and were hospitalized for an average of 17 days at a cost of $12,347 per patient. Forty-eight received allogeneic blood that was filtered and leukocyte reduced. That group was hospitalized for an average of 11 days at a cost of $7,867 per patient. This study supports the concept that allogeneic blood transfusion may in fact be a causative factor rather than a correlative factor in raising infection rates and hospitalization costs.

PAD is not without risk, however. Delays in cardiac surgery for the purpose of collecting PAD units can raise the incidence of cardiac events before surgical intervention. Risk of a serious reaction in an autologous donor is 1:222 if the donor does not meet the usual criteria for allogeneic donation. In total, one out of 17,000 collections of PAD units results in reactions that require hospitalization.

Overall, current economic studies do not allow one to draw definitive conclusions about the cost-effectiveness of PAD. A double-blinded randomized clinical study involving autologous or allogeneic blood is not feasible because of ethical concerns. As long as the public continues to have concerns over the safety of allogeneic blood, autologous donation is likely to remain an option in elective surgical cases.

Marrow Stimulation

Recombinant human erythropoietin (EPO) injection is a well-established and effective treatment for chronic anemia. It has provided great relief to patients suffering from anemia caused by end-stage renal disease, as well as to patients undergoing chemotherapy.[15] Recombinant human EPO has been shown to increase red cell mass by 41% over use of placebo.[16] EPO administration without PAD can reduce by 32% to 48% the number of patients requiring allogeneic transfusions during and after arthroplasties.[17] The cost of treatment with EPO is $840 to produce the equivalent of 1 unit of RBCs.[18] Randomized clinical trials have shown that treatment with EPO at a cost of $1500 to $4500 will allow recipients to avoid receiving 1 unit of allogeneic blood.[10-12] A study produced in Italy[19] demonstrated that patients undergoing EPO for chemotherapy experienced an increase in quality-adjusted life expectancy of 8.4 days at a cost of $4362 more than RBC transfusion. Another study demonstrated that 10% to 29% of patients receiving EPO still required at least 1 unit of allogeneic blood.[20]

A cost-effectiveness study was conducted in Canada on EPO used alone and in conjunction with PAD.[21] The study incorporated the risk of receiving allogeneic blood, the cost of blood products, the risk of developing transfusion-related diseases, the costs of transfusion-related diseases, the impact of transfusion-related diseases on patient morbidity and mortality, and the effect of EPO on the probability of receiving allogeneic blood. For EPO compared with no intervention, the cost of one life year gained was C$66 million (US$67.3 million, at the time of writing). For EPO to augment PAD, the cost per life year gained was C$329 million (US$335.422 million, at the time of writing). On that basis, the authors concluded that the use of EPO to reduce perioperative allogeneic transfusions in orthopedic surgery did not meet criteria conventionally considered financially acceptable. Similar conclusions were drawn by other authors who studied the cost-effectiveness of EPO in elective cardiac surgery[22] and colorectal cancer surgery.[23]

EPO is an effective means of increasing the yield of PAD units and of reducing the degree of exposure to allogeneic blood in a number of settings. In the perioperative arena, current studies have shown that this modality fails to meet the criteria for cost-effective treatment.

Blood Recovery

Blood recovery may reduce the risk of an adverse outcome when compared with allogeneic or PAD transfusions. Because blood recovery results in an autologous unit, the risks and inherent costs of allogeneic transfusion are avoided, including transmission of infectious agents, immune modulation, and higher incidences of postoperative fever, infection, and bed days. Blood recovery also reduces the risks associated with autologous donations—risks such as bacterial contamination resulting from storage, transfusion to the wrong donor, delays in surgery for PAD collection, and adverse events secondary to collection.

Despite the clinical advantages of using recovered blood, there is considerable controversy in the literature regarding the cost-effectiveness of the technique. Some studies report that blood recovery can be quite cost-effective, particularly in cases where heavy blood loss occurs. Others find no cost advantages, and still others cite significant increases in cost. One center reported that blood recovery treatment of patients undergoing repair of abdominal aortic aneurysm reduced the average requirement of allogeneic blood from 5.9 units to 1.7 units.[24] Similar reductions in blood requirements were also reported in a British study involving liver transplantations.[25] That prospective study made blood recovery available to all patients and used blood recovery in 428 of the 660 patients. The mean amount of blood recovered in these patients was 5086 mL. To ensure that recovered blood was equivalent to allogeneic blood concentrate, random samples were taken during the study. Over 5 years, 2366 units of RBCs were recovered for transfusion. Had allogeneic units been used exclusively, a total cost of £503,443 (US$1.026 million, at time of writing) would have been incurred. With blood recovery, the actual cost (including cost of the blood recovery machine, labor, maintenance, and variables, as well as the cost of allogeneic units) totalled £371,542 (US$757,353, at time of writing), a savings of 26%.

A study produced in the United States did not find blood recovery to be cost-effective.[26] In that study, 45 consecutive patients undergoing hip arthroplasty were provided with blood recovery services and were compared to the previous 45 patients who had undergone the same procedure. The cost of blood recovery was a flat fee of $1469, regardless of the number of units transfused. The cost of a single unit of autologous blood, including technical and professional fees, laboratory use, and crossmatching, was $595. If such recovery is to be cost-effective, an average recovery rate of 3 units per patient would be necessary. The control group required an average of 2.2 units of blood. In the experimental group, the addition of blood recovery reduced the need for transfusion to 1.7 units on average. Not surprisingly, blood recovery was not found to be cost-effective because a 2- to 3-liter blood loss is expected in hip arthroplasty, and the price structure for blood recovery would require blood loss of >3 units to break even.

Another study[27] involved patients for whom blood recovery was made available for repair of abdominal aortic aneurysm. The cost for blood recovery at the study facility was $315 per patient, dramatically lower than in the previously described study. Blood loss among these patients was substantial, with a mean loss of 1748 mL. Nevertheless, an average of only 1.6 units of blood was recovered and returned to the patient. Twenty-five of the 136 patients with blood loss of >1000 mL received <250 mL of salvaged blood. A difference in recovery technique may account for the low yield and diminished cost reduction in this study. Overall, only 22% of patients received enough recovered blood to outweigh the cost of providing the service. As in other studies, patients with the highest level of blood loss experienced the greatest economic benefit.

A review of cost-comparison studies was conducted by Ferguson et al.[28] Seven studies compared the cost of blood recovery with the cost of providing allogeneic blood in cardiac, orthopedic, vascular, and liver transplant surgeries. Local costs or charges were used, and the authors note that "with rare exceptions it was impossible to determine how these values were derived or whether they represented fully allocated costs.". . . A minority of studies included the cost of the machine itself and the technician to operate it."[28] The results of the cost comparisons with allogeneic blood varied from a mean savings of $744 per patient to an added cost of $587 per patient.

A recent study conducted at the Cleveland Clinic notes that the cost per unit of recovered blood is highly dependent on the number of units lost and recovered in each blood recovery case. The cost of providing blood recovery was reported as $204.88 per case, with an additional cost of $2.00 for disposables for each unit recovered. In that institution, which has a large number of surgical cases with high levels of blood loss, recovered blood was returned to the patient at an average cost of $89.46 per unit. That figure represented a significant savings over the $200 purchase price of allogeneic blood. Other institutions may not be able to match the efficiency of the Cleveland Clinic's large blood recovery program.[24]

The lack of consistent accounting information in the various cost-comparison studies on blood recovery makes it difficult to assess the technique's cost-effectiveness. In addition to problems of reporting, there are genuine local differences in the cost of providing blood recovery treatment to patients. A recent publication attempted to address that issue by providing a step-by-step formula to determine the cost of setting up an in-house blood recovery program in a given hospital and to determine what loss or gain is likely to occur on an annual basis.[29] A retrospective review of the number of surgical cases and the attendant blood loss is the first step in determining whether blood recovery will be cost-effective. Next, a complete account of all additional expenses incurred by establishing the service is recommended. If the numbers are favorable, a pay-back period can be calculated along with subsequent annual expected returns on the initial investment.

Current data suggest that blood recovery can be cost-effective in cases where the level of expected blood loss is high enough to offset the cost of providing the service. Marked regional variations in the cost of allogeneic blood, autologous blood, and blood recovery services necessitate an individual approach to determining the cost-effectiveness of blood recovery at any given facility.

Acute Normovolemic Hemodilution

ANH is a process by which 2 to 4 units of RBCs are withdrawn from a patient just before surgery and the volume is replaced with acellular fluid. As a result, blood lost during surgery will have a lower concentration of RBCs, and it will be replaced by the withdrawn whole blood at the end of the surgical procedure. The patient receives not only RBCs but also platelets and plasma that can assist in coagulation. One study[30] reports that ANH was highly effective in patients undergoing prostatectomy and was less costly than autologous donation. Disadvantages of ANH include the significant amount of operating room time necessary to initiate the process, fluid shifts, costly central venous pressure lines, and the need for highly trained personnel to manage patients. In addition, mathematical modeling has demonstrated that the technique will avoid little more than 0.6 units of allogeneic RBCs.[31] Futher study is needed to determine the cost-effectiveness of this blood management modality.

Modification of Transfusion Behavior

Perhaps the single most cost-effective modality for blood management is education focused on reducing transfusion thresholds. Recent prospective and randomized controlled trials in critically ill patients indicate that reducing the transfusion trigger for red cell transfusion to a hemoglobin level of 7 g/dL has no effect on survival.[32,33] Reduction in the traditional practice of initiating transfusion from a hemoglobin level of 10 g/dL can have a significant effect on the cost of providing allogeneic blood. Likewise, targeting change of the traditional physician behavior of giving 2 units at a time can also reduce blood use. Through laboratory measurement following each unit of transfused blood, overtransfusion can be avoided. The financial effect of such strategies has been little studied, but they appear to be low-cost, high-yield opportunities.

Conclusion

Blood products account for 1% of the cost of health care in the United States. It is in the interest of patients, caregivers, hospitals, and payors to effectively manage the cost of blood components. A well-documented method to improve cost-effective management of components encompasses education and adherence to current practice standards for transfusion. The use of blood recovery in patients with expected high blood loss also appears to be less costly than transfusion of multiple units of allogeneic blood. Further study is needed to determine whether preoperative autologous donation is truly cost-effective. There have been no studies to date that compare the cost of providing blood recovery with the cost of PAD. The use of ANH may reduce costs in some arenas, but further study is needed in this area as well. Although EPO is an effective means of increasing red cell mass, it is too expensive to be considered a cost-effective alternative to transfusion.

References

1. National health expenditure projections 2006-2016. Baltimore, MD: Centers for Medicare and Medicaid Services, 2007. [Available at [http://www.cms.hhs.gov/NationalHealthExpendData/downloads/proj2006.pdf (accessed October 8, 2007).]

2. Carter TH. Biotechnology, economics, and the business of blood. Biotechnology 1991;19:3-30.

3. Eisenberg JM. Clinical economics. A guide to the economic analysis of clinical practices. JAMA 1989;262:2879-86.

4. Goodnough LT. Blood and blood conservation: A national perspective. J Cardiothorac Vasc Anesth 2004;18(Suppl):6S-11S.

5. Brecher ME, Goodnough LT. The rise and fall of preoperative autologous blood donation. Transfusion 2001;41:1459-62.

6. Blood Safety Act of 1991. New Jersey Permanent Statutes. Title 26. Health and Vital Statistics 26:2A-13,14.

7. Paul Gann blood safety act. California health and safety code. Section 1645. [Available at http://www.leginfo.ca.gov/cgi-bin/displaycode?section=hsc&group=01001-02000&file=1645 (accessed October 8, 2007).]

8. Seed CR, Kiely P, Keller AJ. Residual risk of transfusion transmitted human immunodeficiency virus, hepatitis B virus, hepatitis C virus, and human T lymphotrophic virus. Intern Med J 2005;35:592-8.

9. AuBuchon JP. Blood transfusion options improving outcomes and reducing costs. Arch Pathol Lab Med 1997;121:40-7.

10. McDonald CP. Bacterial risk reduction by improved donor arm disinfection, diversion, and bacterial screening. Transfus Med 2006;16:381-96.

11. Hill GE, Frawley WH, Griffith KE, et al. Allogeneic blood transfusion increases the risk of postoperative bacterial infection: A meta-analysis. J Trauma 2003;54:908-14.

12. Department of Pathology, Massachusetts General Hospital, Harvard Medical School. Allogeneic blood transfusion, hospital charges, and length of hospitalization: A study of 487 consecutive patients undergoing colorectal cancer resection. Arch Pathol Lab Med 1998;122:117-19.

13. Blumberg N, Kirdley SA, Heal JM. A cost analysis of autologous and allogeneic transfusions in hip-replacement surgery. Am J Surg 1996;171:324-30.

14. Jensen LS, Grunnet N, Hanberg-Sorensen F, Jorgensen J. Cost-effectiveness of blood transfusion and white cell reduction in elective colorectal surgery. Transfusion 1995;35:719-22.

15. Cremieux P, Finkelstein S, Berndt E, et al. Cost-effectiveness, quality-adjusted life-years, and supportive care. Recombinant human erythropoietin as a treatment of cancer-associated anaemia. Pharmacoeconomics 1999;16:459-72.

16. Goodnough LT, Rudnick S, Price TH, et al. Increased preoperative collection of autologous blood with recombinant human erythropoietin therapy. N Engl J Med 1989;321:1163-8.

17. Canadian Orthopedic Perioperative Erythropoietin Study Group. Effectiveness of perioperative recombinant human erythropoietin in elective hip replacement. Lancet 1993;431:1227-32.

18. Goodnough LT, Verbrugge D, Marcus RE, Goldberg V. The effect of patient size and dose of recombinant human erythropoietin therapy on red blood cell volume expansion in autologous blood donors for elective orthopedic surgery. J Am Coll Surg 1994;179:171-6.

19. Barosi G, Marchetti M, Liberato NL. Cost-effectiveness of recombinant human erythropoietin in the prevention of chemotherapy-induced anaemia. Br J Cancer 1998;78:781-7.

20. Case DC, Bukowski RM, Carey RW, et al. Recombinant human erythropoietin therapy for anemic cancer patients on combination chemotherapy. J Natl Cancer Inst 1993;85:801-6.

21. Coyle D, Lee KM, Fergusson DA, Laupacis A. Economic analysis of erythropoietin use in orthopaedic surgery. Transfus Med 1999;9:21-30.

22. Coyle D, Lee KM, Fergusson DA, Laupacis A. Cost-effectiveness of epoetin-alpha to augment preoperative autologous blood donation in elective cardiac surgery. Pharmacoeconomics 2000;18:161-71.

23. Benoist S, Panis Y, Pannegeon V, et al. Predictive factors for perioperative blood transfusions in rectal resection for cancer: A multivariate analysis of a group of 212 patients. Surgery 2001;129:433-9.

24. Cali RF, O'Hara PJ, Hertzer NR, et al. The influence of autotransfusion on homologous blood requirements during aortic reconstruction. Cleve Clin Q 1984; 51:143-8.

25. Phillips SD, Maguire D, Deshpande R, et al. A prospective study investigating the cost-effectiveness of intraoperative blood salvage during liver transplantation. Transplantation 2006;81:536-40.

26. Guerra JJ, Cuckler JM. Cost effectiveness of intraoperative autotransfusion in total hip arthroplasty surgery. Clin Orthop Relat Res 1995;315:212-22.

27. Goodnough LT, Monk TG, Sicard G, et al. Intraoperative salvage in patients undergoing elective abdominal aortic aneurysm repair: An analysis of cost and benefit. J Vasc Surg 1996;24:213-18.

28. Fergusson D, van Walraven C, Coyle D, Laupacis A. Economic evaluations of technologies to minimize perioperative transfusion: A systematic review of published studies. Transfus Med Rev 1999;13:106-17.

29. Waters JR, Meier HH, Waters JH. An economic analysis of costs associated with development of a cell salvage program. Anesth Analg 2007;104:869-75.

30. Monk TG, Goodnough LT, Brecher ME, et al. Acute normovolemic hemodilution can replace preoperative autologous blood donation as a standard of care for autologous blood procurement in radical prostatectomy. Anesth Analg 1997;85:953-8.

31. Brecher ME, Rosenfeld M. Mathematical and computer modeling of acute normovolemic hemodilution. Transfusion 1994;34:176-9.

32. Hebert PC, Yetisir E, Martin C, et al. Transfusion requirements in critical care investigators for the Canadian Critical Care Trials Group: Is a low transfusion threshold safe in critically ill patients with cardiovascular diseases? Crit Care Med 2001;29:227-34.

33. Hebert PC, Wells G, Blajchman MA, et al. A multicenter, randomized, controlled clinical trial of transfusion requirements in critical care. Transfusion requirements in critical care investigators, Canadian Critical Care Trials Group. New Engl J Med 1999;340:409-17.

In: Waters JH, ed.
Blood Management: Options for Better Patient Care
Bethesda, MD: AABB Press, 2008

3

Development of a Blood Management Program

SHERRI OZAWA, RN; ELORA THORPE, RN, BSN;
JO VALENTI, RN; AND
JONATHAN H. WATERS, MD

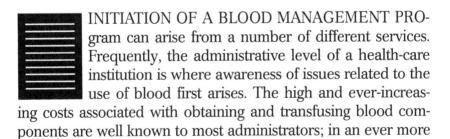 INITIATION OF A BLOOD MANAGEMENT PRO-
gram can arise from a number of different services.
Frequently, the administrative level of a health-care
institution is where awareness of issues related to the
use of blood first arises. The high and ever-increas-
ing costs associated with obtaining and transfusing blood components are well known to most administrators; in an ever more

Sherri Ozawa, RN, Senior Coordinator, Englewood Hospital and Medical Center,
Englewood, New Jersey; Elora Thorpe, RN, BSN, Coordinator, Blood Management,
Saint Luke's Hospital of Kansas City, Kansas City, Missouri; Jo Valenti, RN, Director,
Blood Conservation, Kennedy Health System, Stratford, New Jersey; and Jonathan H.
Waters, MD, Chief and Visiting Associate Professor, Department of Anesthesiology,
Magee-Womens Hospital, University of Pittsburgh Medical Center, Pittsburgh, Penn-
sylvania

cost-conscious health-care system, such expenses generate much concern. Administrators of a hospital may also become aware of the legal and ethical concerns related to patients' refusal of blood transfusion and to the possible litigation related to the inappropriate use of transfusions. Increasing regulatory scrutiny with regard to the use of components may also be generating an increased interest in this area.[1] In some facilities, it is the physician(s) who drives the startup of a program and not the administration—although administrative buy-in is an essential part of the process.[2]

To assess the need for an organized program in an institution, both administrators and physicians should examine a number of factors. These factors include current use and cost associated with the use of blood, physician support, staffing, equipment availability or the cost to acquire it, potential use of outside business consultation, marketing and public relations costs, and the likelihood of increased market share. The existence and success of other programs in surrounding hospitals, particularly in a competitive health-care marketplace, are also factors that are to be considered carefully in planning for a blood management program.

As one proceeds with program development, it is imperative to get the support of hospital senior leadership. This support includes the hospital president or chief executive officer, plus the chief financial officer. It is also important to gain the support of the physician leadership, which includes the chief medical officer, the surgical services committee, the medical executive committee, and the transfusion utilization committee. When one presents the concept of program development to these individuals, it is important to keep the discussion focused on realistic economic benefit. These individuals usually receive incentives according to the financial success of their department and of the hospital so it will be useful to address their own vested interest.

In the development of a program, consideration should be given to outside resources. It might be helpful to arrange for a group to make a site visit to a hospital that has a successful blood management program for a first-hand look. Also, there are consulting firms that will, for a fee, assist an institution in setting up a program. Although this assistance may add considerable cost to the venture, the experience, documentation, and connections that such a consulting entity can provide may prove desirable for a particular hospital. Many institutions, however, successfully forgo the use of outside firms to set up a blood management program. These institutions rely on the experience from within and on assistance from other centers that are already in existence. Careful planning involving many hospital departments is essential to ensure long-term success of a blood management program.

The First Step

When an institution has made the decision to move forward with the implementation of a program, one of the first considerations is securing suitable staff members to handle the daily responsibilities of program development and management. Integral to this process is the selection of a medical director early in the process. The medical director should be someone who can interact between the blood bank and the operating room. In addition, ancillary support will be needed to drive the program forward. In many hospitals, a nurse will take on the role of blood management coordinator. The blood management coordinator will manage the day-to-day operations of the program with the medical director acting as the executive leader. After all staff members have been secured, implementation of the actual program can take place more efficiently.

The following steps represent the many factors and entities that must be considered in the creation of an organized blood management program. These steps are not necessarily presented in a chronological order because each institution must address these issues within the context of institutional culture.

Assembly of a Task Force

To ensure that all hospital services have a voice in the process of program development, one should develop a task force so that early buy-in and support are gained. Representation from the following departments is imperative:
1. Administration.
2. Nursing.
3. Surgical Services.
4. Performance Improvement.
5. Blood Bank.
6. Pharmacy.
7. Risk Management.
8. Information Technology.
9. Admissions.
10. Emergency Room.
11. Department of Medicine.
12. Hematology.
13. Critical Care/Intensive Care Unit (ICU).
14. Anesthesiology.
15. Finance.

All of these departments should meet to discuss the feasibility of a blood management program from their perspectives. Initial concerns should be addressed at a level that satisfies departmental chairs and directors. From this group, a steering committee can be formed—perhaps with department designees whose job it will be to present a final recommendation about developing a program.[3]

Steering Committee

The initial task of the steering committee will be to research the topic. The program's medical director should serve as chair of this committee and steer it toward manageable goals and successes. An audit of current blood usage in the institution should be completed to assess the volume of components being used, the actual costs of this blood use, and the breakdown of blood use by hospital services. The committee should focus on areas where there is evidence of room for improvement. The committee should determine where a blood management program fits into the overall strategic plan of the hospital. For instance, is there an opportunity for reduction of costs that will affect the hospital's financial standing? Identifying the patient population that will be served by the program will be part of the research. A blood management program can represent an opportunity to serve. An active Jehovah's Witness community that may be in the hospital locality, for example, might bring business to the hospital that is not currently optimized.

Early meetings should create a framework for the program by involving many departments and by discussing how each will be affected as well as how each will interface for program success. Medical and nursing staff as well as the Operating Room, Laboratory, Administration, Social Work, Pharmacy, and Admitting Departments are all examples of key groups that must be included in such a steering committee.

It is recommended that the committee meet on a regular basis—monthly or quarterly—to ensure that program development is progressive and that obstacles are managed promptly. The steering committee should assign various members to create necessary program policies, which include—but are not limited to—an administrative policy for blood management, outpatient anemia management, severe acute anemia management, guidelines for use of erythropoietics, blood transfusion order sets, transfer of patients between institutions, and nutrition guidelines. Policies that already exist in some form in the institution need not be recreated, but they should be examined and updated as needed in the context of the blood management program.[4]

All of this due diligence will serve to identify the feasibility for the development of a blood management program. It will illustrate what work needs to be done and will focus the group on the many reasons that proper blood management is a rational approach to patient care.[5]

Choice of a Medical Director

One of the most successful models for program implementation involves two key positions: a medical director driving the program and a program director/coordinator. Experience has shown that a physician-driven program is more effective than an administration-driven one. Certainly, selecting the right medical director can be one of the most challenging and important decisions to be made in developing a program. Most importantly, a medical director must be a true champion of blood management. Not only must medical directors understand the science behind blood management, they must also be convinced that it is "best practice" medicine and that it can provide the best cost savings for the hospital. Of course, a high degree of respect among peers for the medical director can be a great impetus for the program.

An important goal for the program is for blood management to be viewed as a specialty by the medical community, just as nephrology and cardiology are specialties. Therefore, it is important that the medical director be an expert in blood management. To that end, he or she must keep abreast of current literature on the subject and must know how to effectively reduce the need for blood transfusions preoperatively, intraoperatively, and postoperatively. The specialty from which the medical director comes may vary, depending on the hospital. Some facilities choose to have an anesthesiologist as their medical director. Others choose a surgeon, an internist, a family practice physician, or a hematologist. Occasionally, a facility will choose not to have a medical director at all. More often than not, though, such absence greatly hampers the development of an effective program.

Whatever the background of the medical director, it is important to keep in mind that the program director/coordinator needs to have full access to the medical director for patient consultations, for consultation with physicians and hospitals, or even for handling the occasional confrontation that inevitably occurs. The medical director, along with the program director, should be able to face these responsibilities and challenges with courage and discretion.[6]

Blood Management Program Director

A blood management program requires execution of programmatic change. The medical director can implement these programmatic changes; however, most physicians are typically limited in their capacity to devote time to this activity by a busy medical practice. For this reason, a program director is often hired to perform the day-to-day tasks necessary to implement and maintain a program. Some of the most successful blood management programs are run by professional nurses. Others are run by administrators, pharmacologists, and medical scientists. The knowledge of blood component use, the ability to interpret laboratory values, and the capacity to understand medications are all essential functions. The individual also should have excellent organization and communication skills, and should be a team leader and team player. (A sample job description is attached as Appendix 3-1.) However, care should be taken to ensure that details about the expected function of the program director, the program's place in the hospital structure, and the program director's immediate supervisor are specifically adapted to the hospital.

Development of a Business Plan

Formulating an effective business plan can increase the likelihood that the program will be successful. In fact, the plan can make the difference between success and failure. Development of an effective business plan should be an ongoing endeavor throughout the entire research process. The plan will help to focus attention on what is truly important, and it will prevent a hospital from spending unnecessary time on strategies that are not going to be productive. The plan should ultimately define the actions, serve as a road map, and act as a sales tool.

The plan should be written as clearly and concisely as possible and should be easy to read. For the plan to be credible, it must be accurate. Enthusiasm can be generated by being realistic and professional. One should include both the things that can make the plan a success and the obstacles that can prevent it from succeeding. For validation, the plan could be sent to several trusted colleagues to make sure that it includes all necessary elements.

In general, every plan should include a cover sheet; an executive summary, which is a clear and effective overview of the plan; a statement of purpose, which should be clear and concise; and a description of the program. The description should include the following:

1. The strategic plan of the institution. (The plan should follow and strengthen the vision of the institution as well as support the strategic plan.)
2. The tangible and intangible advantages to the organization.
   - Identification of the current status.
   - Identification of the challenges.
   - Improvement of the quality of care.
   - Response to community needs.
3. Market analysis.
   - Identification of the demographic trends of the facility.
   - Identification of the market and economic trends.
   - Identification of any other programs or competitors.
4. Operating plan.
   - Effect on nursing staff and ancillary personnel.
   - Outcome measures.
   - Staffing.
     - Program director.
     - Assignments of medical staff.
     - Support of medical staff.
     - Administrative assistant.
     - Other.
5. Capital expenditures, equipment, and budget.
6. Marketing plan.

7. Educational plan.
8. Financial plan (cost savings vs revenue generation).

An example of a business plan may be found as Appendix 3-2. This business plan was developed to consolidate blood recovery services within a single institution. The plan illustrates the comprehensive nature of this undertaking and helps formulate ideas around financial return. The process of writing such a plan forces a full conceptualization of the program.

Components of a Blood Management Program

Blood management can take place over the entire spectrum of a patient's hospital care. Blood management does not involve just one activity but covers a wide spectrum of activities that, when combined, can reduce or eliminate the need for allogeneic blood transfusion. These activities span the gamut of complexity ranging from simple monitoring of crossmatching to transfusion ratios and to the more complex process of perioperative apheresis. Appendix 3-3 provides a list of some of the components of a blood management program that can be used in each perioperative phase.

Education and Roll-Out

In general, when implementing change, one should take small incremental steps so immediate and tangible success can be measured. By doing so, success generates momentum to build on the success. Many hospitals start with a pilot in a particular high blood-use area, such as orthopedics. Others "go live" with a physician's order set in an ICU setting to see how the order set can affect anemia management and allogeneic blood utilization. Appendixes 3-4 and 3-5 are samples of order sets that can be used. An audit of transfusion practice may prove helpful in identifying the efficacy of a blood management program. The benefits derived from preoperative anemia management may also be assessed. A first step in program implementation could be the development of a preoperative anemia management clinic. Education should be the top priority no matter which avenue is pursued first.

Although facilities will need to provide an abundance of blood management education for physicians, it may not be physicians who are the best catalysts for change. Nursing education often yields some of the best results. For example, one hospital tried to institute change related to diabetes and acute myocardial infarction. When physicians initiated the orders, there was only 9% compliance. However, when nurses initiated the orders, compliance increased to the 90th percentile range (J Spertus, personal communication). It is uncertain whether such results may point to any clear cause.

Education for both physicians and nurses can be in the form of conferences that provide continuing medical education/continuing education units (CME/CEUs), national conferences, grand rounds, nursing orientation, resident orientation, or one-on-one instruction, which often works the best. Regardless of the form of the education, the important thing is to build enthusiasm for conserving and managing allogeneic blood appropriately.

Another group to be considered—and not to be underestimated—when it comes to education is the ancillary staff. From the kitchen to housekeeping and to the engineering staff, the goal is to create a hospital-wide culture of blood management.

Marketing

Although excellent clinical care is the most important aspect of a successful blood management program, there is also a need for supervision of public relations and marketing as it relates to the program. Internal communication is vital to promote a cultural awareness of issues concerning blood use within the health-care organization. Nurses and physicians may benefit from direct educational sessions, as discussed earlier, but ancillary personnel should also be educated as appropriate in the development of the program.

Additionally, the uniqueness of such a program within the community often attracts attention of the media, and this attention should be anticipated and managed. Patients who refuse blood transfusion in surrounding communities will also undoubtedly take a great deal of interest in the development of such a program, and they will most likely seek out further information on services provided. This interest can lead to increased market share of this patient population, which is an important measure of success in the current competitive health-care marketplace. Communication to the community can involve newsletters, public information sessions, health fairs, direct advertising, and use of the media.

Conclusion

Regardless of the order in which the steps are taken, the process can result in the development and operation of a successful blood management program. The program will enable the hospital to achieve improved patient outcomes through reduction of inappropriate blood transfusions. Incorporating current evidence-based clinical guidelines for blood use, casting a critical eye on areas where blood use is high, and developing strategies for performance improvement are all part of the process. These things do not take enormous financial commitment. Buying equipment and hiring experts are not necessary. Changing practice *does* take team effort. Because transfusions take place in virtually all hospital services, a buy-in across these services is critical to success. With some clinicians, it will take more convincing than others. It can be a surprise as to which of the players step up to the plate and become early champions. But as the benefits of better blood management are realized, more and more clinicians will become convinced that the effort was worthwhile. When a hospital is surveyed by various regulatory agencies, a best-practice blood utilization culture is an advantage—another tangible benefit.

Every year—but also on a monthly basis in the beginning—hospital administrators should evaluate the viability of the program. Markers of success include, but are not limited to, the following: decreased use of donor blood, improved use of autologous blood, increased market share, added physician and patient satisfaction, greater positive media attention, and improved patient outcomes.

References

1. Vernon S, Pfeifer GM. Are you ready for bloodless surgery? Am J Nurs 1997; 97:40-6.
2. Ratcliffe CJ. Development and implementation of a bloodless medicine and surgery program. J Health Manag 2004;49:405-9.
3. Cogliano J, Kisner D. Bloodless medicine and surgery in the OR and beyond. AORN J 2002;76:830-7.
4. Ozawa S, Shander A, Ochani TD. A practical approach to achieving bloodless surgery. AORN J 2001;74:34-40.
5. Ratcliffe CJ. Development and implementation of a bloodless medicine and surgery program. J Health Manag 2004;49:405-9.
6. Goodnough LT, Shander A, Spence R. Bloodless medicine: Clinical care without allogeneic blood transfusion. Transfusion 2003;43:668-76.

Appendix 3-1. Sample Job Description for Program Director

JOB DESCRIPTION

POSITION TITLE:
Director of Blood Management Program

REPORTS TO:
Medical Director, Blood Management Program

DEPARTMENT AND DIVISION:
Blood Management

I. MAJOR RESPONSIBILITIES

A. *Patient Care Activities*
  1. Completes patient rounds with emphasis on the following:
     a. Service as liaison among patient, family, staff, physician, and other disciplines as needed.
     b. Patient/family teaching.
     c. Provision of appropriate physician referrals.
     d. Entry of progress notes relative to blood management aspects of patient's care.
     e. Assistance with transportation, accommodations, and arrangements for patient, family, or both.
     f. Recommendations for discharge planning.
  2. Attends patient care conferences as appropriate.
  3. Acts as resource person for staff.
     a. Provides services regularly and as needed.
     b. Answers questions when necessary.
     c. Addresses orientation classes.
  4. Works closely with Social Service and/or Case Management on discharge planning.

    5.   Takes the lead in developing policies and guidelines that facilitate best practices with regard to blood management, such as the following:
        a.   Policy for blood-refusal patients.
        b.   Guidelines for prehospital optimization for elective surgery.
        c.   Anemia treatment protocol.
        d.   Blood component order set.

B.   *Statistical Information*
    1.   Keeps complete and appropriate statistics for reports and distribution.
        a.   Patient census.
        b.   Communications.
        c.   Personnel records.
        d.   Expenses or budgets when appropriate.
        e.   Unit or staff conferences.

C.   *Marketing Activities*
    1.   Maintains current mailing list.
    2.   Responds to all correspondence and forwards the response through appropriate parties.
    3.   Works with appropriate departments to further the image of the program within the community through regular newsletters, institution Web site, and community outreach programs.

D.   *On-Call Activity*
    1.   Screens all calls.
        a.   Referral to appropriate physician as necessary.
        b.   Coordination of physician-to-physician contact.
        c.   Coordination of patient transfers.
        d.   Appropriate handling of all inquiries regarding the program.
    2.   Is available to all patients and families for emergencies on a 24/7 basis.

3. Acts as a liaison between patient and medical staff to promote quality communication and professional relationship.

E. *Physician Referral*
   1. Maintains accurate information regarding physicians, physicians' office locations, hours, specialties, and insurance.
   2. Encourages physician participation in the program by providing educational opportunities to physicians.
   3. Develops and maintains a participating physician roster.
   4. Maintains a record of referral transactions and follow-ups.

II. DEPARTMENTAL RESPONSIBILITIES

A. *Staffing*
   1. Adheres to scheduling policies; requests time off appropriately.
   2. Fulfills role in the staffing plan; complies with sick time policies; consistently reports on- and off-duty time.
   3. Functions independently.

B. *Policy and Procedures*
   1. Practices within approved unit policies and procedures, as well as those of the department and organization.
   2. Clarifies unfamiliar policies and procedures when indicated.
   3. Reads intradepartmental and interdepartmental directives and communication to keep abreast of new or revised policies and procedures.

C. *Blood Management Program Advisory Panel*
   1. Cochairs advisory panel along with Medical Director.

    2.   Coordinates and schedules monthly meetings for members.

    3.   Prepares and distributes meeting agenda.

    4.   Participates in meetings as a member.

    5.   Records minutes that are forwarded to the medical staff office.

    6.   Follows through on actions as recommended by the committee.

D. *Consultation*

    1.   Is available to outside facilities and organizations for consultation or presentation to assist in establishing a similar program.

    2.   Charges hosting facility according to the established rate; reports to Senior Nursing Officer.

    3.   Represents [ ] Medical Center in a manner appropriate to the situation.

III. RELATIONSHIPS AND KEY CONTACTS

A. *Responsible to Medical Director*

B. *Key Contacts*

    1.   Patients.

    2.   Patient's family.

    3.   Physicians.

    4.   Unit managers.

    5.   Nursing staff.

    6.   Ancillary personnel.

    7.   Administration.

IV. DESIRABLE EDUCATION AND EXPERIENCE

A. Graduation from an accredited professional school of nursing; current nursing license.

B. Clinical experience of at least 3 years (preferred).

C. Experience in patient relations, business management, and marketing.

D. Good communication skills.
E. Familiarity with the beliefs and organization of Jehovah's Witnesses.
F. Good mental and physical health that is sufficient to meet position demands.

Appendix 3-2. Sample Business Plan for a Medically Directed Intraoperative Blood Management Service

Executive Summary

Rationale

The blood management service discussed in this business plan proposes to organize related blood and coagulation services under medical direction, to make autotransfusion available to all patients with medically documented need, to implement quality improvement and quality control processes, and to do so in a fashion that is cost-effective to the institution.

Autotransfusion offers the potential for improved perioperative outcomes through the following:

- Decreased hospital length-of-stay (0.75-1.25 days, per preliminary data).
- Decreased risk of postoperative infection.
- Decreased risk of recurrence of cancer.
- Decreased risk of pulmonary complications and disseminated intravascular coagulation (DIC).

Autotransfusion services can return positive net income while presenting the institution with a lower-cost blood therapy alternative for a selected population.

Resource Needs

Technical support needs for autotransfusion are estimated to require 0.4 full time equivalents (FTEs) of an anesthesia equipment specialist (AES). Required skills for technical support of the service are consistent with the division's objectives for AES involvement in anesthesia equipment setup and operation.

Autotransfusion resources will be managed for optimal utilization by adherence to the clinical indications protocol already developed.

Organization and Control

The program leadership will be accomplished by the program director, whose responsibilities will include adherence to clinical indications, patient safety, technical personnel supervision, quality improvement, research, and education.

Financial Complications

Pro forma analysis of the program demonstrates favorable financial results, featuring net income of $43,696, including professional, technical, and point-of-care testing net income.

Recommendation

The program's quality improvement effect on preoperative blood management will be to break even under the best financial scenario. It is realistically expected that benefits to the institution will include a reduction of length of stay by 1 day.

Recommendations:

1. Approve the blood management service to become officially operational within the scope of the clinical indications protocol incorporated herein.
2. Authorize AES technical support of the service.
3. Authorize management of the service's supply inventory through the institution's main storeroom, which will achieve the supply continuity through par levels. Clinical Engineering will monitor supplies usage, with routine reports to the service's medical director.

Blood Management Service Definition and Cost/Benefit Overview

Definition

The clinical practice of autotransfusion is defined as the collection and intraoperative processing of blood for return to the patient as red cells, plasma, or platelets. Autotransfusion procedures include red cell recovery and washing, apheresis, and production of platelet gel as a biologic sealant. The benefits of autotransfusion procedures include reduced reliance on allogeneic blood supplies, reduced risk of complication related to allogeneic blood, and reduced cost compared to allogeneic blood components. This business plan proposes an autotransfusion service to provide intraoperative blood component therapy for a defined range of indications. (See section titled "Indications for Use of Recovered Blood.")

Cost/Benefit Highlights

Blood management services have demonstrated additional cost savings—in addition to revenue generated for the Department of Anesthesiology—through decreases in hospital stay, infection rates, and autologous predonation use. Results from an ongoing retrospective study arc presented below to give the reader an overview of the additional savings.

An internal (unpublished) retrospective study is evaluating the effect of autotransfusion services on a single surgeon performing radical retropubic prostatectomies. The surgeon averages 2208 ±1039 mL of blood loss per procedure. Previous to the institution of the program, either his patients were presenting to the operating room with autologous units predonated or he relied purely on allogeneic blood components from the blood bank. On average these patients received 0.7 ±1.6 units (with autologous predonation) and 2.3 ±1.7 units (without pre-donation) of allogeneic Red Blood Cells (RBCs) from the blood bank. By comparison, medically directed blood management patients have received 0.1 ±0.3 units of allogeneic blood.

The hospital stay for each of the groups is 4.07 ±1.22 days, 4.55 ±1.49 days, and 3.25 ±0.46 days for the autologous pre-donation (AP) group, allogeneic blood only (HT) group, and blood management patients, respectively. Thus, these study data, for more than 100 patients, would suggest that 0.8 hospital days are saved for this patient population for this procedure when compared to autologous predonation, and 1.3 days are saved when compared to allogeneic blood use only. This difference appears to relate to a greater incidence of infection and postoperative fever.

The figure below illustrates the cost savings effect of autotransfusion on blood bank use and hospital length of stay.

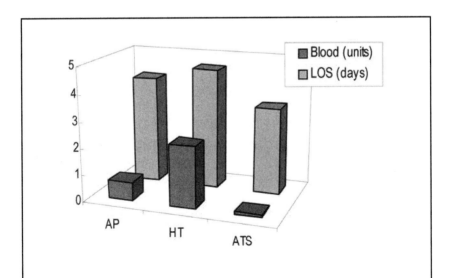

Cost savings effect of autotransfusion on bank blood use and length of stay. AP = autologous predonation; ATS = autotransfusion service; HT = homologous (allogeneic) transfusion; LOS = length of stay.

Blood Recovery vs Autologous Predonation

Many patients presenting to the general operating room have predonated their own blood. Of these units, approximately 80% are never used. The cost to the hospital of donation and storage is significant. The figure below illustrates how the cost of autologous blood donation compares to blood recovery, depending on how many units of blood are harvested. The validity of these data is currently being tested.

Blood Recovery vs Allogeneic Blood

The modification of immune function attributable to allogeneic transfusion is thought to relate to the leukocytes. Leukocyte-reduced blood has been advocated and is currently the primary type of allogeneic blood transfused in Canada and Europe. The figure below depicts the direct cost of this type of blood compared to blood recovery. As is readily seen, the larger the transfusion requirements, the larger the savings. This is because most costs of blood recovery relate to the setup cost. Thus, it is important to appropriately identify the patients who use this

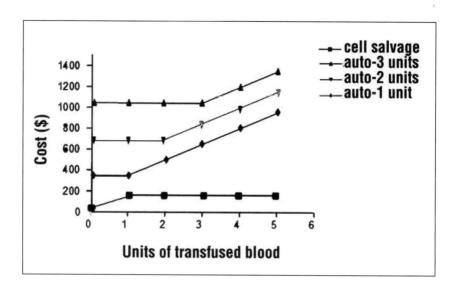

service. The blood recovery standby setup is an attempt to reduce the costs of setup ($55.00) by opening a reservoir for blood collection, with washing of the blood occurring only if a clinical indication exists for transfusion. This arrangement would increase the basic cost to $134.00. In addition, well-defined indications for blood recovery have been developed (see section "Indications for Use of Recovered Blood").

Service Objectives

The service will be guided by the following objectives:
1. Provide intraoperative blood component therapy services of the highest clinical quality.
2. Improve cost-effectiveness and perioperative outcomes through the following:
   - Decreased hospital length of stay (0.75–1.25 days, per preliminary data).[1,2]
   - Decreased risk of postoperative infection.[3,4]
   - Decreased risk of recurrence of cancer.[5-7]
   - Decreased risk of pulmonary complications and DIC.[8-11]
   - Decreased mortality following myocardial infarction.[12]
   - Capture of appropriate professional and technical revenue.
   - Promotion of the service as a marketing tool for surgery.
   - Development of a blood management technician training program.
   - Incorporation of medical direction training for the service into the anesthesiology residency in conjunction with the Section of Blood Banking, and establishment of the service as a center of excellence for clinical and research aspects of perioperative blood management.

Current Practice

Current hospital autotransfusion services are threefold:
- Blood recovery by the operating room (OR) nurses.

- Hemodilution by anesthesia personnel.
- Off-site (blood bank) blood recovery.

The volume of these services in 1997 was approximately 300 surgical cases. The advantages and disadvantages of each practice are outlined next.

Operating Room Blood Recovery by Nurses

Advantages
- Current practice.

Disadvantages
- Billing inadequacy.
- No record keeping, contradictory to the requirements of the AABB and The Joint Commission.
- No standardized policy and procedure for machine and blood handling; no clinical indications for services.
- No quality improvement or quality control.
- Documented inadequate blood washing and concentration (per testing of random samples obtained from nursing).
- Documented poor quality of recovered blood as performed by the nursing service is described by O'Hara et al.[13] In their experience, an average recovered blood unit had a hematocrit of 31.6%. A random survey revealed hematocrits as low as 14%. Recovered blood units should reflect concentrations of red cells equivalent to those of allogeneic blood from the blood bank (ie, hematocrits in the 60% range). If low hematocrit blood is administered, the patient will become hemodiluted, lowering his or her hematocrit rather than the intended goal of raising the hematocrit.
- No physician supervision.
- Limited to vascular surgery.
- Not suitable for Jehovah's Witness patients.
- Not suitable for pediatric patients.

Hemodilution by Anesthesia Personnel

Advantages
- Current practice.
- Inexpensive ($6 supply cost; labor performed by staff providing anesthesia).
- Minimal training needed for the practice.

Disadvantages
- No policy and procedures.
- Little documented clinical efficacy.
- Not suitable for anemia.
- Not suitable for Jehovah's Witness patients.
- Not suitable for pediatric patients.

Off-Site Blood Recovery

(OR nursing collects; blood bank processes)

Advantages
- Current practice.
- Inexpensive.

Disadvantages
- Limited blood recovery because of the suction canister size.
- Blood transported away from patients, leading to the possibility of ABO incompatibilities or clerical error and transfusion reaction risk.
- Blood recovery yield that is <50% because of inadequate labeling and container contamination.
- Return of blood from the blood bank that is slow and sometimes does not occur. For instance, one patient (S.S.) was undergoing a major spine instrumentation. A reservoir of blood was sent to the blood bank for processing, but the blood was discarded because the container top was open and leaking. Another case of note (B.W.) was undergoing a spine procedure with the container being

sent to the blood bank for processing. The blood was washed, taking approximately 25 minutes, but the blood bank was then unable to find the patient. The patient was eventually located in the intensive care unit (ICU) where she no longer had a need for the blood.

- Low hematocrit (lowest random sample, 14%) of washed blood, leading to patient hemodilution.
- Blood return to the patient typically takes 1 to 2 hours because of handling and processing. This results in patients receiving unnecessary allogeneic blood components or having severe hemodilution as they wait for blood processing.
- Incompatible with Jehovah's Witness patients.
- Incompatible with pediatric patients.

Point-of-Care Testing

Basic hematology testing is an important intraoperative diagnostic component of the service. Point-of-care testing is already being performed by the liver and vascular sections of the department with a proposal for initiation of a hematology-testing site, which would enable billing for these services. Currently, prothrombin time (PT), partial thromboplastin time (PTT), sonoclot, thromboelastography (TEG), and hemoglobin testing are being performed as a part of the BCM care. These tests are performed at various intervals throughout a surgical procedure to assess coagulation status and hemoglobin level.

- Each blood recovery case would have a minimum of two hemoglobin checks.
- Each plasmapheresis case would have a minimum of one PT/PTT assessment.
- Each plasmapheresis case would have a minimum of one sonoclot or TEG assessment.
- Each plasmapheresis case would have a minimum of two hemoglobin checks.
- Each platelet glue case would have a minimum of two hemoglobin checks.

Financial Overview

Projected 1999 Blood Management Case Activity

Case activity projections for the autotransfusion service for 1999 have been made and were based on a combination of the service's actual experience in 1998 and a modest expansion of blood management services to several surgical disciplines in 1999. Activity count projections for 1999 for professional and technical services are listed in the table below.

Activity Count Projections for 1999

Service	Count/Yr	Basis for Estimation
Blood recovery cases	319	Projected from 1998 experience
Blood recovery blood units produced	968	Avg 3 units* per patient
Blood recovery standby cases	100	+ 30% of blood recovery cases
Pheresis cases	183	Projected from 1998 experience
Pheresis blood product units produced	1496	Avg 8.2 units* per patient
Professional consultations	215	100% apheresis patients + 10% blood recovery patients
Intraoperative professional services	199	100% apheresis patients + 5% blood recovery patients

*unit = one unit of Red Blood Cells, Fresh Frozen Plasma, or Platelets.

Professional Revenue and Expense

Professional fees will be charged for two circumstances:

- Intraoperative services, where the clinical care standard requires a second anesthesiologist for longer and more complex blood recovery cases. Special clinical indications requiring a second anesthesiologist for blood management services include high blood loss surgery cases, tumor filtration, or contamination of blood. Such circumstances are expected to occur in approximately 5% of blood recovery cases. The professional charge will be determined by the amount of time spent directly providing services for the case. The estimated average time to be spent by the staff anesthesiologists in both blood recovery and pheresis cases is 1 hour. Clinical services provided and time spent in the case will be documented in the anesthesia record and the green clinical notes to support billing of fees for professional services.
- All apheresis cases will be billed under current procedural terminology code 36520. Response to an inquiry to the medical director of the Medicare carrier yielded verbal confirmation that billing for the services is appropriate when clinically indicated and when documented in the medical record. Documentation will feature a signed note in the green clinical sheets identifying the staff who requested the consultation, the clinical indication for the services provided, the pertinent laboratory data, and an assessment and plan. The anesthesia record will also contain a signed notation regarding apheresis services.

Thus, the professional fee structure is as in the table below.

Professional Charge Basis	Charge per Occurrence
Intraoperative services—5% of blood recovery cases	$320
Apheresis cases	$575

Professional expenses are exclusively related to physician time spent providing blood management services. Physician time assumptions incorporated in the pro forma operating statement are 6 minutes per blood unit produced while providing intraoperative autotransfusion services.

The pro forma operating statement for professional revenue and expense calculates revenue from the volume estimates and charge structure explained earlier. The statement incorporates a net revenue ratio of 48% derived from the anesthesiology professional cost center. Professional expenses are shown and calculated using an average physician salary figure. Indirect expenses are applied at the same percentage (11% of contribution margin) as in the general anesthesiology professional cost center.

The professional pro forma operating statement for 1999 projects a net revenue of $53,049, a net income of $7,608, and a net-income-to-net-revenue ratio of 33%. For a project go-or-no-go decision, however, the relevant financial return figure is $53,049 net revenue, because no personnel additions are planned.

Point-of-care testing professional services, in support of the service, adds a contribution margin of $5,765 and net revenue of $5,073.

Technical Revenue and Expense

Revenue for technical services and supplies will be charged according to services provided (see table below).

Technical Charge Basis	Charge
Blood recovery—base fee	$250
Blood recovery—per blood unit produced	80
Blood recovery—standby	160
Pheresis—base fee	125
Pheresis—per blood component unit produced	30

This technical charge structure incorporates costs for standard blood management supplies and for technician staffing. Structuring the technical charges on a base fee per case, plus a charge per blood unit generated, permits billing in relation to the supply costs and technical personnel costs incurred. The provision for a standby charge reflects an important operating efficiency whereby a case in which services are possible but not certain is set up with the minimum supplies required to immediately initiate blood recovery, if necessary. A case that proceeds to full blood recovery services will be charged the full blood recovery base fee and a per blood unit fee.

Technical charges will be assessed directly for additional supplies used per case, including leukocyte reduction filters and suction anticoagulation lines. The general anesthesiology technical billing ticket has been revised to include all blood management charge options. A reconciliation process for technical billing has been designed and successfully tested that will facilitate a patient-level verification that charges from the service have been processed correctly through the hospital billing system. The individual patient records will be reconciled to specific patients' technical charge data extracted from the operating room information system and in aggregate to the hospital revenue and statistics report.

Technical expenses for the service include supply costs and technician personnel costs. Blood recovery and apheresis supply expenses are detailed in the pro forma operating statement that is based on the case activity projections outlined earlier. Personnel expense is calculated at $13.50 per hour for an AES, applying the assumption of AES labor at 15 minutes per blood management setup and per 15 minutes for each blood unit produced. Total AES technical personnel support is projected to be 721 hours for the case activity level anticipated in 1999. This figure equates to 39% [721 of 1856 non-paid time off (PTO) work hours] of one FTE AES.

The technical pro forma operating statement calculates revenue from the volume estimates and technical charge structure explained earlier. The statement incorporates a net revenue ratio of 52% derived from the anesthesiology professional cost center. Technical expenses for supplies and personnel are calculated as discussed earlier. Indirect expenses are applied at the same percentage (75% of contribution margin) as in the general anesthesiology technical cost center. The technical pro forma operating statement for 1999 projects net income of $11,717 and a net-income-to-net-revenue ratio of 9%.

Point-of-care testing technical services, in support of the service, will yield a contribution margin of $53,622 and net income of $13,406.

Combined service net income is projected at $43,696, or a net-income-to-net-revenue ratio of 11%. However, for project decision making, the relevant financial return figure is the $98,185 contribution margin, because no additional resources will be needed to support the program.

Resources

Professional Personnel

Dr. Bleedalot, MD, will direct the service. Two other professional staff have completed blood management training. This number of professional staff should be sufficient for the needs of the service.

Technical Personnel

Technical staffing is an essential resource for successful and efficient operation of the autotransfusion service. Two AES personnel were trained in 1998 to support the initial limited case activity. The estimate for 1999 is 641 case-hours of involvement by AES personnel. The objective in 1999 will be to train two additional AES personnel as certification-eligible technicians. Thus, technician support will be available from any of the four technicians. Having four AESs trained will increase flexibility in covering support requirements with minimal adverse effect on their productivity in routine anesthesia support functions. Training additional AESs will not directly increase technician manhours in support of the service but will assist in flexibility for covering simultaneous blood management cases and evening cases requiring support or cleanup and take-down.

Certification training for the technicians is available through the American Board of Autotransfusion Technology (ABAT). Requirements involve 20 hours of classroom training and approximately 10 supervised cases. Certification is achieved through written examination. ABAT certification will serve as the credential qualifying AES team members to work on the service.

Case scheduling will be arranged where possible to schedule blood management cases early in the day, thus reducing the need for evening technician coverage. The objective of training an increasing proportion of the AES team complement is consistent with the plan to increase the skill base, certification status, and job codes of the AES technicians.

Responsibilities of AESs for the service will include the following:

- Respond to assignments and direction from the service's staff anesthesiologists.
- Provide intraoperative autotransfusion technical assistance, including equipment and supply setup and operation of equipment.
- Maintain autotransfusion supplies inventory.
- Maintain quality control documentation.

Implementation Strategy

The service's experience during 1998 has constituted a pilot implementation for the following:
- Anterior-posterior spinal fusion.
- Radical retropubic prostatectomy.

The service will initiate support to the following surgical services:
- Orthopedics, for revision total joint replacements.

- Vascular, for major procedures, including abdominal and thoracic aortic aneurysms.

Objectives of operations in 1999 will include demonstrating the cost-effectiveness of autotransfusion relative to banked blood and demonstrating effective record-keeping, data management, quality control, and quality improvement activities and reports.

Research, Education, and Quality Management

Research

A center of excellence is intended as the ultimate goal for research encompassing blood and fluid management. Contained within the arena of blood management would be autotransfusion and hemoglobin substitutes. The research plan for autotransfusion currently encompasses projects that are designed to determine how best to allocate resources by identifying high-risk blood loss procedures (clinical indications) and by evaluating outcome differences that result from application of these technologies.

Projects

Currently, the following projects are ongoing or in various approval stages:
1. Clinical indications
    - Clinical indications for blood recovery in radical retropubic prostatectomy: Retrospective analysis of all radical retropubic prostatectomies performed since 1995 is ongoing with the intent to determine variables associated with large blood loss. The importance of this study is to maximize resource utilization by performing blood recovery only in patients expected to incur large blood loss.

2. Outcome
- Retrospective outcome study of major spine surgery with autotransfusion services: Perioperative plasmapheresis and platelet glue have now been used in more than 50 cases of major spine instrumentation. The intent of this study is to determine if short-term outcome is affected by this service.
- Randomized trial of autologous predonation vs intraoperative blood recovery in radical prostatectomy: The allogeneic avoidance and cost-effectiveness will be compared in two common methods of preventing allogeneic blood transfusion.

3. Other
- Amniotic fluid removal in recovered blood in the peripartum period: The second leading cause of peripartum death is hemorrhage. The intent of this study is to determine if recovered blood can be cleansed to a degree similar to the contamination of circulating maternal blood leaving the uterus.
- Blood recovery in the peripartum patient: According to the outcome of the earlier study, administration of recovered blood to patients who require blood components will be monitored and studied with respect to its effect on coagulation and hemodynamics.

4. Planned projects include the following:
- Randomized trial of perioperative plasmapheresis in combination with blood recovery vs blood recovery alone in major instrumentation spine surgery: Perioperative plasmapheresis is an additional adjunct to blood recovery that can be used for allogeneic avoidance. No data have been published to date concerning the benefits of this technique.
- Randomized trial of platelet glue and its effect on bone growth in major spine surgery: Platelet glue offers the advantages of fibrin glue without the allogeneic exposure. Additionally, platelet-derived growth factors have been isolated that may enhance bone healing.

- Blood recovery efficiency in varying surgical procedures: Accurate assessment of blood loss depends on accurate determination of blood recovery rates. This study is intended to determine how this rate relates to the type of procedure.

Research Funding

- Corporate sponsorship for projects has been requested from autotransfusion device makers. To date, one has been forthcoming with support. That gift included 155 sets of blood recovery bowls and tubing, 30 sequestration kits, and a blood recovery machine, with a total value of approximately $70,000.
- Funding has been sought for two of the projects discussed earlier.
- Additional grant support is being sought from the National Blood Foundation and the American Heart Association.

Education

Education encompasses four levels: technicians, attending staff, house staff, and patients.

Technicians

Development of technician support is crucial to the success of the service. As part of training for an AES, successful completion of national certification by the American Board of Clinical Autotransfusion is planned. The following expectations for proficiency are raised:

A. Basic Technique (3-day didactic course followed by written proficiency exam):
  - Define the role of the autotransfusion technician in the OR.
  - Teach basic hematology cell types and function.

- Discuss the advantages and disadvantages of blood recovery and banked blood.
- Examine the physics of the Latham bowl.
- Discuss how differing conditions in the OR affect the final blood recovery product.
- Learn basic quality assurance procedures and record-keeping.
- Participate in wet labs (bovine blood) to examine machine functionality.

B. Advanced Technique (additional classroom training followed by written proficiency exam):
  - Discuss transfusion medicine theory.
  - Learn point-of-care testing of TEG studies, hemoglobin, PT, and PTT for intraoperative use.
  - Learn basic component pheresis.

Following the didactic instruction, the technician must serve a period of internship under supervision. This period involves a minimum of 10 cases and possibly more depending on the volume of processed blood.

Attending Staff

An introductory course in autotransfusion techniques was held in the department on November 24, 1998. This course introduced six staff members to the basic principles of autotransfusion including the following:
- The physics of the centrifuge bowl.
- Theoretical advantages of autotransfusion.
- An introduction to the Haemonetics Cell Saver 5 and the Medtronic Sequestra-Bovine blood, which will be used to train staff in the function of these devices.

House Staff

A 1-month elective rotation in autotransfusion is planned as part of the third-year anesthesia resident curriculum, which is on an advanced clinical track. This rotation is intended to cover the many aspects of autotransfusion while using the textbook *Autotransfusion: Therapeutic Principles and Trends*, by Roy Lawson Tawes Jr., as a reference source.

Patients

Patient awareness of alternatives to banked blood will be developed through various media.

- A **pamphlet** describing the autotransfusion services will be developed for use in the preoperative anesthesia clearance and evaluation clinic and for distribution in community speaker engagements. This pamphlet will be transformed into an electronic form and posted on the Web site. It will be developed in collaboration with patient education. Approximate cost is $0.11 per pamphlet.
- An educational **videotape** will be developed for the hospital's closed circuit television system. This tape will be developed in collaboration with the TV coordinator. Approximate cost is $1000.
- Dr. Bleedalot has been added to the **Speaker's Bureau** list of lecturers for community organizations with "Alternatives to Blood Transfusion" as the title of the lecture.

Clinical Documentation, Data Management, and Quality Improvement

Clinical Documentation

- **Written protocols** defining who is responsible for the service, the hours of service, the scheduling procedures, and the qualifications of the operator will be developed. Cleaning procedures for the autotransfusion equipment will be developed in consultation with the institutional Infection Control Department.

- **Patient record-keeping** is required by the AABB and The Joint Commission. Currently, data for each case are generated and stored in a password-protected program written in FileMaker 4.0. These data include the date of service, patient name, patient hospital ID, operative procedure, surgeon, autotransfusion technician, and supervising physician. In addition, the products generated, volume, and hematocrit are recorded.

Data Management

Monthly activity records will be generated from the automated clinical records. These management reports will provide documentation to support supply replenishment and inventory control. This information will be reported to the Transfusion Utilization Committee.

Quality Improvement

The autotransfusion service will develop a method of incorporating the program into the department's quality improvement plan. Review mechanisms will include patient-specific medical record reviews and system review.

- **System review** will include the number of procedures performed, the appropriateness of patient selection (compliance with the developed list of clinical indications), the chart documentation of the procedures performed, and the necessity for allogeneic transfusion in patients receiving autologous blood.
- **Patient-specific review** will include unexplained renal insufficiency, postoperative temperature elevation, sepsis, respiratory insufficiency, coagulopathy, and positive blood cultures.

The quality of recovered blood will also be monitored by determination of the hematocrit for every unit of blood processed. Periodic measurement of heparin levels, free hemoglobin, and blood cultures may be performed. However, this practice is not universal and would not be performed unless the quality indicators suggested a need to do so.

Indications for Use of Recovered Blood

The AABB recommends the following general indications for use of recovered blood (1997)[14]:
- The anticipated blood loss is 20% or more of the patient's estimated blood volume, or
- Blood would ordinarily be crossmatched, or
- More than 20% of patients undergoing the procedure require transfusion, or
- Mean transfusion for the procedure exceeds two units.

Specific Surgical Cases

Specific types of surgery for which the technique is especially useful include open heart[15-19] and vascular surgery,[20-23] total joint replacements,[24-28] spine surgery,[29-31] liver transplantation,[32,33] ruptured ectopic pregnancy,[34,35] and selected neurosurgical procedures[36] such as resection of arteriovenous malformations.

Orthopedics

The table at the top of the next page represents the Toronto classification system, which is based on retrospective hospital data from Orthopedic section members.

Based on that classification scheme and the criteria in said table, patients undergoing Class III and IV type procedures would

Major Spine Surgery—A Classification System[37]

Class	Cases	Predicted Blood Loss (mL)	Patients at Risk for Transfusion (%)
I	Discectomy Laminectomy (1 level) Tumor biopsy	<250	2
II	Laminectomy (>2 level) Fusion (1 level) Hardware removal	250-750	15
III	Fusion (>2 level) Instrument correction Kyphosis correction	>750	67
IV	Fusion-anterior/posterior Scoliosis or congenital surgery Tumor decompression Infection debridement or fusion	unpredictable	87

Note: Developed at the University of Toronto and based on 455 cases.

be candidates for blood recovery. Data collected from the hospital database during the last 6 months are shown in the table below.

Procedure	Mean ±SD	95% CI
Anterior/posterior spinal fusion	4,404 ±3,064	−3,207-12,010
Spine tumors	2,702 ±406	1,409-3,994
Multilevel fusion	2,166 ±2,329	1,183-3,149

SD = standard deviation; CI = confidence interval.

These data would support implementation of the stratification from Toronto. In addition, the following cases are thought by the Orthopedic section head to be associated with high blood loss:

- Bilateral knee replacements.
- Hip replacement revision.
- Hemipelvectomy.

Urology

(Source: Diaspirin cross-linked hemoglobin study,[38] retrospective hospital data, Urology section members)

- Radical retropubic prostatectomy
- Recent retrospective data collection at this institution demonstrates an average blood loss of 2645 ± 1821 for one surgeon. Currently, data collection of all radical retropubic prostatectomies is being performed. This data collection is aimed at developing more specific criteria for using recovered blood similar to that for major spine surgery.
- Cystectomy.
- Limited to patients with prior radiation therapy to the pelvis.
- Nephrectomy with inferior vena cava thrombus.

Cranial Neurosurgery

(Source: Neurosurgery section head)

- Giant (>3 cm) and basilar aneurysm resection.
- Arteriovenous malformations [must be complex type (ie, deep and extensive)].

Vascular Surgery

(Source: Neurosurgery section head)

- Thoraco-abdominal aneurysm repair.
- Ruptured aortic aneurysm repair.[39]

Liver Transplant

(Source: Liver Transplant section head)
- Patients undergoing liver transplant whose liver failure is related to primary biliary sclerosis or idiopathic autoimmune chronic hepatitis would be candidates for perioperative blood recovery.
- Patients with liver failure related to hepatitis A, B, or C are not candidates.

Other

- Jehovah's Witnesses undergoing major surgical procedures with significant blood loss expected (assuming the patient consents to the procedure).
- Emergent use for surgical procedures that have unexpected, massive blood loss.
- Patients with rare blood types where allogeneic blood is difficult to obtain.[39]
- Ectopic pregnancy.[40]
- Patient request (only with prepayment).

Indications for Blood Recovery Plus Perioperative Component Sequestration

Devices designed for removal of platelet-rich plasma immediately before surgery are currently marketed. It has been suggested that they may be beneficial if used before open-heart surgery.[41] At this time, insufficient data are available to document the usefulness of this technique.

References

1. Blumberg N, Kirkley SA, Heal JM. A cost analysis of autologous and allogeneic transfusions in hip-replacement surgery. Am J Surg 1996;171:324-30.

2. Vamvakas EC, Carven JH. Allogeneic blood transfusion, hospital charges, and length of hospitalization. Arch Pathol Lab Med 1998;122:145-51.

3. Blumberg N. Allogeneic transfusion and infection: Economic and clinical implications. Semin Hematol 1997;34:34-40.

4. ensen LS, Andersen AJ, Christiansen PM, et al. Postoperative infections and natural killer cell function following blood transfusion in patients undergoing elective colorectal surgery. Br J Surg 1992;79:513-6.

5. Schreimer PA, Longnecker DE, Mintz PD. The possible immunosuppressive effects of perioperative blood transfusion in cancer patients. Anesthesiology 1988;68:422.

6. Heiss MM, Mempel W, Delanoff C, et al. Blood transfusion-modulated tumor recurrence: First results of a randomized study of autologous versus allogeneic blood transfusion in colorectal cancer surgery. J Clin Oncol 1994;12:1859-67.

7. Creasy TS, Veitch PS, Bell PR. A relationship between perioperative blood transfusion and recurrence of carcinoma of the sigmoid colon following potentially curative surgery. Ann R Coll Surg Engl 1987;69:100-3.

8. Sieunarine K, Lawrence-Brown MM, Drennan D, et al. The quality of blood used for transfusion. J Cardiovasc Surg (Torino) 1992;33:98-105.

9. Bull BS, Bull MH. Hypothesis: Disseminated intravascular inflammation as the inflammatory counterpart to disseminated intravascular coagulation. Proc Natl Acad Sci U S A 1994;91:8190-4.

10. Sieunarine K, Langton S, Lawrence-Brown MM, et al. Elastase levels in salvaged blood and the effect of cell washing. Aust N Z J Surg 1991;61:612-16.

11. Sieunarine K, Wetherall J, Lawrence-Brown MM, et al. Levels of complement factor C3 and its activated product, C3a, in operatively salvaged blood. Aust N Z J Surg 1991;61:302-5.

12. Sprung J, Abdelmalak B, Gottlieb A, et al. Analysis of risk factors for myocardial infarction and cardiac mortality after major vascular surgery. Anesthesiology 2000;93:129-40.

13. O'Hara PJ, Hertzer NR, Santilli PH, Beven EG. Intraoperative autotransfusion during abdominal aortic reconstruction. Am J Surg 1983;145:215-20.

14. Stowell P, ed. Guidelines for blood recovery and reinfusion in surgery and trauma. Bethesda, MD: AABB, 1997:1.

15. Ottesen S, Froysaker T. Use of Haemonetics cell saver for autotransfusion in cardiovascular surgery. Scand J Thorac Cardiovasc Surg 1982;16:263.

16. Young JN, Edker RR, Moretti RL, et al. Autologous blood retrieval in thoracic, cardiovascular, and orthopedic surgery. Am J Surg 1982;144:48.

17. Breyer RH, Engelman RM, Rousou JA, Lemeshow S. Blood conversation for myocardial revascularization: Is it cost-effective? J Thorac Cardiovasc Surg 1987;93:512.

18. McCarthy PM, Popovsky MA, Schaff HV, et al. Effect of blood conservation efforts in cardiac operations at the Mayo Clinic. Mayo Clinic Proc 1988;63:225.

19. Giordano GF, Goldman DS, Mammana RB, et al. Intraoperative autotransfusion in cardiac operations: Effect on intraoperative and postoperative transfusion requirements. J Thorac Cardiovasc Surg 1988;96:382.

20. Cali RF, O'Hara PJ, Hertzer NR, et al. The influence of autotransfusion on allogeneic blood requirements during aortic reconstruction. Cleve Clin Q 1983; 51:143.

21. Tawes RL, Scribner RG, Duval TB, et al. The cell saver and autologous transfusion: An underutilized resource in vascular surgery. Am J Surg 1986;152:105.

22. Hallett JW Jr, Propovsky M, Ilstrup D. Minimizing blood transfusions during abdominal aortic surgery: Recent advances in rapid autotransfusion. J Vasc Surg 1987;5:601.

23. Stanton PE, Shannon J, Rosenthal D, et al. Intraoperative autologous transfusion during major aortic reconstructive procedures. South Med J 1987;80:315.

24. Bovil DF, Moulton CW, Jackson WS, et al. The efficacy of intraoperative blood salvage and induced hypotension on transfusion in major orthopedic surgery: A regression analysis. Orthopedics 1986;9:1403.

25. Wilson WW. Intraoperative autologous transfusion in revision total hip arthroplasty. J Bone Joint Surg 1989;71A:8.

26. Goulet JA, Bray TJ, Timmerman LA, et al. Intraoperative autologous transfusion in orthopaedic patients. J Bone Joint Surg Am 1989;71:3-8.

27. Bovill DF, Norris TR. The efficacy of intraoperative autologous transfusion in major shoulder surgery. Clin Orthop Relat Res 1989;240:137.

28. Semkiw LB, Schurman DJ, Goodman SB, Woolson ST. Postoperative blood salvage using the cell saver after total joint arthroplasty. J Bone Joint Surg 1989;71A:823.

29. Flynn JC, Metzger CR, Csencistz TA. Intraoperative autotransfusion (IAT) in spinal surgery. Spine 1982;7:432.

30. Kruger LM, Colbert JM. Intraoperative autologous transfusion in children undergoing spinal surgery. J Pediatr Orthop 1985;5:330.

31. Lennon RL, Hosking MP, Gray JR, et al. The effects of intraoperative blood salvage and induced hypotension on transfusion requirements during spinal surgical procedures. Mayo Clin Proc 1987;62:1090.

32. Dzik WH, Jenkins R. Use of intraoperative blood salvage during orthotopic liver transplantation. Arch Surg 1985;120:1946.

33. Williamson KR, Taswell HF. Intraoperative autologous transfusion: Its role in orthotopic liver transplantation. Mayo Clin Proc 1989;64:340.

34. Merrill BS, Mitts DL, Rogers W, Weinberg PC. Autotransfusion: Intraoperative use in ruptured ectopic pregnancy. J Reprod Med 1980;24:14.

35. Silva PD, Beguin EA Jr. Intraoperative rapid autologous blood transfusion. Am J Obstet Gynecol 1989;160:1226.

36. Keeling MM, Gray LA, Brink MA, et al. Intraoperative autotransfusion: Experience in 725 consecutive cases. Ann Surg 1983;197:536.

37. Callum JL, Hall GA, Kraetschmer BG, et al. A clinical classification scheme and an audit of blood to optimize transfusion practice utilization in patients undergoing spinal surgery (abstract). Blood 1997;90(Suppl 1, pt 2 of 2):128b.

38. Schubert A, Przybelski RJ, Eidt JF, et al. Perioperative Avoidance or Reduction of Transfusion Trial (PARTT) Study Group. Diaspirin-crosslinked hemoglobin reduces blood transfusion in noncardiac surgery: A multicenter, randomized, controlled, double-blinded trial. Anesth Analg 2003;97:323-32.

39. Williamson KR, Taswell HF. Indications for intraoperative blood salvage. J Clin Apher 1990;5:100-3.

40. Keeling MM, Gray LA Jr, Brink MA, et al. Intraoperative autotransfusion: Experience in 725 consecutive cases. Ann Surg 1983;197:536-41.

41. Giordano GF, Rivers SL, Chung GKT, et al. Autologous platelet-rich plasma in cardiac surgery: Effect on intraoperative and postoperative transfusion requirements. Ann Thorac Surg 1988;46:416-19.

Appendix 3-3. Components of a Perioperative Blood Management Program

Blood management should be addressed over the entire perioperative course. Components for each stage of the perioperative period are listed below.

Preoperative Period
1. Erythropoietin.
2. Iron, folate, vitamin B_{12} supplements.
3. Avoidance of anticoagulant drugs.
    a. Nonsteroidal anti-inflammatory drugs.
    b. Herbal supplements.
    c. Antiplatelet drugs.
    d. Heparin/warfarin.

Intraoperative Period
1. Red cell avoidance.
    a. Normovolemic hemodilution.
    b. Blood recovery.
2. Coagulation system avoidance.
    a. Component sequestration.
    b. Normovolemic hemodilution.
3. Adjuncts.
    a. Point-of-care testing.
    b. Microsampling.
    c. Drug therapy: desmopressin, aprotinin, ε-aminocaproic acid, recombinant Factor VIIa.
    d. Deliberate hypotension.
    e. Maintenance of normothermia.
    f. Avoidance of normal saline.
    g. Appropriate positioning.

Postoperative Period
1. Washed or unwashed recovered blood.
2. Erythropoietin.
3. Hyperbaric oxygen therapy.

Appendix 3-4. Sample Order Set for Preoperative Anemia Management

		PHYSICIAN'S PLANS (ORDERS)	
DATE	TIME	ANOTHER MEDICATION SIMILAR IN FORM AND ☐ ACTION MAY BE DISPENSED PER MEDICAL STAFF POLICY UNLESS CHECKED.	"✓" Read Back
		Anemia Management Order Set	
		Call Blood Conservation Office at 932-6183 or the **Blood Conservation Coordinator at 440-8131** for assistance.	
		To be used in conjunction with Anemia Prevention Protocol	
		1. Determine etiology of anemia	
		2. Please draw the following labs:	
		[ ] Draw today and once weekly: CBC	
		[ ] Draw today: iron transferrin and ferritin	
		[ ] 72 hours after initiation of erythropoietin: draw reticulocyte count	
		[ ] Draw transferrin receptor [soluble transferring receptor (STFR)] if ferritin greater than 600	
		*** PHARMACY WILL HOLD A COPY OF THIS ORDER AND SEND MEDS AS APPROPRIATE WHEN LAB RESULTS ARE AVAILABLE***	
		3. Iron store replacement:	
		If ferritin <100 or TSAT <20%, or if STFR is above the upper limit of normal, replace iron stores as follows:	
		[ ] Venofer (iron sucrose) 300 mg over 1-2 hours once weekly	
		[ ] Folic acid 1 mg PO daily (if NPO, give 1 mg daily in IV fluid or subcutaneously	
		[ ] Multivitamin 1 tablet PO daily (if NPO, give 10 mL in IV fluid daily)	
		[ ] Consult dietician regarding foods rich in iron	
		DO NOT GIVE IRON IF TSAT >45% OR FERRITIN >600 UNLESS STFR ELEVATED	

Affix patient label to **ALL** pages (including carbon copies)	ALLERGIES / INTOLERANCES Height _____ Weight _____ ☐ kg ☐ lbs Latex allergy Yes ☐ No ☐
	Page 1 of 2 PO-XXX (MM/YY)

PHYSICIAN'S PLANS (ORDERS)

DATE	TIME	ANOTHER MEDICATION SIMILAR IN FORM AND ☐ ACTION MAY BE DISPENSED PER MEDICAL STAFF POLICY UNLESS CHECKED.	"✓" Read Back
		Anemia Management Order Set (cont.)	
		4. Erythropoietin therapy:	
		The following criteria must be met before erythropoietin is initiated:	
		• Hb <10 or Hct <30	
		• Iron stores checked and replaced as needed	
		If patient meets above criteria, initiate treatment:	
		[ ] Erythropoietin 40,000 units subcutaneous weekly (may IV push, but subcutaneous preferred)	
		[ ] Continue iron replacement as directed above throughout erythropoietin therapy	
		Discontinue erythropoietin and iron therapy when Hb 12 or Hct 36 (May restart erythropoietin if levels fall again)	
		5. Red Blood Cell Transfusion Refer to "Red Blood Cell Transfusion Order Set" for indication and instructions	
		Physician's signature _____	

Affix patient label to **ALL** pages (including carbon copies)	ALLERGIES / INTOLERANCES Height _____ Weight _____ ☐ kg ☐ lbs Latex allergy Yes ☐ No ☐ Page 2 of 2 PO-XXX (MM/YY)

CBC = complete blood count; PO = by mouth; NPO = nothing by mouth; IV = intravenous; TSAT = transferring saturation; Hb = hemoglobin; Hct = hematocrit.

Appendix 3-5. Sample Order Set for Blood Transfusion

		PHYSICIAN'S PLANS (ORDERS)	
DATE	TIME	ANOTHER MEDICATION SIMILAR IN FORM AND ACTION MAY BE DISPENSED PER MEDICAL STAFF POLICY UNLESS CHECKED. ☐	"✓" Read Back
		Red Blood Cell Transfusion Order Set	
		1. Choose one (1) of the following: (Indications/consent must be completed by MD):	
		[ ] Type and crossmatch (#)_____units and transfuse today	
		[ ] Type and crossmatch (#)_____units to hold for surgery	
		[ ] Type and crossmatch (#)_____units and hold	
		2. Hemoglobin/hematocrit:_____	
		3. Indications for Red Blood Cell transfusion (physician must check one or more boxes)	
		A. Anemia	
		• Patients should be **symptomatic and normo-volemic** • Crystalloid or colloid infusion should be used initially to correct hypovolemia	
		Please check which symptoms are present:	
		[ ] Dyspnea	
		[ ] Tachycardia	
		[ ] Hemodynamic instability	
		(Physician must check one or more boxes)	
		I. Acute:	
		[ ] Acute massive blood loss (Example: loss of 3 units or more of blood in 12 hours **or** a drop in hemoglobin >3.0 g/dL in 12 hours)	
		[ ] Hemoglobin <7 g/dL without evidence of acute coronary syndrome	
		[ ] Hemoglobin <10 g/dL in patients with **acute coronary syndrome**	

Affix patient label to **ALL** pages (including carbon copies)

ALLERGIES / INTOLERANCES
Height _____
Weight _____ ☐ kg ☐ lbs
Latex Allergy Yes ☐ No ☐

Page 1 of 2
PO-XXX (Rev. MM/YY)

		PHYSICIAN'S PLANS (ORDERS)	
DATE	TIME	ANOTHER MEDICATION SIMILAR IN FORM AND ☐ ACTION MAY BE DISPENSED PER MEDICAL STAFF POLICY UNLESS CHECKED.	" ✓ " Read Back
		Red Blood Cell Transfusion Order Set (cont.)	
		II. Chronic (Consider the following before you transfuse):	
		• Treatable causes of anemia should be ruled out first, including iron, folate, or vitamin B_{12} deficiencies.	
		• Review "Anemia Management Physician Order Set" to treat anemia.	
		• Young healthy adults can tolerate hemoglobin levels as low as 5.0 g/dL.	
		[ ] Patient is symptomatic with hemoglobin <7 g/dL.	
		B. Perioperative Use—Individualize treatment plan based on patient's risk assessment. Consider the following:	
		• Consider preoperative dosing with anemia management order set to stimulate bone marrow production:	
		[ ] Preoperative hemoglobin <8 g/dL with an operative procedure associated with major blood loss >1000 mL in an individual without evidence of acute coronary syndrome	
		[ ] Intraoperative patients with hemoglobin <10 g/dL in patients with acute coronary syndrome	
		C. Prophylactic Use	
		[ ] Sickle Cell disease with sickle cells >20%	
		Consent: Prior to the time of the transfusion above described, I explained to the patient named below (or to any person who has consented to the transfusion on the patient's behalf) the nature, purpose, benefits, risks, and possible consequences of the transfusion as stated, as well as possible alternative options.	
		Physician's signature:	

Affix patient label to **ALL** pages (including carbon copies)	ALLERGIES / INTOLERANCES Height _____ Weight _____ ☐ kg ☐ lbs Latex allergy Yes ☐ No ☐
	Page 2 of 2 PO-XXX (Rev. XX/03)

In: Waters JH, ed.
Blood Management: Options for Better Patient Care
Bethesda, MD: AABB Press, 2008

4

Transfusion Triggers

LAWRENCE TIM GOODNOUGH, MD;
MINH-HA TRAN, DO; AND
MARK H. YAZER, MD, FRCP(C)

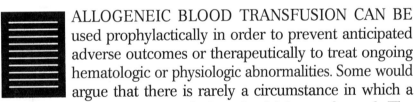 ALLOGENEIC BLOOD TRANSFUSION CAN BE used prophylactically in order to prevent anticipated adverse outcomes or therapeutically to treat ongoing hematologic or physiologic abnormalities. Some would argue that there is rarely a circumstance in which a prophylactic allogeneic transfusion should be performed. The decision to transfuse a patient prophylactically is based on transfusion triggers. Such a trigger is a point at which a laboratory test result is obtained that is thought to be associated with potential adverse patient outcomes. This chapter discusses

Lawrence Tim Goodnough, MD, Professor of Pathology and Medicine, Stanford University, Stanford, California; Minh-Ha Tran, DO, Assistant Professor of Pathology, University of Pittsburgh, Pittsburgh, Pennsylvania; and Mark H. Yazer, MD, FRCP(C), Medical Director, RBC Serology Reference Laboratory, The Institute for Transfusion Medicine, and Assistant Professor of Pathology, University of Pittsburgh, Pittsburgh, Pennsylvania transfusion triggers as they relate to red cell, platelet, and plasma transfusion (see Table 4-1).

Red Cell Transfusion

The therapeutic goal of a red cell transfusion is to improve oxygen delivery according to the physiologic need of the recipient. The usual response to an acute reduction in hemoglobin in the normovolemic state is an increase in cardiac output to maintain adequate oxygen delivery.[1] The heart is therefore the principal organ at risk in acute anemia. Myocardial anaerobic metabolism, indicating inadequate oxygen delivery, occurs when lactate metabolism in the heart converts from lactate uptake to lactate production. The normal whole-body oxygen-extraction ratio (the ratio of oxygen consumption to oxygen delivery) is 20% to 25%. The oxygen-extraction ratio approaches 50%

Table 4-1. Transfusion Triggers for Blood Components

Component	Situations	Transfusion Trigger
Red cells	All	Hb <7 g/dL
Platelets	Surgery	$<50 \times 10^9$/L generally indicated; $\geq 50 \times 10^9$/L and $\leq 100 \times 10^9$/L when bleeding
Platelets	Hematologic malignancy and hematopoietic stem cell transplantation	$\leq 10 \times 10^9$/L in stable patients; $\leq 20 \times 10^9$/L in patients with unstable features
Plasma	All	INR ≥ 1.6 or PT >1.5 times greater than the midpoint of the reference range

Hb = hemoglobin; INR = international normalized ratio; PT = prothrombin time.

when myocardial lactate production occurs, thereby indicating anaerobic metabolism. In a normal heart, lactate production and an oxygen-extraction ratio of 50% occur at a hemoglobin level of approximately 3.5 to 4 g/dL.[2] In a model of coronary stenosis, the anaerobic state occurs at a hemoglobin level of approximately 6 to 7 g/dL.[3]

No single number, neither the extraction ratio nor hemoglobin, can serve as an absolute indicator of transfusion need. However, the use of such a physiologic value in conjunction with clinical assessment of the patient's status permits a rational decision regarding the appropriateness of transfusion before the onset of hypoxia or ischemia.[4]

The Benefit of Red Cell Transfusion

If a transfusion is appropriate, a benefit should result. In a literature assessment of the benefit of red cell transfusion, data on mortality are the clearest. In a review of 16 reports of the surgical outcomes in Jehovah's Witnesses who underwent major surgery without red cell transfusion, mortality associated with anemia occurred in 1.4% of the 1404 operations.[5] In one large study, the risk of death was found to be higher in patients with cardiovascular disease than in those without.[6] A subsequent analysis[7] found that, although the risk of death was low in patients with postoperative hemoglobin levels of 7.1 to 8 g/dL, morbidity occurred in 9.4%. The odds of death in patients with a postoperative hemoglobin <8.0 g/dL increased 2.5 times for each gram decrease in hemoglobin level. Those data suggest that, in surgery-induced anemia, survival in patients at risk is improved with blood transfusion. However, in a large retrospective study of elderly patients who underwent surgical repair of hip fracture, the use of perioperative red cell transfusion in patients with hemoglobin levels as low as 8 g/dL did not appear to influence 30-day or 90-day mortality.[8]

Anemia is a common problem in critical care patients, with two-thirds of patients receiving blood transfusions.[9-12] There is an epidemiologic association between transfusions and diminished organ function as well as between transfusions and mortality.[13,14] A multi-institutional study[15] was conducted to evaluate the effects of a "liberal" vs a "conservative" transfusion threshold on mortality in critically ill patients. A total of 418 critical care patients received red cell transfusions when the hemoglobin dropped below 7 g/dL, with hemoglobin maintenance in the range of 7 to 9 g/dL. Another 420 patients received transfusions when the hemoglobin declined below 10 g/dL, with hemoglobin levels maintained in the range of 10 to 12 g/dL. The 30-day mortality rates were not different in the two groups (18.7% vs 23.3%; p = 0.11), thus indicating that a transfusion threshold as low as 7 g/dL is as safe as a higher transfusion threshold of 10 g/dL in critical care patients.

A follow-up analysis[16] found that the more restrictive strategy of red cell transfusion appeared to be safe in most patients with cardiovascular disease. Among a subgroup of 257 patients with ischemic heart disease, however, there was an insignificant (p >0.30) decrease in overall survival among the patients treated according to the restrictive transfusion strategy. Only a fraction of eligible patients actually participated in that trial, thus raising the question of selection bias (ie, patients may not have entered into the study if their physicians anticipated that they may not do well if they were randomly assigned to be maintained between a hemoglobin of 7 and 9 g/dL). Clearly, more data are needed to determine when transfusion in such a setting is beneficial, particularly when patients are known to have risk factors for ischemic heart or cerebral disease.

A study by Wu et al[17] analyzed the relationships among anemia, red cell transfusion, and mortality in a retrospective analysis of nearly 80,000 elderly (>65 years) patients hospitalized for acute myocardial infarction. First, lower hematocrit values on admission were associated with higher 30-day mortality rates. Second, anemia (defined as hematocrit <39%) was present on hospital admission in nearly half (43.7%) of patients and was clinically significant (ie, 33% or lower) in 10.4% of patients. Finally, red cell transfusion in patients with hematocrit levels <33% at admission was associated with significantly lower 30-day mortality.

Data on the relationship between red cell transfusion and morbidity are less clear. A reduction in morbidity may be possible with transfusion in critically ill patients, especially those with hypoxia or sepsis, by optimizing oxygen delivery and minimizing the frequency of potential complications. In one study,[18] hemodynamic and oxygen transport measurements were examined in five severely burned male patients who did not receive red cell transfusions for 36 to 48 hours after the operative incision. The hemoglobin level was then raised 3 g/dL with multiple transfusions. Although red cell transfusion raised the red cell mass significantly and increased oxygen delivery, the physiologic benefit seemed marginal. The oxygen extraction ratio in particular was not markedly deranged before the transfusion, which indicates that the compensation for the anemia was quite adequate. In addition, there was no change in oxygen consumption, which suggests that red cell transfusion may not benefit critically ill patients without known risk factors.

A report by Babineau et al[19] examined the benefit of red cell transfusion in 30 surgical patients who were in intensive care and were normovolemic and hemodynamically stable. Once again, transfusion increased the hemoglobin level and total oxygen delivery but had a negligible effect on oxygen consumption. There were no important hemodynamic benefits in that group of patients. One can conclude from the data that the assumed benefit of an increase in the red cell mass does not always translate into a true benefit in terms of oxygen transport in critically ill patients.

Silent perioperative myocardial ischemia has been observed in patients undergoing noncardiac[20] as well as cardiac[21] surgery. A study[22] of elderly patients who were undergoing elective, noncardiac surgery found that intraoperative or postoperative myocardial ischemia was more likely to occur in patients with hematocrits below 28%, particularly in the presence of tachycardia. Hemoglobin levels ranging from 6 to 10 g/dL—a range in which indicators other than hemoglobin may identify patients who may benefit from blood—therefore need to be the most closely scrutinized.[4,23] In the absence of a physiologic need or known risk factors in a stable, nonbleeding patient, a decline in hemoglobin level alone is not a good reason to give a transfusion.[24]

Erythropoietin therapy has been shown to effectively increase hemoglobin levels and to reduce the mean number of red cell units transfused in critical care patients.[25] A subsequent multicenter trial of erythropoietin therapy in critical care patients showed a reduction in the percentage of patients transfused, but it did not demonstrate any benefit for a rise in hemoglobin levels when analyzed for time on a ventilator, duration of stay in intensive care, or days in a hospital.[26] Whether blood transfusion is associated with a clinically significant immunomodulatory effect (eg, perioperative infections) has been the subject of debate.[27,28] A single-institution study in a prospective randomized trial found no effect on length of hospital stay or health-care costs when leukocyte-reduced blood transfusions were compared to non-leukocyte-reduced transfusions.[29]

Guidelines for Transfusion

Guidelines for red cell transfusion have been issued by several organizations, including a National Institutes of Health consensus conference on the perioperative transfusion of red cells,[30] the American College of Physicians,[31] the American Society of Anesthesiologists,[23] and the Canadian Medical Association.[32] Those guidelines recommend that blood not be transfused prophylactically, and they further suggest that, in patients who are not critically ill, the threshold for transfusion should be a hemoglobin level of 6 to 8 g/dL. A hemoglobin of 8 g/dL seems an appropriate threshold for transfusion in surgical patients with no risk factors for ischemia, whereas a threshold of 10 g/dL can be justified for patients who are considered at risk. A mathematical analysis[33] suggests that surgical blood losses that exceed 70% to 120% (eg, 3500 to 6000 mL in a 70-kg patient with a 5-L blood volume) of a patient's baseline estimated blood volume are necessary before any blood transfusion, but this model assumes a perisurgical red cell transfusion trigger of a hematocrit between 18% and 21%. Reports by Hebert et al[15,16] of two different transfusion triggers concluded that critically ill patients could tolerate hemoglobin levels as low as 7 g/dL. However, no conclusion could be made for patients with risk factors for cardiac or cerebral ischemia. The evidence reviewed here indicates that patients with known risk factors may very well benefit from higher hemoglobin transfusion thresholds.[34]

With substantial improvements in blood safety,[35,36] concern has been expressed that patients are now at risk for undertransfusion.[37,38] A study by Wu et al[17] provides evidence for the first time that patients with an ischemic organ at risk are affected adversely by the underuse of transfusion. Results of that study have prompted recommendations that hematocrit levels be maintained above 33% in patients who present with acute myocardial infarction.[38]

In summary, increasing evidence indicates that patients who are known to have cardiovascular risk factors and who are anemic should be managed differently from patients now known to be at risk. Clinical studies of patients who are in critical care units, patients who have acute myocardial infarction and are in cardiac care units, and Jehovah's Witness patients who are undergoing surgical procedures have demonstrated that patients at risk suffer adverse clinical consequences with moderate to severe anemia. Studies in a number of clinical settings indicate that morbidity and mortality can be reduced with aggressive management of anemia.

Platelet Transfusion

Although most blood components can be stored for extended periods, platelets, due to their 7- to 10-day circulating life span and need for room temperature storage, have only a limited shelf life (currently 5 days in most blood banks) and are particularly susceptible to inventory shortages. The elucidation of optimal physical conditions for preparation and storage of platelet concentrates—including centrifugation steps, container characteristics, anticoagulant preparation, and storage conditions—have made possible modern platelet transfusion practice.[39-42]

With the addition of apheresis platelet collection and HLA typing methods, transfusion support for refractory patients has improved. Leukocyte reduction, both via nylon-fiber filters and through in-process leukocyte reduction in the case of apheresis collection, reduces the incidence of febrile, nonhemolytic transfusion reactions, cytomegalovirus transmission, and allosensitization.[43-46]

In the absence of other coagulation defects, bleeding risk appears to increase as thrombocytopenia declines to below 30 × 10^9/L.[47] A number of testing methods have been developed to measure platelet function. Although platelet testing can aid in the diagnosis of a qualitative platelet defect, abnormal results are only variably predictive of surgical bleeding.[48] Clinical history of ongoing antiplatelet and other anticoagulation medications and response to previous hemostatic challenges remains a powerful tool in predicting bleeding risk.[49,50] Although indications for platelet transfusion vary, platelet transfusion practice remains an area in need of further clinical trial data to further expand the evidence-based pool of data upon which treatment decisions can be made.

Thrombocytopenia and Bleeding Risk

Absolute thrombocytopenia, even to severe degrees, does not appear to reliably predict bleeding. Risk for mild spontaneous hemorrhage and excessive surgical bleeding begins to rise at counts below 30 × 10^9/L, though, and serious spontaneous bleeding risk rises substantially at counts below 10 × 10^9/L. In a report of 92 patients with acute leukemia, any type of hemorrhage was observed on 92% of days spent at platelet counts <1.0 × 10^9/L. Grossly visible bleeding was observed on 31% of such days and on <1% of days spent at platelet counts above 20 × 10^9/L. Intracerebral hemorrhage was rare (0.76% of days) at counts below 1 × 10^9/L when blast crisis was absent.[47] Such findings have been echoed in patients with autoimmune thrombocytopenic purpura (AITP) as well, where counts of >30 × 10^9/L have generally not been associated with bleeding or increased mortality.[51] Bleeding appears to increase significantly as counts fall below the $10 \times 10^9/L$ threshold.[52] Even before line placement, a number of retrospective studies failed to identify a count that is clearly predictive for postprocedural bleeding. Instead, operator skill, the presence of concomitant severe coagulopathy, and other high-risk features such as sepsis appear to be present in patients with significant bleeding.

Bleeding Risk and Qualitative Platelet Defects

Qualitative platelet defects include inherited and acquired abnormalities. Inherited defects include defects of granule processing and packaging (delta storage pool defect, gray platelet syndrome, and Quebec platelet syndrome), defects of membrane receptors (including Bernard Soulier syndrome and Glanzman's thrombasthenia), and defects in circulating proteins that assist in platelet function [von Willebrand disease (vWD) and congenital afibrinogenemia]. Many other congenital platelet defects are recognized, but an exhaustive review is beyond the scope of this chapter.

The acquired platelet defect that is most commonly encountered in a clinical setting results from antiplatelet agent use in coronary artery bypass graft (CABG) surgery. Here, qualitative platelet defects are routinely imposed through anticoagulation strategies. The qualitative platelet defect imposed by aspirin and thienopyridines—even in the face of normal platelet counts—results in a significantly higher risk of postoperative bleeding. In 40 patients on aspirin with or without thienopyridine therapy within 7 days of undergoing CABG surgery, blood loss was measured via chest tube drainage and transfusion need. In treated patients, regardless of regimen, blood loss and transfusion requirements were significantly greater than either control patients who had not received antiplatelet agents within 8 days or patients whose antiplatelet drug-free interval was 2 days or more.[53]

Chu et al[54] prospectively reviewed the operative course of 312 patients ($\approx$70%-80% received aprotinin) undergoing urgent or emergent on-pump coronary bypass surgery and found that the use of clopidogrel within 4 days of surgery was an independent predictor of transfusion and increased length of stay. Leong et al[55] found no difference in blood loss or hospital stay in clopidogrel-exposed, off-pump CABG patients, but statistically significant differences emerged in the clopidogrel-exposed on-pump patients. This group had a greater degree of blood loss via surgical drains, an increased number of red cell transfusions, and an overall increase in length of stay. Antifibrinolytic therapy was not routinely used in this study. Similar trends were found for the group on both aspirin and clopidogrel. Hekmat and colleagues[56] found similar results in a study examining anti-platelet agent exposure within 5 days of on-pump CABG despite antifibrinolytic coverage; mediastinal drainage, need for blood, and platelet and FFP transfusion were all greater among the exposed patients when compared to nonexposed controls.

Shim and colleagues[57] followed 106 patients divided into 3 groups by time of exposure to surgery (aspirin and clopidogrel continued up to 6 days prior, 3-5 days prior, and 2 days prior, respectively). None of the patients were given antifibrinolytics. There were no differences between groups comparing hematocrit before and after, thrombelastogram parameters, Red Blood Cell unit infusion, or hospital stay. The numbers were small, however, with 33, 50, and 20 patients in each group, respectively. A meta-analysis comprising 10 studies, 913 aspirin-treated patients, and 835 control patients reported an increased amount of mediastinal tube drainage and an increased blood component transfusion rate among patients who were undergoing CABG and were last exposed to aspirin 4 to 10 days before surgery.[58]

In the setting of CABG, a critical issue appears to be whether the surgery is done on-pump or off-pump. Exposure to the artificial surfaces of the bypass circuit leads to platelet activation, consumption, thrombocytopenia, and qualitative platelet defects. Studies assessing the effect of antiplatelet agents on blood loss in general show no increase when an off-pump strategy is used but increased blood transfusion when on-pump procedures are undertaken. The second critical variable is the exposure period: in general, 4 days or more of an antiplatelet agent-free period before surgery appears to limit blood loss more than exposure up to and within 2 days of surgery. One conclusion that can be drawn from these observations is that antiplatelet therapy, in addition to defects induced by the bypass circuit, combine to produce a more severe degree of platelet inhibition than antiplatelets alone. With patients in whom operative bleeding is a concern because of ongoing antiplatelet therapy, consideration could be given to performing off-pump CABG, if possible.

Among other medications with platelet inhibitory function are the glycoprotein (GP) IIb/IIIa inhibitors, which include abciximab [ReoPro (Centocor Pharmaceuticals, Horsham, PA)] and eptifibitide [Integrillin (Millenium Pharmaceuticals, Cambridge, MA)]. The former is a monoclonal antibody directed against GP IIb/IIIa; the latter, a small-molecule inhibitor. These medications are associated with significant bleeding that may be only partially responsive to platelet transfusion.

Platelet Function Testing

The hemostatic competence of platelets in a patient with a convincing history of platelet-type bleeding can be evaluated using testing methods that evaluate platelet function. In the absence of a personal or family history of bleeding, the results are difficult to interpret and detectable abnormalities may be clinically insignificant. Functional testing seeks to measure the platelet response following exposure to a platelet agonist. Markers of platelet activation include release of granular contents, aggregation, and shape change. Commonly used functional tests include the Platelet Function Analyzer [PFA-100 (Dade Behring, Miami, FL)], Plateletworks (Helena Laboratories, Beaumont, TX), platelet aggregometry, and lumiaggregometry. Under research settings or in specialized laboratories, electron microscopy and flow cytometry can also be used to further elucidate a platelet defect. The initial step is to ensure that the patient has a normal platelet count; thrombocytopenia may produce abnormal functional testing results in the absence of a qualitative defect. Platelet satellitism can result from EDTA used as an anticoagulant in the sample and can spuriously lower platelet counts.

Platelet Function Analyzer

PFA-100 is a test accomplished using a specialized test system that simulates high-shear conditions by drawing citrated whole blood up a capillary tube and through an aperture in a membrane situated at the proximal end. The membrane is saturated with platelet agonists leading to activation of platelets whose adhesion and aggregation eventually occlude the aperture. The time it takes to occlude the aperture is measured in seconds and referred to as the closure time. Two cartridges are used: in one, the membrane contains collagen and epinephrine; in the other, collagen and adenosine diphosphate (ADP). Prolongation of the closure time in the nonthrombocytopenic patient is a nonspecific indicator of qualitative platelet dysfunction. Aspirin and nonsteroidal anti-inflammatory drug (NSAID) use commonly results in isolated prolongation of the collagen/epinephrine closure time. Patients with vWD, most of whom express abnormal von Willebrand factor (vWF) production rather than abnormal platelets, may also express prolonged closure time results.

Plateletworks

The Plateletworks system uses a two-step process. The kit provides three tubes: a baseline tube (containing EDTA) and two agonist tubes (both containing citrate and either ADP or collagen). Into each tube, 1 mL of blood is dispensed and, following mixing, a platelet count is performed on each using any hematology analyzer that uses impedance methodology for platelet count determination. In agonist tubes, aggregation (of uninhibited platelets) will be induced by collagen (as an initial screen), ADP (to detect ADP inhibitor or anti-IIb/IIIa effect) or arachidonic acid (to detect aspirin/NSAID effect), and only nonaggregated (ie, inhibited and therefore nonresponsive) platelets will be counted by the analyzer.[59] The following formula can then be applied:

$$\% \text{ aggregation} = \frac{(\text{baseline platelet count} - \text{agonist platelet count})}{\text{baseline platelet count}} \times 100$$

Platelet inhibition may be present as a result of cardiopulmonary bypass circuit, aspirin, thienopyridines, GPIIb/IIIa inhibitors, or other medications. Inhibition may lead to a falsely interpreted platelet count because many of these platelets may not be functional. In a bleeding patient with preoperative exposure to aspirin, a baseline platelet count of $90 \times 10^9/L$, and a collagen agonist platelet count of $40 \times 10^9/L$, the inhibition would be 44%. The equation $0.44 \times 90 \times 10^9/L$ results in a functional platelet count of $39.6 \times 10^9/L$, which gives a value that may theoretically be more meaningful than the baseline count of $90 \times 10^9/L$ in a bleeding patient.

Platelet Aggregometry

Cuvettes of platelet-rich plasma (PRP) containing magnetic stirbars are placed in an aggregometer along with appropriate control samples. Light transmission through the cloudy PRP is measured and set at zero. Alternatively, absorbance of light by the sample can be registered and set at 100%. Following the addition of various platelet agonists, the change in transmission or absorbance of light is measured and graphed in a time-dependent fashion. As platelets are activated and they agglutinate, they fall out of suspension and the sample becomes more translucent, leading to less absorbance or increased transmittance. The aggregometer measures the amount of light passing through the cuvette following addition of an agonist, and a graph of either absorbance or transmission per unit of time measured is produced.

A typical response representing strong platelet activation and aggregation is described by a biphasic line curve representing both reversible and irreversible platelet activation. The latter phase represents complete degranulation of vesicular contents of the platelet with strong activation. Abnormal results can be demonstrated in the setting of antiplatelet therapy, inherited receptor defects, Bernard Soulier syndrome (where dysfunctional, deficient, or completely absent surface expression of GP Ib or GP IX receptors leads to adequate aggregation with all agonists except for ristocetin), or Glanzman's thrombasthenia (where dysfunctional, deficient, or completely absent GP IIb or IIIa leads to adequate aggregation with ristocetin but abnormal aggregation with all other agonists). Although aggregometry appears to provide a relatively sensitive method of describing qualitative platelet defects,[60] it is time consuming, dependent upon operator expertise, and not available at all centers.

Lumiaggregometry and Electron Microscopy

Lumiaggregometry employs various methods to detect platelet granular contents released following platelet activation with various agonists. Although this test is not widely available, it is geared toward detecting inherited or acquired defects. Acquired defects may involve dysfunctional packaging of platelet granules that results in a qualitative, postreceptor defect in platelet function. Detectable abnormalities include delta storage pool defects, gray platelet syndrome, Quebec platelet syndrome, and others. Myelodysplastic syndrome and other hematologic disorders can be accompanied by a storage-pool defect. Further confirmation of such defects requires demonstration of the absence or paucity of specific or several types of platelet granules using electron microscopy.

Indications for Platelet Transfusion

Platelet transfusion is indicated for the bleeding patient strongly suspected to have either thrombocytopenia or qualitative platelet defects. Another subset of patients who might benefit from platelet transfusion includes nonbleeding hematology patients with hypoproliferative thrombocytopenia receiving prophylactic platelet transfusion at predetermined platelet-count thresholds.

Platelet transfusion before bedside procedures to prevent procedural bleeding is a common but non-evidence-based practice. In this situation, it may be more desirable to reserve transfusion for the rare patient who bleeds, as opposed to arbitrarily transfusing all patients. Platelet counts of $\geq 50 \times 10^9$/L and 100×10^9/L are generally recommended before general surgery and neurosurgery/ophthalmic surgery, respectively.[61,62]

Some disease processes [thrombotic thrombocytopenic purpura (TTP) and heparin-induced thrombocytopenia and thrombosis (HITT)] represent relative contraindications to platelet transfusion in the nonbleeding patient. Situations in which platelet transfusions are unlikely to result in meaningful increments include the transfusion of non-HLA-matched platelets to highly HLA-alloimmunized patients, the use of non-antigen-negative platelets in the setting of posttransfusion purpura and neonatal alloimmune thrombocytopenia, and the transfusion of platelets in nonbleeding patients with AITP.

Hematologic Malignancy and Hematopoietic Stem Cell Transplantation

Literature-supported thresholds for prophylactic transfusion in the hematopoietic stem cell transplant patient are generally set at 10×10^9/L in stable patients and 20×10^9/L in patients with unstable features (active bleeding, planned procedure, fever/sepsis, etc).

A number of studies have established the overall safety of a restrictive platelet transfusion policy in the setting of a nonbleeding hematology patient. Trials examining outcomes of prophylactic platelet transfusion have found no significant differences between minor or major bleeding, whether a threshold of 20×10^9/L or 10×10^9/L is used. In addition, the overall platelet usage is significantly lower[62-64] and there tends to be no difference between total units of red cells transfused.[65,66]

In general, patients who experienced major bleeding tended to have other identifiable risk factors for bleeding [fever, sepsis, disseminated intravascular coagulation (DIC) with or without heparin therapy, anatomic lesions, other coagulopathies, increased platelet consumption, mucositis, etc], often in the face of non-critical thrombocytopenia (>10 to $20 \times 10^9/L$) and despite increased intensity of platelet transfusion.

Prophylactic Platelet Transfusion Before Bedside Procedures

A retrospective review of 608 patients was reported by McVay and Toy,[67] using change in hemoglobin as a marker of blood loss. For simple procedures such as thoracentesis and paracentesis, the authors found no increased bleeding in patients with prothrombin time (PT) or partial thromboplastin time (PTT) up to twice the midpoint of normal or platelet counts of 50 to 99 $\times 10^9/L$. The only predictor of bleeding was a creatinine level above 6 g/dL. Only 0.2% of patients required transfusion because of bleeding.

A retrospective analysis of 490 intensive care patients, in whom 938 arterial and venous catheters were placed,[68] found at least one hemostatic defect in 41% and severe abnormalities in 27%. Coagulation abnormalities were scored [based on presence and degree of abnormalities in PT, international normalized ratio (INR), PTT, platelet count, and creatinine] from 0 to 15. The complication rate was 0.25%, 2.87%, and 22% in patients with bleeding scores of 0, 1 to 7, and >7, respectively. Only 2% (16 patients) had excessive bleeding with line placement, whereas 10 had oozing managed with dressing changes and local care. Preprocedural transfusion did not appear to impact complication rate; in fact, it was found to be inappropriately prescribed in 18 of 57 patients in whom transfusion was given specifically to prevent bleeding associated with line placement. The authors suggest that the low rate of bleeding complications results from the inherently thrombogenic physiology of line placement with tissue injury and activation of thrombogenic mediators leading to reduction in hemorrhagic sequelae. Interestingly, a higher rate of bleeding was found in medical patients (9%) as opposed to trauma (1.4%) or surgery (0.6%) patients and was attributed to operator inexperience (line placement by medical residents who had a far lower number of procedures per resident when compared to anesthesia or surgery residents). Results of this inexperience did not seem to be ameliorated by the greater rate of preprocedural transfusion in the medical service group.

In a report of 1000 attempts at internal jugular vein cannulations, predominantly in patients with coagulopathy of liver disease (which includes derangements in PT, PTT, and platelet count), hemorrhagic complications occurred in only 10. All of these were hematomas with only one being severe enough to require surgical drainage.[69]

A report of 104 central venous catheterizations in 76 patients with hemostatic abnormalities[70] described bleeding in 7 cases (6.5%), all of which responded to local pressure, except one patient who received platelet transfusion for prolonged oozing at the site of insertion and did not respond to direct compression alone. This patient had Kaposi's sarcoma and a platelet count of $6 \times 10^9/L$. According to the report, 11 catheters were placed with platelet counts below $20 \times 10^9/L$; 30 with counts between 20 and $50 \times 10^9/L$, and 22 with counts above $50 \times 10^9/L$. Many of these patients also had other hemostatic derangements as well. Patients were not actively transfused before line placement, and the majority did not develop bleeding despite the presence of one or more hemostatic derangements.

Most series examining transfusion before line placement in patients with thrombocytopenia (with or without other coagulopathy) report a low incidence of bleeding complication ($\leq 1\%$-6%). In terms of bleeding-related complications, laboratory parameters tended to be unreliable at describing at-risk patients, or they demonstrated severe coagulopathy (ie, platelet count $\leq 10 \times 10^9/L$ and/or INR ≥ 3). In several series, the greatest predictor of bleeding complication was operator inexperience. In summary, it appears that preprocedural or prophylactic platelet transfusion has little impact on subsequent bleeding complications.

Transfusion of the Bleeding Patient

Active bleeding represents a clear indication for component therapy in a patient with thrombocytopenia or coagulopathy, in whom transfusion will replace the deficient factors. If a drug-induced coagulopathy is present, a specific antidote should be administered (protamine sulfate completely reverses unfractionated heparin and reverses 60% of the anticoagulant effect of low-molecular-weight heparin). No antidote exists for fondaparinux or direct thrombin inhibitors, although some can be partially dialyzed. Many reports are surfacing regarding the off-label use of recombinant activated Factor VII for massive hemorrhage. Additional clinical trial data are needed to better define the use of this agent in such scenarios.

Monitoring the Response to Platelet Transfusion

Following platelet transfusion, clinicians can evaluate for response both by clinical evaluation and by obtaining a posttransfusion platelet count. Thresholds for appropriate corrected count increments (CCI) include $\geq 7.5 \times 10^9$/L at 10 to 60 minutes and $\geq 4.5 \times 10^9$/L at 24 hours in a stable patient (see Fig 4-1). Alternatively, one study considered a CCI of 13,500 ±6000 following transfusion as adequate and a CCI ≤ 5000 following two sequential transfusions of ABO-compatible platelets as refractoriness.[71] Responses at either time point indicate differing etiologies for poor response to transfusion and highlight the practical use of obtaining a 1-hour post-count. Platelet transfusions may precipitate any type of transfusion reaction, but because of room temperature storage, bacterial contamination becomes a concern.

For the average adult with thrombocytopenia, a typical platelet dose would comprise a pool of 4 to 6 units of whole-blood-derived platelets or a single apheresis unit. Knowledge of the patient's height, weight, and pre- and posttransfusion platelet count allow for the calculation of the CCI:

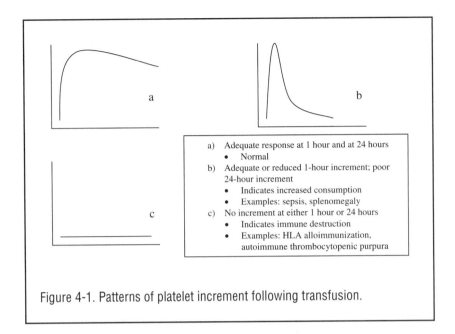

a) Adequate response at 1 hour and at 24 hours
    • Normal
b) Adequate or reduced 1-hour increment; poor
    24-hour increment
    • Indicates increased consumption
    • Examples: sepsis, splenomegaly
c) No increment at either 1 hour or 24 hours
    • Indicates immune destruction
    • Examples: HLA alloimmunization,
      autoimmune thrombocytopenic purpura

Figure 4-1. Patterns of platelet increment following transfusion.

$$CCI = [(\text{postcount}/\mu L - \text{precount}/\mu L) \times \text{body surface area} / \text{platelets transfused}] \times 10^{11}$$

For example, a patient with a body surface area of 1.30 m² is transfused for bleeding at a platelet count of 15,000/μL. The platelet count increases to 40,000/μL when measured 60 minutes following transfusion with an apheresis platelet component containing 3×10^{11} platelets. The CCI would be 10,833, suggesting an adequate response to platelet transfusion.

In a stable, previously transfused patient without splenomegaly, the lack of increment at 1 hour after transfusion is suggestive of HLA alloimmunization. If HLA alloimmunization is suspected, enzyme-linked immunosorbent assay-based testing for the presence of HLA alloantibodies can describe panel-reactive antibodies (PRA) expressed as a percentage. In general, PRA of 10% or more, coupled with clear refractoriness (lack of increment at 1 hour after transfusion) to whole-blood-derived platelet transfusion is strongly suggestive of HLA alloimmunization, particularly when other causes have been ruled out. For these patients, the provision of HLA-matched components may provide improved increment. Patients with sepsis or fever may exhibit a normal or mildly suboptimal 1-hour posttransfusion increment, but because of increased peripheral destruction, they often demonstrate limited survival of transfused platelets and exhibit a rapid decline in platelet count over the next 24 hours. Increased platelet sequestration in the setting of splenomegaly may also lead to suboptimal platelet increments.

Special Scenarios

Administration of antithymocyte globulin (ATG) can lead to quantitative declines in all cell lines. If ATG is administered before drawing the posttransfusion count, one may falsely conclude that the poor increment is the result of HLA alloimmunization rather than destruction by ATG. Administration of GP IIb/IIIa inhibitors in the cardiology setting may be associated with transient thrombocytopenia. Drug-induced TTP/hemolytic-uremic syndrome has been reported following initiation of clopidogrel therapy and during the course of calcineurin inhibitor therapy. The development of HITT is typically seen between days 5 and 10 of unfractionated heparin therapy in the previously heparin-naïve patient. In HITT, a significant hypercoagulable state is initiated—despite declining platelet counts—and bleeding tends not to be a feature. In fact, thrombosis is more imminently a concern, and, if clinically suspected, all sources of heparin should be stopped and a direct thrombin inhibitor started and maintained until the platelet count returns to normal. In this setting, platelet transfusion would appear to be contraindicated.

Platelet transfusion in the setting of TTP is a controversial issue because it is thought to exacerbate ongoing microvascular thrombosis. Scattered case reports report both decompensation and apparent lack of complication following platelet transfusion. Until further data are available, it is prudent to avoid platelet transfusion in this condition unless there is a convincing indication or active bleeding that is clearly caused by thrombocytopenia. If TTP is strongly considered, a plasma exchange regimen should be initiated as soon as possible.

Plasma Transfusion

Numerous plasma components are listed in the *Circular of Information for the Use of Human Blood and Blood Components*.[72] This section will focus on the most commonly used plasma components: Fresh Frozen Plasma (FFP), Thawed Plasma, and Plasma Frozen Within 24 Hours After Phlebotomy. A brief discussion of the appropriate uses of Cryoprecipitated Antihemophilic Factor (AHF) will follow after. As these plasma components are considered equivalent in reversing an elevated INR, the generic term *plasma* will be used to describe their application.

Recommendations for the Use of Plasma

All three types of plasma named above are equivalent components for reversing significant coagulopathies. Emerging evidence suggests that many perioperative patients with slightly elevated PT/INRs do not suffer from major bleeding at a higher rate than those without coagulopathies, although further study is required to delineate when correction is required. The generally employed threshold for plasma transfusion is INR ≥ 1.6 or PT >1.5 times greater than the midpoint of the reference range, because at higher levels the concentration of clotting factors begins to approach critical levels where hemostasis might be negatively affected. The routine administration of small quantities of plasma to perioperative patients with minor coagulopathies probably confers very little hemostatic benefit and potentially subjects the recipients to numerous adverse reactions, including volume overload and transfusion-related acute lung injury (TRALI). Conversely, higher doses of plasma than are currently recommended might be necessary to reverse a significant coagulopathy.

Dose of Plasma

The most commonly used dose of plasma that is thought to reverse a coagulopathy is 10 to 15 mL/kg. When the INR starts to exceed 1.6 (the commonly employed threshold mentioned earlier), factor levels begin to drop below 30%, which for many of them is the threshold for normal hemostasis (Fig 4-2, point A). Factor VII has a short half-life (4-6 hours); therefore, if FFP is administered more than 8 to 10 hours before the planned

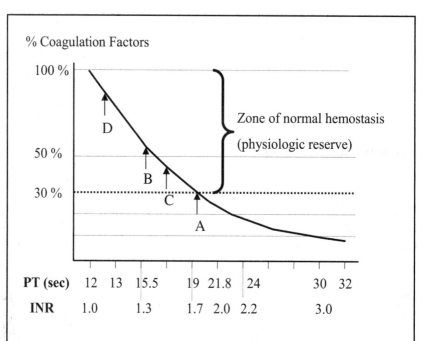

Figure 4-2. Theoretical relationship between concentration of coagulation factors and prothrombin time/international normalized ratio (PT/INR). Experience with single-factor deficiencies has shown that coagulation proceeds normally until the concentration of factors drops below 30%. Thus, nature has provided a significant reserve of clotting factors (the physiologic reserve). Of note, abnormal clotting times can occur while the levels of clotting factors are still within the physiologic reserve—another reason that the PT/INR does not necessarily predict perioperative bleeding. Refer to text for explanation of the labels. Modified with permission from Dzik.[73]

procedure, it will have gone through at least 2 half-lives, thus reducing its hemostatic efficacy at the time of surgery. On the other hand, once plasma is transfused, like all blood products, it is almost completely intravascular volume; unlike crystalloids that distribute themselves between the intra- and extravascular spaces, plasma remains nearly entirely in the circulation. Consequently, it should not be administered too close to the time of the procedure where fast infusion rates (to facilitate the administration of the entire dose of plasma before the start of the surgery) could tip a susceptible patient into volume overload.

Clinical Use of Plasma

The use of plasma in the United States is growing. In 2005, approximately 4 million units were transfused,[74] which is several orders of magnitude higher than in several other developed countries.[75] The indications for plasma transfusion include 1) reversal of a coagulopathy in a bleeding patient or one who is about to undergo a surgical procedure, 2) bleeding in the setting of multiple factor deficiencies or in a patient with a deficiency of a factor for which there is no viral-inactivated/recombinant concentrate available, 3) bleeding associated with massive transfusion, and 4) as a replacement fluid for therapeutic apheresis in TTP patients. But when is a coagulopathy significant enough for the benefits of plasma transfusion to outweigh its potential adverse events, such as TRALI and volume overload?

To answer this question, two important meta-analyses have been performed. Segal and Dzik analyzed 25 studies of variably coagulopathic patients undergoing a variety of minor procedures, including liver biopsy, kidney biopsy, central vein cannulation, paracentesis, and others and asked whether the perioperative PT/INR predicts the risk of major bleeding during these procedures.[76] The vast majority of the reports included in this meta-analysis were observational studies, and only one was a clinical trial. The authors concluded that the strongest evidence suggesting that the preprocedure INR does not likely predict the bleeding risk lies with central vein cannulation, although just how coagulopathic patients can still tolerate the procedure safely has not been elucidated.

As for the literature on the other procedures, the variability in study size and quality makes drawing firm conclusions about the bleeding risk difficult. In 14 of the 25 studies included in the meta-analysis, a control group of patients with normal laboratory parameters of coagulation were also included in the report. In these studies, the risk of bleeding between the two groups of patients undergoing the same procedure could be estimated.[76] Although the confidence intervals of some of these comparisons were relatively large due to the small number of patients in these studies, there was no significant difference in the risk of major bleeding between the patients who underwent the various procedures with and without coagulopathies. While further study is required, especially for coagulopathic patients undergoing kidney biopsy, overall it would appear that patients with mild coagulopathies undergoing various surgical procedures might not require normalization of their laboratory coagulation parameters with plasma to reduce their risk of bleeding.[76] For further discussion of why the PT/INR does not necessarily predict the risk of perioperative bleeding, see Dzik.[73]

The second meta-analysis can shed some light on this question: If plasma is administered to perioperative patients, does it have a beneficial effect in reducing transfusion requirements or surgical blood loss? Stanworth and colleagues searched various medical publication databases looking exclusively for randomized controlled trials where FFP was the therapeutic intervention.[77] Of 57 such trials identified, 19 were focused on surgical or potentially surgical patients: 11 studies based on cardiovascular surgery in children and adults, three studies on liver disease with or without gastrointenstinal bleeding, and one study each on warfarin reversal with intracerebral hemorrhage, massive transfusion, hip surgery, hysterectomy, and renal transplantation. In only 12 of these 19 studies (10 cardiovascular surgery studies, one liver disease study, and the lone study on hysterectomy) did the patients in the control arm receive either no FFP or a colloid volume expander, thus allowing a true evaluation of the effect of the FFP administration. Most of these studies concluded that FFP administration did not reduce blood loss or transfusion requirements.[77]

To understand why prophylactic plasma administration does not reduce perioperative bleeding, it is helpful to consider a study of 22 nontrauma patients who received a total of 68 units of FFP (500-mL units).[78] On average, each recipient received approximately 2 units of FFP, and this dose was >10 mL/kg for each recipient. The average pretransfusion INR was 1.37 (range = 1.1-1.6), and the average decrease in INR was a clinically insignificant 0.03 per unit of FFP transfused. Figure 4-2 demonstrates a theoretical relationship between PT/INR and the concentration of clotting factors; a recipient with an INR of 1.37 would likely have clotting factor concentrations in excess of 50% of normal (Fig 4-2, point B). From the experience with patients with single clotting factor deficiencies such as hemophilia A and B, levels of clotting factors >30% are sufficient for normal hemostasis. Thus, the recipients with INRs of 1.37 were unlikely to bleed even in the absence of FFP transfusion, and the slight reduction in INR did not confer any improvement in the recipient's hemostatic potential. Furthermore, given that some FFP units can have INRs approaching that of these recipient's INRs,[78] it is not surprising that the decreases in the posttransfusion INRs were quite modest.

Abdel-Wahab and colleagues studied FFP recipients from a wide variety of hospital wards and with an assortment of clinical diagnoses.[79] In this retrospective study, 324 FFP units were transfused to 121 recipients who had relatively low pretransfusion INRs (1.1-1.85) and who had posttransfusion INRs performed within 8 hours of the transfusion (the approximate duration of effect of plasma). Once again, only small reductions in the posttransfusion PT and INR were seen: 0.20 and 0.07 seconds, respectively. Only one of the 324 recipients completely corrected their PT/INR, and only 15% of patients corrected their PT/INR to 50% of normal. It is not surprising that patients with lower INRs (1.1-1.5) were no more likely to correct their coagulation parameters than those with slightly higher INRs (1.5-1.85). These authors did not find a correlation between the magnitude of the change in the INR and the dose of FFP administered; that is, recipients of 2 units of FFP were no more likely to correct their INR by 50% than those who received 1 unit.[79]

The latter finding can be understood by considering that 1 unit of FFP (approximately 225 mL), when administered to a 70-kg recipient, translates into a dose of 3.2 mL/kg. Receipt of 2 units of FFP by a 70-kg recipient would amount to a dose of 6.4 mL/kg—both doses are significantly below the recommended 10 to 15 mL/kg of plasma to correct a coagulopathy. Furthermore, each recipient in this study received, on average, 2.7 units of FFP, and assuming each recipient weighed 70 kg, the average dose of FFP would have been only 8.7 mL/kg. Thus, the low rate of correction could be attributable to the small volume of FFP transfused. Additionally, it is useful to consider that the plasma volume of a 70-kg recipient with a hematocrit of 0.40 is approximately 3000 mL. Transfusing 450 mL of plasma (2 regular units) would increase the concentration of clotting factors by 15%; according to Fig 4-2, a 15% increase in clotting factors in a recipient with an INR of 1.5 would amount to only a small decrease in INR (Fig 4-2, point C). A recipient with an INR of 1.5 still has a considerable reserve of clotting factors, and a slight increase in their concentration is unlikely to be important for hemostasis.

This might explain the popular perception of the success of prophylactically administering plasma to recipients with modestly elevated INRs. At one of the authors' institutions, it is a fairly common practice to administer 2 units of plasma to recipients with INRs of 1.3 to 1.5 immediately before or during minor surgical or interventional radiological procedures. Surgeons often comment afterwards that the patient did not bleed excessively during the procedure, which they attribute to the plasma transfusion, when instead the recipient was unlikely to have had a coagulopathic bleed because of the significant reserve of clotting factors (even with the slightly elevated INR). Another study of plasma recipients in Canada also found a minimal response in INR when mildly coagulopathic patients were transfused with small quantities of FFP.[80]

A study of patients with liver cirrhosis who were transfused with FFP was performed in two parts: 1) a retrospective review of the charts of 80 patients who received FFP to reverse a PT prolonged by >3 seconds and 2) a prospective analysis of 20 patients who received FFP with the same laboratory abnormality.[81] The indications for FFP ranged from preprocedure prophylaxis to acute bleeding or prophylactic reversal of a prolonged PT in nonbleeding recipients. The etiology of the cirrhosis in the majority of these patients was either alcohol use or a combination of hepatitis C and alcohol use. The investigators found only a small number of FFP recipients who corrected their PT to within 3 seconds of normal after FFP transfusion (12/100). Interestingly, the two recipients with the highest pretransfusion PTs (PT = 23.8 s and 22.9 s), who received 6 units of FFP, demonstrated, on average, a 9.75-second reduction in their PTs after transfusion. The two recipients with the lowest PT who also received 6 units of FFP (both had PT of 15.5 s) demonstrated only a 0.4-second reduction after transfusion.[81] Although the authors did not convert PT into INR, a PT of 15.5 seconds roughly translates into an INR of approximately 1.3 to 1.5, depending on the sensitivity of the PT reagent, once again indicating that in patients with a relatively mild coagulopathy, minimal correction is expected after FFP transfusion.

It might be hypothesized that the low rates of PT/INR correction after plasma infusion are related to the fact that the patients in these studies have been quite sick. However, a different type of study evaluating the recovery of Factor VII in normal FFP compared to a pathogen-inactivated (S-59 + UVA light) form of FFP in healthy volunteers showed a similar magnitude of PT correction as the earlier studies.[82] In this study, 27 healthy volunteers donated approximately 2.5 L of autologous plasma over time and were then administered warfarin to deplete their levels of vitamin K-dependent clotting factors, which include Factor VII. After they were anticoagulated to levels between 1.5 and 2.0, they were reinfused with 1 L of either their unaltered plasma or their plasma once it had undergone pathogen inactivation after one final dose of warfarin (Fig 4-3, point

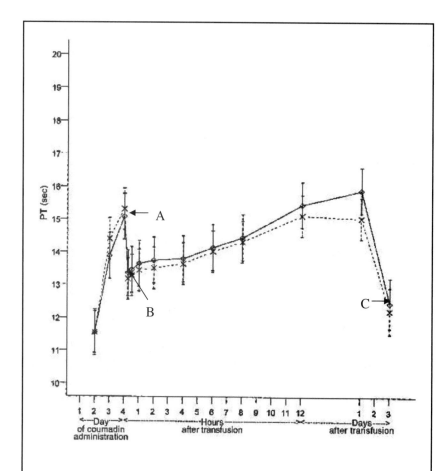

Figure 4-3. Prothrombin time (PT) values in healthy individuals who first received oral anticoagulation, then 1 L of autologous plasma, then oral vitamin K. The Fresh Frozen Plasma (FFP) produced only a partial correction of the elevated PT (B), whereas the vitamin K completely reversed the coagulopathy (C). The therapeutic effect of FFP lasted for approximately 7 to 8 hours. Modified with permission from Hambleton et al.[82]

A). This dose of plasma was, on average, 12 mL/kg for all study participants. The investigators then measured a series of pharmacokinetic parameters of Factor VII, along with a PT. Immediately before FFP administration, the average PT was 15 seconds, and within 1 hour after FFP administration it had dropped to approximately 13 seconds (Fig 4-3, point B). This 2-second decrease in PT represents only about 50% correction compared to the average preanticoagulation baseline PT of 11.5 seconds. At the end of the study period, all volunteers were given oral vitamin K, which resulted in a rapid and complete reversal of their PT prolongation (Fig 4-3, point C). This result should serve as a reminder that, in situations when reversal of a coagulopathy is not urgent, nonhuman-source medications such as vitamin K could be employed.[82]

Interestingly, whereas only 15% of the sick patients in the study by Abdel-Wahab et al[79] corrected their PT/INR by 50%, the average PT correction by the healthy volunteers in this study was 50%.[82] This 50% correction of the PT could have been predicted from Fig 4-2. Again, if the average plasma volume of the healthy recipients was 3000 mL, and they received 1 L of FFP, their clotting factors should have been increased by 33%. A 33% increase in clotting factors is consistent with a decrease of about 2 seconds (from 15 to 13 seconds; see Fig 4-2, from point B to point D). Although these healthy volunteers received,[82] on average, about 3 mL/kg more FFP than those reported by Abdel-Wahab et al,[79] perhaps other factors are involved in determining a recipient's propensity to correct their PT/INR after FFP infusion.

Perhaps the currently employed dose of plasma to reverse coagulopathies is insufficient to effect a significant reduction in the PT/INR. A small Welsh study extensively evaluated the laboratory parameters of hemostasis, including factor levels, PT, and PTT in intensive care patients before and after receiving a median dose of either 12.2 mL/kg (n = 10) or 33.5 mL/kg (n = 12) of FFP.[83] The researchers found much larger increases in the posttransfusion factor levels and decreases in the PT and PTT (especially the PTT) in the recipients of the higher dose of FFP. Although this study did not investigate the clinical impact of higher levels of clotting factors or lower PT and PTT values on these recipients, it is possible that the currently recommended dose of 10 to 15 mL/kg is insufficient to reverse a coagulopathy.[83]

Cryoprecipitated AHF

Cryoprecipitated AHF (Cryo) is prepared by thawing FFP in a water bath from 1 to 6 C and freezing the small mass that precipitates out within 1 hour. The minimum amount of Factor VIII in a unit of Cryo is ≥80 international units (IU), and ≥150 mg of fibrinogen is also required to be present.[72] Cryo also contains vWF and Factor XIII. The total volume of a unit of Cryo is quite small, often 15 to 20 mL. Although the actual amount of fibrinogen per unit of Cryo is probably higher, this discussion will assume that each unit contains 150 mg, as this is the lowest amount that is required to be present. Cryo is a very concentrated form of fibrinogen (150 mg ÷ 15 mL = 10 mg/mL). In contrast, plasma normally contains between 2 and 4 mg/mL of fibrinogen. However, given that the average unit of plasma contains 225 mL, 1 unit of plasma is equivalent to the fibrinogen content in 3 or 4 units of Cryo.

As stated, although Cryo contains Factor VIII and vWF, which are used to treat hemophilia A and vWD, respectively, the first line of treatment of these bleeding disorders should always be viral-inactivated or recombinant factor concentrates, if available. Thus, the main application of Cryo is to correct the hypofibrinogenemia that can occur secondary to numerous disease states, including DIC, massive bleeding, congenital deficiencies, etc. To calculate the amount of fibrinogen required to achieve a hemostatic level—often 100 mg/dL—the following formula can be used:

desired fibrinogen increment (mg/dL) × plasma volume (dL)

For a 70-kg person with a 0.40 hematocrit, the plasma volume is 30 dL; thus, to raise the fibrinogen level by 100 mg/dL, 3000 mg of fibrinogen is required. To calculate the approximate number of Cryo units required to provide the desired amount of fibrinogen, simply divide by the amount of fibrinogen in a unit of Cryo. Therefore, a 70-kg recipient would require 20 (3000 mg ÷ 150 mg) units of Cryo, where 150 mg is the minimum amount of fibrinogen per unit of Cryo. If the patient has already received plasma or platelets (which are suspended in plasma), the number of Cryo units required to reach the threshold is lower. In the above example, what would be the effect of administering 2 units of plasma (450 mL) before the Cryo? Because plasma contains 2 mg/mL of fibrinogen, 900 mg of fibrinogen would have already been transfused. The patient would then require 2100 mg (3000 mg − 900 mg) of fibrinogen or 14 (2100 mg ÷ 150 mg) units of Cryo. These calculations are intended to be a starting point in estimating how much fibrinogen the recipient will require. Close monitoring of the patient's fibrinogen levels and clinical status is recommended.

Acknowledgments

Thanks to Darrell Triulzi, MD, for thoughtful discussion and critical review of the manuscript and to Walter Dzik, MD, for kindly providing Fig 4-2.

References

1. Finch CA, Lenfant C. Oxygen transport in man. N Engl J Med 1972;286:407-15.
2. Levy PS, Chavez RP, Crystal GJ, et al. Oxygen extraction ratio: A valid indicator of transfusion need in limited coronary reserve? J Trauma 1992;32:769-74.
3. Levy PS, Kim SJ, Eckel PK, et al. Limit to cardiac compensation during acute isovolemic hemodilution: Influence of coronary stenosis. Am J Physiol 1993;265:H340-9.
4. Goodnough LT, Despotis GJ, Hogue CW. On the need for improved transfusion indicators in cardiac surgery. Ann Thorac Surg 1995;60:473-80.
5. Kitchens CS. Are transfusions overrated? Surgical outcome of Jehovah's Witnesses (editorial). Am J Med 1993;94:117-19.
6. Carson JL, Duff A, Poses RM, et al. Effect of anaemia and cardiovascular disease on surgical mortality and morbidity. Lancet 1993;348:1055-60.
7. Carson JL, Novock H, Berlin JA, Gould SA. Mortality and morbidity in patients with very low postoperative hgb levels who decline blood transfusion. Transfusion 2002;42:812-18.

8. Carson JL, Duff A, Berlin JA, et al. Perioperative blood transfusion and postoperative mortality. JAMA 1998;279:199-205.
9. Corwin HL, Surgenor SD, Gettinger A. Transfusion practice in the critically ill. Crit Care Med 2003;31(Suppl):S668-71.
10. Corwin HL, Krantz SB. Anemia of the critically ill: "Acute" anemia of chronic disease. Crit Care Med 2000;28:3098-9.
11. Hobisch-Hagen P, Wiederman F, Mayr A, et al. Blunted erythropoietin response to anemia in multiply traumatized patients. Crit Care Med 2001;29:5157-61.
12. Von Ahsen N, Muller C, Serkes F, et al. Important role of nondiagnostic blood loss and blunted erythropoietin response in the anemia of medical intensive care patients. Crit Care Med 1999;27:2630-9.
13. Vincent JL, Baron JL, Reinhart K, et al. Anemia and blood transfusion in critically ill patients. JAMA 2002;288:1499-526.
14. Corwin HL, Gerringer A, Pearl RG, et al. The CRIT study: Anemia and blood transfusion in the critically ill—current clinical practice in the United States. Crit Care Med 2004;32:39-52.
15. Hebert PC, Wells G, Blajchman MA, et al. A multicenter, randomized, controlled clinical trial of transfusion requirements in critical care. N Engl J Med 1999;340:409-17.
16. Hebert PC, Yetisir E, Martin C, et al. Is a low transfusion threshold safe in critically ill patients with cardiovascular disease? Crit Care Med 2001;29:227-34.
17. Wu WC, Rathore SS, Wang Y, et al. Blood transfusion in elderly patients with acute myocardial infarction. N Engl J Med 2001;345:1230-6.
18. Gore DC, DeMaria EJ, Reines HD. Elevations in red blood cell mass reduce cardiac index without altering the oxygen consumption in severely burned patients. Surg Forum 1992;43:721-3.
19. Babineau TJ, Dzik WH, Borlase BC, et al. Reevaluation of current transfusion practices in patients in surgical intensive care units. Am J Surg 1992;164:22-5.
20. Mangano DT, Browner WS, Hollenberg M, et al. Association of perioperative myocardial ischemia with cardiac morbidity and mortality in men undergoing noncardiac surgery. N Engl J Med 1990;323:1781-8.
21. Rao TLK, Montoya A. Cardiovascular, electrocardiographic and respiratory changes following acute anemia with volume replacement in patients with coronary artery disease. Anesth Dev 1985;12:49-54.
22. Hogue CW Jr, Goodnough LT, Monk TG. Perioperative myocardial ischemic episodes are related to hematocrit level in patients undergoing radical prostatectomy. Transfusion 1998;38:924-31.
23. Practice guidelines for blood component therapy: A report by the American Society of Anesthesiologists Task Force on Blood Component Therapy. Anesthesiology 1996;84:732-47.
24. Welch HG, Mehan KR, Goodnough LT. Prudent strategies for elective red blood cell transfusion. Ann Intern Med 1992;116:393-40.
25. Corwin HL, Gettinger A, Rodriquez RR, et al. Efficacy of recombinant human erythropoietin in the critically ill patient: A randomized, double-blind, placebo-controlled trial. Crit Care Med 1999;27:236-40.

26. Corwin HL, Gettinger A, Pearl RG, et al. Efficacy of recombinant human erythropoietin in critically ill patients: A randomized controlled trial. JAMA 2002; 288:2827-35.

27. Blajchman MA. Transfusion-associated immunomodulation and universal white cell reduction. Are we putting the cart before the horse? Transfusion 1999;39: 667-70.

28. Goodnough LT. The case against universal leukoreduction (and for the practice of evidence-based medicine). Transfusion 2000;40:1522-7.

29. Dzik S, Anderson JK, O'Neill M, et al. A prospective randomized clinical trial of universal WBC reduction. Transfusion 2002;42:1114-22.

30. Consensus conference: Perioperative red blood cell transfusion. JAMA 1988; 260:2700-3.

31. American College of Physicians. Practice strategies for elective red blood cell transfusion. Ann Intern Med 1992;116:403-6.

32. Expert Working Group. Guidelines for red blood cell and plasma transfusions for adults and children. Can Med Assoc J 1997;156(Suppl 11):S1-S24.

33. Weiskopf RB. Efficacy of acute normovolemic hemodilution assessed as a function of fraction of blood volume lost. Anesthesiology 2001;94:439-46.

34. Goodnough LT, Brecher ME, Kanter MH, Aubuchon JP. Medical progress: Transfusion medicine, part I. Blood transfusion. N Engl J Med 1999;340:438-47.

35. Goodnough LT, Shander A, Brecher ME. Transfusion medicine, looking to the future. Lancet 2003;361:161-9.

36. Valeri CR, Crowley JP, Loscalzo J. The red cell transfusion trigger: Has a sin of commission now become a sin of omission? Transfusion 1998;38:602-10.

37. Lenfant C. Transfusion practices should be audited for both undertransfusion and overtransfusion (letter). Transfusion 1992;32:873-4.

38. Goodnough LT, Bach RG. Anemia, transfusion, and mortality. N Engl J Med 2001;345:1272-4.

39. Mourad N. A simple method for preparing platelet concentrates free of aggregates. Transfusion 1968;8:48.

40. Slichter SJ, Harker LA. Preparation and storage of platelet concentrates. Transfusion 1976;16:8-12.

41. Slichter SJ, Harker LA. Preparation and storage of platelet concentrates. I. Factors influencing the harvest of viable platelets from whole blood. Br J Haematol 34:395-402.

42. Slichter SJ, Harker LA. Preparation and storage of platelet concentrates. II. Storage variables influencing platelet viability and function. Br J Haematol 34:403-19.

43. Heddle NM, Klama L, Singer J, et al. The role of plasma from platelet concentrates in transfusion reactions. N Engl J Med 1994;331:625-8.

44. Yazer MH, Podlosky L, Clarke G, Nahirniak SM. The effect of prestorage WBC reduction on the rates of febrile nonhemolytic transfusion reactions to platelet concentrates and RBC. Transfusion 2004;44:10-5.

45. Bowden RA, Slichter SS, Sayers M, et al. A comparison of filtered leukocyte-reduced and cytomegalovirus (CMV) seronegative blood products for the prevention of transfusion-associated CMV infection after marrow transplant. Blood 1995;86:3598-603.

46. Seftel MD, Growe GH, Petraszko T, et al. Universal prestorage leukoreduction in Canada decreases platelet alloimmunization and refractoriness. Blood 2004;103:333-9.

47. Gaydos LA, Freireich EJ, Mantel N. The quantitative relation between platelet count and hemorrhage in patients with acute leukemia. N Engl J Med 1962;266:905-9.

48. Bracey AW, Grigore AM, Nussmeier NA. Impact of platelet testing on presurgical screening and implications for cardiac and noncardiac surgical procedures. Am J Cardiol 2006;98(Suppl):25N-32N.

49. Koscielny J, Ziemer S, Radtke H, et al. A practical concept for preoperative identification of patients with impaired primary hemostasis. Clin Appl Thromb Hemost 2004;10:195-204.

50. Koscielny J, von Tempelhoff GF, Ziemer S, et al. A practical concept for preoperative management of patients with impaired primary hemostasis. Clin Appl Thromb Hemost 2004;10:155-66.

51. Stasi R, Provan D. Management of immune thrombocytopenic purpura in adults. Mayo Clin Proceed 2004;79:504-22.

52. Lacey JV, Penner JA. Management of idiopathic thrombocytopenic purpura in the adult. Semin Thromb Hemost 1977;3:160-74.

53. Picker SM, Kaleta T, Hekmat K, et al. Antiplatelet therapy preceding coronary artery surgery: Implications for bleeding, transfusion requirements, and outcome. Eur J Anaesthesiol 2007;24:332-9.

54. Chu MWA, Wilson SR, Novick RJ, et al. Does clopidogrel increase blood loss following coronary artery bypass surgery? Ann Thoracic Surg 2004;78:1536-41.

55. Leong JY, Baker RA, Shah PJ, et al. Clopidogrel and bleeding after coronary artery bypass graft surgery. Ann Thoracic Surg 2005;80:928-33.

56. Hekmat K, Menzel C, Kroener A, et al. The effect of preoperative antiplatelet therapy in coronary artery surgery: Blood transfusion requirements for patients on cardiopulmonary bypass. Curr Med Res Opin 2004;20:1429-35.

57. Shim JK, Choi YS, Oh YJ, et al. Effects of preoperative aspirin and clopidogrel therapy on perioperative blood loss and blood transfusion requirements in patients undergoing off-pump coronary artery bypass graft surgery. J Thorac Cardiovasc Surg 2007;134:59-64.

58. Alghamdi AA, Moussa F, Fremes SE. Does the use of preoperative aspirin increase the risk of bleeding in patients undergoing coronary artery bypass grafting surgery? Systematic review and meta-analysis. J Cardiac Surg 2007;22: 247-56.

59. Helena Laboratories Point of Care. Plateletworks ADP and Collagen (package insert). Beaumont, TX: Helena Laboratories, 2006. [Available at http://www.helena.com/Procedures/Pro190Rev5.pdf (accessed January 2, 2008).]

60. Rebulla P, Finazzi G, Marangoni F, et al. The threshold for prophylactic platelet transfusions in adults with acute myeloid leukemia. New Engl J Med 1997; 337:1870-5.

61. Stroncek DF, Rebulla P. Platelet transfusions. Lancet 2007;370;427-38.

62. Slichter SJ. Platelet transfusion therapy. Hematol Oncol Clin North Am 2007; 697-729.

63. Wandt H, Frank M, Ehninger G, et al. Safety and cost effectiveness of a $10 \times 10^9/L$ trigger for prophylactic platelet transfusions compared to the traditional

20×10^9/L: A prospective comparative trial in 105 patients with acute myeloid leukemia. Blood 1998;91:3601-6.

64. Gmur J, Burger J, Schanz U, et al. Safety of stringent prophylactic platelet transfusion policy for patients with acute leukemia. Lancet 1991;338:1223-6.

65. Zumberg M, Luz U, del Rosario M, et al. A prospective randomized trial of prophylactic platelet transfusion and bleeding incidence in hematopoietic stem cell transplant recipients: 10,000/µL vs 20,000/µL trigger. Biol Blood Marrow Transplant 2002;8:569-76.

66. Nevo S, Fuller A. Acute bleeding complications in patients after hematopoietic stem cell transplantation with prophylactic platelet transfusion triggers of 10×10^9 and 10×10^9 per L. Transfusion 2007;47:801-81.

67. McVay PA, Toy PT. Lack of increased bleeding after paracentesis and thoracentesis in patients with mild coagulation abnormalities. Transfusion 1991;31:164-71.

68. DeLoughery TG, Liebler JM, Simonds V, Goodnight SH. Invasive line placement in critically ill patients: Do hemostatic defects matter? Transfusion 1996;36:827-31.

69. Goldfarb G, Lebrec D. Percutaneous cannulation of the internal jugular vein in patients with coagulopathies: An experience based on 1000 attempts. Anesthesiology 1982;56:321-3.

70. Doerfler ME, Kaufman B, Goldenberg AS. Central venous catheter placement in patients with disorders of hemostasis. Chest 1996;110:185-8.

71. The Trial to Reduce Alloimmunization to Platelets Study Group. Leukocyte reduction and ultraviolet B irradiation of platelets to prevent alloimmunization and refractoriness to platelet transfusions. N Engl J Med 1997;337:1861-9.

72. AABB, America's Blood Centers, American Red Cross. Circular of information for the use of human blood and blood components. Bethesda, MD: AABB, 2002.

73. Dzik WH. Component therapy before bedside procedures. In: Mintz PC, ed. Transfusion therapy: Clinical principles and practice. 2nd ed. Bethesda, MD: AABB Press, 2005.

74. US Department of Health and Human Services. The 2005 nationwide blood collection and utilization survey report. Washington, DC: DHHS, 2006:20. [Available at http://www.aabb.org/Content/Programs_and_Services/Data_Center/NBCUS/nbcus.htm (accessed January 3, 2008).]

75. Wallis JP, Dzik S. Is fresh frozen plasma overtransfused in the United States? Transfusion 2004;44:1674-5.

76. Segal JB, Dzik WH. Paucity of studies to support that abnormal coagulation test results predict bleeding in the setting of invasive procedures: An evidence-based review. Transfusion 2005;45:1413-25.

77. Stanworth SJ, Brunskill SJ, Hyde CJ, et al. Is fresh frozen plasma clinically effective? A systematic review of randomized controlled trials. Br J Haematol 2004;126:139-52.

78. Holland LL, Foster TM, Marlar RA, et al. Fresh frozen plasma is ineffective for correcting minimally elevated international normalized ratios. Transfusion 2005;45:1234-5.

79. Abdel-Wahab OI, Healy B, Dzik WH. Effect of fresh-frozen plasma transfusion on prothrombin time and bleeding in patients with mild coagulation abnormalities. Transfusion 2006;46:1279-85.

80. Cheng CK, Sadek I. Fresh-frozen plasma transfusion in patients with mild coagulation abnormalities at a large Canadian transfusion center. Transfusion 2007; 47:748.

81. Youssef WI, Salazar F, Dasarathy S, et al. Role of fresh frozen plasma infusion in correction of coagulopathy of chronic liver disease: A dual phase study. Am J Gastroenterol 2003;98:1391-4.

82. Hambleton J, Wages D, Radu-Radulescu L, et al. Pharmacokinetic study of FFP photochemically treated with amotosalen (S-59) and UV light compared to FFP in healthy volunteers anticoagulated with warfarin. Transfusion 2002; 42:1302-27.

83. Chowdhury P, Saayman AG, Paulus U, et al. Efficacy of standard dose and 30 mL/kg fresh frozen plasma in correcting laboratory parameters of haemostasis in critically ill patients. Br J Haematol 2004;125:69-73.

In: Waters JH, ed.
Blood Management: Options for Better Patient Care
Bethesda, MD: AABB Press, 2008

5

Blood Management Strategies to Treat Anemia and Thrombocytopenia in the Cancer Patient

PATRICIA A. FORD, MD

THIS CHAPTER OUTLINES STRATEGIES THAT optimize the use of erythropoietic agents and iron as well as other non-blood medical techniques to treat anemia and thrombocytopenia, especially as they relate to the oncologic patient. Cancer-related anemia and thrombocytopenia are still frequently treated with transfusion support, resulting in subsequent reduction or delay of radiation or chemotherapy dosages, which may lead to suboptimal treatment.

The pathophysiology of anemia and thrombocytopenia directly caused by malignancy and subsequent treatment is multifactorial (see Table 5-1). The anemia of cancer is characterized,

Patricia A. Ford, MD, Director, Center for Bloodless Medicine and Surgery, Pennsylvania Hospital, Joan Karnell Cancer Center, Philadelphia, Pennsylvania

---

Table 5-1. Factors in Cancer-Related Anemia and Thrombocytopenia

---

Malignancy-associated
- Bone marrow infiltration
- Humoral inhibitors of hematopoiesis
- Reduced levels of hematopoietic growth factors
- Nutritional deficiency
- Blood loss
- Hypersplenism
- Autoimmune hemolysis
- Disseminated intravascular coagulopathy

Therapy-associated
- Bone marrow fibrosis or necrosis
- Committed progenitor cell death (short-term myelosuppression)
- Stem cell death (long-term myelosuppression)
- Blockage or delay of hematopoietic precursor proliferation
- Long-term myelodysplasia
- Immune-mediated destruction

Surgery-associated
- Perioperative blood loss
- Reduced levels of hematopoietic growth factors after surgery

---

like the anemia of chronic disease, by reduced red cell production coupled with impaired iron use despite adequate stores of bone marrow iron. Malignant tumors also produce inflammatory cytokines, such as interleukin 1 and tumor necrosis factor, that directly suppress marrow function and impair iron absorption.

A non-blood-therapy approach would be desirable to avoid infections and further immunosuppression in individuals with cancer. Interventions to avoid anemia allow cancer therapy to be given on time, and they potentially decrease cancer recurrence[1,2] and improve quality of life.[3-5] Many of the strategies learned from the care of Jehovah's Witness patients to reduce transfusions have proved useful in many medical, surgical, and obstetric settings. This chapter's approach to anemia and thrombocytopenia focuses on simultaneous interventions to enhance hemostasis, stimulate erythropoiesis, control ongoing blood losses, and maintain hemodynamic stability.

Treatment of Anemia

Erythropoietic Agents

Erythropoiesis-stimulating agents (ESAs) should be started as soon as the hemoglobin begins to decline from baseline rather than when significant anemia is present. The two recombinant ESAs that have been approved for the treatment of chemotherapy-induced anemia are epoetin alfa [Procrit (Ortho Biotech, Bridgewater, NJ) or Epogen (Amgen Inc, Thousand Oaks, CA)] and darbepoetin alfa [Aranesp (Amgen Inc)]. Endogenous erythropoietin (EPO) is a glycoprotein that is produced in the kidney and that stimulates red cell production by exerting its effect on committed erythroid progenitors in the marrow. Epoetin alfa (epoetin) is a recombinant glycoprotein that contains the identical amino acid sequence that is biologically indistinguishable from EPO. Darbepoetin alfa (darbepoetin) is a newer drug that is classified as a novel erythropoiesis-stimulating protein. It activates the same receptors as recombinant human erythropoietin but has a serum half-life that is two to three times longer. That phenomenon has been attributed to its higher carbohydrate content, which also creates the potential for prolonging its dosing interval.

A thorough anemia evaluation should be performed at the initiation of therapy and again if an inadequate response occurs. Causes other than cancer treatment may coexist, including iron deficiency, occult blood losses, or hemolysis. Baseline laboratory studies should include complete blood count (CBC) with review of the peripheral smear, reticulocyte count, EPO level, and ferritin, vitamin B_{12}, and folate levels, as well as a full metabolic panel to assess renal and liver function.

Administration of epoetin in subcutaneous weekly injections of 40,000 international units (IU) has become standard because that schedule was found to produce efficacy similar to the original three-times-per-week dosing.[6,7] Weekly CBC and reticulocyte counts are obtained to assess response. In general, patients with lower baseline EPO levels have better responses. A review of multiple studies showed an expected increase in hemoglobin after 4 weeks, ranging from 1.8 to 2.8 g/dL.[8] If there is no improvement at that point, dosages are increased to 60,000 IU and additional iron is administered. Subsequently, if there is no response in 8 weeks, administering more epoetin may not be beneficial. Once a target hemoglobin has been achieved, less frequent maintenance dosing can be attempted for patient convenience and cost-effectiveness, especially in the nononcologic setting.

For darbepoetin in cancer patients, the package insert recommends a starting dose of 2.25 µg/kg every week.[9] For inadequate responses (hemoglobin increases <1 g/dL), the dose can be increased to 4.5 µg/kg. Darbepoetin has been found to have a dose-response relationship, with greater efficacy seen with increasing doses.[10] Darbepoetin is supplied as either vials or prefilled syringes of 200, 300, or 500 µg. To avoid wasting unused drug, most patients in community settings receive 200 µg, with an increase to 300 µg at Week 4 for inadequate responses. Recently published results of randomized trials suggest using a front-loading approach as an effective method to achieve and maintain hemoglobin levels during chemotherapy: weekly darbepoetin until the target hemoglobin level is reached, followed by administration every 2 or 3 weeks.[11]

Both agents are well tolerated, although adverse effects such as constipation, edema, myalgia, headache, pyrexia, vomiting, dyspnea, and pruritus have been reported. All erythropoietic agents are contraindicated in patients with hypersensitivity to albumin or other mammalian-derived products and in patients with uncontrolled hypertension. There does not appear to be any direct effect on blood pressure, but blood pressure can elevate during administration of epoetin and darbepoetin. Therefore, blood pressure should be adequately controlled before therapy and closely monitored throughout treatment. EPO receptors are expressed in various cancer cell lines, including breast and endometrial lines; however, it is not known if those receptors are functional or if they have any clinical implications.[12,13]

On November 8, 2007, the Food and Drug Administration approved new boxed warnings and other safety-related product labeling changes for the ESAs Epogen, Procrit, and Aranesp because of adverse events in recent trials. Patients with renal failure experienced greater risks for death and serious cardiovascular events when administered ESAs to target higher hemoglobin levels.[14] ESAs shortened overall survival and/or time-to-tumor progression in clinical studies in patients with advanced breast, head and neck, lymphoid, and non-small-cell malignancies when dosed to target a hemoglobin of 12 g/dL.[15-18] The risks of shortened survival and tumor progression have not been excluded when ESAs are dosed to such a target. When used preoperatively, ESAs increased the rate of deep venous thromboses in patients not receiving prophylactic anticoagulation.[19]

To minimize these risks, the following guidelines should be followed. Medical personnel should always use the lowest dose of ESA that will gradually increase the hemoglobin concentration to the lowest level sufficient to avoid the need for red cell transfusion. Target hemoglobin level should be 11 to 12 g/dL to decrease risk of complications. In cancer patients, ESAs should be used only for treatment of anemia resulting from concomitant myelosuppressive chemotherapy, and it should be discontinued following the completion of a chemotherapy course. And finally, antithrombotic prophylaxis should be considered with preoperative use.

Regarding cost, very limited pharmacoeconomic data exist. Cost reimbursement varies widely, and there is a lack of direct comparison for epoetin vs darbepoetin. Because each insurance carrier has different guidelines and policies, all patients at the author's practice meet with a billing specialist at the initiation of therapy to review their coverage options.

Iron Therapy

Iron deficiency is categorized as being either "absolute," as evidenced by inadequate iron stores, or "functional," where the provision of iron is insufficient to meet the increased demands of erythropoiesis. There are numerous reasons for a high prevalence of iron deficiency among cancer patients, including inadequate dietary intake, impaired iron reabsorption, occult blood loss, phlebotomy, and blood loss attributed to repeated laboratory testing or surgery. Concurrent administration of iron is essential with ESA therapy because the effectiveness of ESAs is limited when any degree of iron deficiency is present (ferritin <100 µg/L and transferrin saturation <20%). A diagnosis of absolute iron deficiency can be made when the ferritin level is <12 µg/L; however, a level between 12 and 100 µg/L can be difficult to interpret in the context of underlying inflammatory processes such as malignancy.

Although various oral iron formulations are available (most providing approximately 200 mg/day of elemental iron), their use is limited by intolerable gastrointestinal side effects and an inability to meet the demands of ESA-induced accelerated erythropoiesis. For instances in which oral iron therapy is desirable, tolerability can be improved by gradually escalating the dosage and administering it with meals. Taking oral iron in conjunction with vitamin C has the potential to increase absorption. Iron and vitamin supplementation (folate, vitamin B-complex, and vitamin C) necessary for red cell production should be started concurrently. Dietary goals should also be reviewed, as shown in Tables 5-2 and 5-3.

Some patients who do not respond to ESAs alone will respond when supplemental intravenous (IV) iron is added to the regimen. IV iron dextran [INFeD Pharma (Watson Inc, Corona, CA) and Dexferrum (American Regent Inc, Shirley, NY)] has been available for decades, and two dextran-free preparations were recently introduced in the United States: sodium ferric gluconate [Ferrlecit (Watson Nephrology, Morristown, NJ)] and iron sucrose [Venofer (American Regent)] (see Table 5-4). Of the three IV iron formulations available in the United States,

Table 5-2. Dietary Sources of Iron*

High	Medium	Low
Cereals (eg, Cream of Wheat,[†] Total,[‡] Product 19[§])	Blackstrap molasses	Blackberries
	Dried apricots and peaches	Black-eyed peas
Farina (enriched)	Dried beans	Bread
Heart	Lean meat and turkey	Eggs
Kidney	Lima beans	Green peas
Liver	Liverwurst	Strawberries
	Nuts (eg, cashews, Brazil nuts, walnuts)	Watermelon
	Oysters and clams	
	Prunes	
	Raisins	
	Spinach	

*Iron dietary goals:
1. Eat at least one food high in iron at each meal.
2. Limit consumption of coffee and tea because they decrease iron absorption.
3. Use cast-iron cookware.
4. Eat more fortified and enriched grain products.
[†]B&G Foods, Parsippany, NJ.
[‡]General Mills, Minneapolis, MN.
[§]Kellogg, Battle Creek, MI.

iron dextran is the only one that requires a test dose to help avoid anaphylactic reactions that have been attributed to the dextran component.

Iron dextran preparations are the only products that can be given as total dose infusions even though additional adverse events have been associated with them. An extensive review by Faich and Strobos[20] compared the safety profile of sodium ferric gluconate used in Germany and Italy (2.7 million doses per year from 1992 to 1996) with the safety profile of iron dextran used in the United States (3 million doses per year in 1995) during a 20-year period (1976-1996). During the period reviewed, there was a rate of 3.3 allergic reactions per million doses of sodium

Table 5-3. Dietary Sources of Vitamin C and Vitamin K		
Vitamin C	**Vitamin K**	
Broccoli	Beef	Oats
Citrus fruits and juices	Broccoli	Pork
Green leafy vegetables	Brussels sprouts	Spinach
Potatoes	Cabbage	Strawberries
Tomatoes	Cauliflower	Swiss chard
	Cheese	Turnip greens
	Green tea	Vegetable oil
	Milk	

ferric gluconate (74 reactions with no deaths) and a rate of 8.7 allergic reactions per million doses for IV iron dextran (196 reactions with 31 deaths). More recently, a US safety study[21] found that the incidence of life-threatening reactions was 0.04% for sodium ferric gluconate vs 0.61% for IV iron dextran (p = 0.0001), with incidences of other adverse events of 0.44% and 2.47%, respectively (p <0.0001). In postmarketing surveillance of iron sucrose from 1992 to 2002, a total of 83 non-life-threatening anaphylactic reactions were reported, based on an estimated use in more than 2 million patients.[22] Of note, in a study by Kosch et al,[23] the iron sucrose regimen evaluated (250 mg once a month) was determined to be as effective and well tolerated as once-weekly sodium ferric gluconate, thus possibly representing an alternative to the usual iron sucrose weekly schedule. Although not currently FDA-approved, third generation IV irons are undergoing clinical trials with the hope that they will provide a safer, better-tolerated option with total dose infusion potential.

Parenteral iron may not be appropriate for some patients, including those with underlying autoimmune disease, malnourishment, and active infections or those who are at risk for iron overload. Some evidence suggests that parenteral iron can stim-

Table 5-4. Comparison of Parenteral Iron Formulations

Drug	Dosing	Premedications
Iron dextran (INFeD*)	Test dose: 0.5 cc IV push in free-flowing NSS; wait ½ hour; 500 mg in 500 cc NSS over 1½ to 2 hours	Tylenol 650 mg PO Decadron 10 mg IV Benadryl 25 mg IV
Sodium ferric gluconate (Ferrlecit†)	125 mg in 100 cc NSS over 1 hour weekly × 4 doses	None
Iron sucrose (Venofer‡)	300 mg weekly × 3 doses/week	None

*Watson Inc, Corona, CA.
†Watson Nephrology, Morristown, NJ.
‡American Regent Inc, Shirley, NY.
IV = intravenous; PO = by mouth; NSS = normal saline solution.

ulate bacterial virulence, thereby potentially leading to increased infections.[24]

Treatment of Thrombocytopenia

Platelet disorders can be either qualitative or quantitative. Cancer patients most commonly suffer from thrombocytopenias that stem from chemotherapy- and radiation-therapy-induced megakaryocyte depletion, although some malignancies do directly infiltrate the bone marrow. The classifications of thrombocytopenia are listed in Table 5-5. The major concern in individuals with profound thrombocytopenia is the risk for spontaneous cerebral hemorrhage or life-threatening gastro-intestinal bleeding. Among the many reasons to limit platelet transfusions are avoidance of infection and avoidance of a platelet refractory state. A liberal prophylactic platelet transfusion policy can lead to production of alloantibodies in approximately one-third of patients, thereby creating a state in which future transfusions to control bleeding will no longer result in significant increases in platelet numbers for those patients.

Table 5-5. Classifications of Thrombocytopenia

Type	Cause
Ineffective thrombopoiesis	Vitamin B_{12} or folate deficiency
Immune-mediated peripheral destruction of platelets	• Autoimmunity • Drug-induced antibodies
Consumption of platelets	• Disseminated intravascular coagulation • Thrombotic thrombocytopenic purpura
Sequestration of platelets	Splenomegaly
Platelet loss	Extracorporeal circulation

Prophylactic Platelet Transfusions

It is difficult to determine the risk of bleeding in any individual patient with thrombocytopenia, although platelet counts above 100,000/μL are generally associated with normal hemostasis and are considered adequate for most invasive or surgical procedures. The direct relationship between the absolute platelet count and bleeding occurrences was first observed in acute leukemic patients in 1962 by Gaydos and colleagues.[25] It was observed that, when the platelet count was above 20,000/μL, major bleeding episodes rarely occurred. More recent studies have attempted to determine the platelet level at which prophylactic transfusions should be administered. For adults who have leukemia and who are receiving therapy, the American Society of Clinical Oncology (ASCO) recommends that platelet transfusions be given at a level of 10,000/μL.[26] The recommendation is based on multiple randomized trials, which showed that such an approach was equivalent to transfusing at 20,000/μL. The ASCO guidelines suggest maintaining a higher platelet count in certain high-risk groups such as neonates and patients with hemorrhage, high fevers, hyperleukocytosis, rapidly declining platelet counts, or coagulopathy. A recent review by Slichter[27] reports that a platelet count of 5000/μL may be adequate for hemostasis in nonbleeding individuals. The author's practice has not had any significant bleeding episodes in any high-risk, autologous stem cell transplantation patients when platelet counts were maintained at 5000/μL, if the patients were also empirically placed on vitamin K and antifibrinolytics to enhance hemostasis.[28]

Platelet transfusions are still considered the standard of care in patients with bleeding or platelet counts under 10,000/μL. Several types of platelet transfusions, which differ in how the platelets are collected and matched to patients, can be administered. Random-donor platelet concentrates are collected from several whole blood donations, increasing the likelihood of alloimmunization, whereas single-donor apheresis platelets are collected from single individuals and can be crossmatched to the patient's own human leukocyte antigens to avoid alloimmunization.

Pharmacologic Agents and Blood Components

There are multiple reasons to use alternatives to platelet transfusion, including patient refusal of blood components, refractoriness, and anticipation of a significant number of future transfusions (especially among stem cell transplant and leukemic patients). In some clinical situations, such as thrombotic thrombocytopenic purpura, platelet transfusions can cause thrombosis and can actually worsen the clinical state. The author's approach to basic non-blood therapy for thrombocytopenia is outlined in Table 5-6.

The backbone of non-blood therapy for thrombocytopenic individuals consists of antifibrinolytic agents and vitamin K. A few types of antifibrinolytic agents include aminocaproic acid and tranexamic acid. Aminocaproic acid binds to plasminogen, thereby blocking the binding of plasminogen to fibrin and precluding fibrin activation. Studies have shown that aminocaproic acid decreases mucosal bleeding in patients with thrombocytopenia[29] and reduces blood loss in cardiac surgery.[30] Aminocaproic acid is available in injection, syrup, or tablet form (supplied as 500 mg and 1000 mg tablets).

To treat acute bleeding, intravenous aminocaproic acid is administered as 4 g to 5 g in 250 mL of diluent during the first hour of treatment, followed by a continuous infusion at a rate of 1 g/hour to 1.25 g/hour until bleeding has subsided. If therapy is given orally, 5 g should be administered during the first hour of treatment for acute bleeding, then 1 g/hour. In the author's autologous stem cell transplant population, patients empirically received aminocaproic acid at a total daily dose of 12 g (2 g every 4 hours), starting when the platelet count fell below 30,000/µL. The dose was increased to a daily maximum of 24 g (4 g every 4 hours) for bleeding or platelet counts under 10,000/µL. The IV form was often required when mucositis and other gastrointestinal side effects were present. Aminocaproic acid should be avoided in patients with upper urinary tract bleeding because it can cause intrarenal obstruction.

Phytonadione (vitamin K) is necessary for hepatic production of coagulation Factors II, VII, and IX, which are essential in nor-

Table 5-6. Management of Thrombocytopenia

Nonbleeding

- Calcium supplementation
- Vitamin K (10 mg)
- Antifibrinolytic agents, such as aminocaproic acid (Amicar, Wyeth-Ayerst, Madison, NJ) (12 g/24 hours)
- Progestational agents (cessation of menses)
- GI prophylaxis with protein pump inhibitors/stool softeners

Bleeding (in addition to above)

Medical techniques
- Increased dose of aminocaproic acid (24 g/24 hours)
- Epistaxis: vasoconstrictors (nasal sprays)/humidified air
- Desmopressin acetate
- Cyroprecipitated AHF
- Factor concentrates
- Recombinant Factor VIIa

Invasive techniques
- Transcutaneous arterial embolization or balloons
- Vessel ligation
- Inferior vena cava filters (when anticoagulation is contraindicated)

GI = gastrointestinal; AHF = Antihemophilic Factor.

mal hemostasis. It is also needed for adequate function of proteins C and S, which are anticoagulants. Vitamin K levels are measured indirectly by depletion of Factor VII according to the protime or international normalized ratio values. The recommended dietary allowance used only once for vitamin K is 80 µg/day for the adult male and 65 µg/day for the adult female. Dietary sources of vitamin K are shown in Table 5-3. Excessive vitamin E can inhibit vitamin K activity and can precipitate signs of deficiency. A portion of the body's vitamin K is supplied by normal bacteria that reside in the intestine. Vitamin K depletion can occur from warfarin, antibiotics that deplete intestinal flora, and poor nutrition. Vitamin K should be given empirically in the thrombocytopenic patient because the lab values will not reveal abnormalities until 70% of vitamin K has been depleted. Vitamin K doses range from 2.5 to 10 mg and can be administered intravenously, subcutaneously, and orally. High-dose IV treatments tend to be the most effective. Table 5-7 lists other over-the-counter medications that can increase bleeding risk.

Progestational agents are used to control uterine bleeding episodes and to prevent the onset of menses in premenopausal women with thrombocytopenia. One to two tablets of medroxyprogesterone acetate or norethindrone per day should stop uterine bleeding in 72 hours.[31] If not, 25 mg intravenous premarin should control it in 6 to 24 hours.

Other agents such as blood fractions or NovoSeven (Novo Nordisk Inc, Princeton, NJ) can enhance hemostasis by affecting platelets or coagulation proteins when vitamin K and aminocaproic acid are inadequate. Desmopressin, an analog of arginine vasopressin, has also been used to control bleeding. The mechanism of action may be formation of ultralarge multimers of von Willebrand factor, which increase platelet adhesion to the vascular subendothelium. Desmopressin is administered at a dose of 0.3 µg/kg intravenously, with the potential for repeat dosing when maximal doses of aminocaproic acid are not effective in

---

Table 5-7. Over-the-Counter Medications and Nutritional Supplements to Avoid 2 Weeks Before Surgery

Alcohol	Ginseng
Aspirin (or aspirin-containing medications)	Kava kava
	Licorice root
Feverfew	Mahuang
Fish oil caps	Medications containing ibuprofen
Garlic	Melatonin
Ginger	St. John's wort
Ginkgo	Vitamin E

controlling bleeding. Common side effects include hyponatremia, flushing, headaches, diarrhea, and water retention.

Cryoprecipitated Antihemophilic Factor (AHF) is prepared from a unit of Fresh Frozen Plasma and is indicated for the treatment of bleeding or the prevention of bleeding before an invasive procedure in patients with hypofibrinogenemia (fibrinogen level <100 mg/dL). The dose for the treatment of hypofibrinogenemia should be computed on the basis of the patient's plasma volume and the initial vs desired fibrinogen levels.

NovoSeven is made up of recombinant human coagulation Factor VIIa (rFVIIa).[32] Its purpose is to promote hemostasis by activating the extrinsic pathway of the coagulation cascade. It is vitamin-K-dependent and similar in structure to human-plasma-derived Factor VIIa. NovoSeven is indicated for the treatment of hemophilia with inhibitors, but it has been used off-label for cases of refractory and life-threatening bleeding.

Oprelvekin [Neumega (Genetics Institute Inc, Cambridge, MA)] is a recombinant human interleukin-11 (IL-11) cytokine that stimulates the production of platelets by enhancing the size and ploidy of megakaryocytes. It is typically used following chemotherapy treatment in patients who have a high thrombocytopenic risk. IL-11 can promote platelet production to reduce or eliminate the need for platelet transfusions, to improve the platelet count, and to shorten the duration of severe thrombocytopenia. In a randomized, multicenter, placebo-controlled, IL-11 Phase II clinical trial, 93 patients who had received at least one platelet transfusion during a prior chemotherapy cycle demonstrated a reduction in need for platelet support.[33]

Conclusion

Care of the oncologic patient often involves management of anemia and thrombocytopenia with transfusion support. Exposure to blood components may be reduced by the early initiation of growth factors, elimination of absolute transfusion triggers, and more liberal use of non-blood therapy techniques.

Correction of anemia may lead to better patient outcomes in addition to improvements in quality of life.

References

1. Bohlius J, Langensiepen S, Schwarzer G, et al. Recombinant human erythropoietin and overall survival in cancer patients: Results of a comprehensive meta-analysis. J Natl Cancer Inst 2005;97:489-98.

2. Caro JJ, Salas M, Ward A, Goss G. Anemia as an independent prognostic factor for survival in patients with cancer: A systematic, quantitative review. Cancer 2001;91:2214-21.

3. Glaspy J, Bukowski R, Steinberg D, et al. Impact of therapy with epoetin alfa on clinical outcomes in patients with nonmyeloid malignancies during cancer chemotherapy in community oncology practice. J Clin Oncol 1997;15:1218-34.

4. Demetri GD, Kris M, Wade J, et al. Quality-of-life benefit in chemotherapy patients treated with epoetin alfa is independent of disease response or tumor type: Results from a prospective community oncology study. J Clin Oncol 1998;16:3412-25.

5. Crawford J, Cella D, Cleeland CS, et al. Relationship between changes in hemoglobin level and quality of life during chemotherapy in anemic cancer patients receiving epoetin alfa therapy. Cancer 2002;95:888-95.

6. Cheung W, Minton N, Gunawardena K. Pharmacokinetics and pharmacodynamics of epoetin alfa once weekly and three times weekly. Eur J Clin Pharmacol 2001;57:411-18.

7. Gabrilove JL, Cleeland CS, Livingston RB, et al. Clinical evaluation of once-weekly dosing of epoetin alfa in chemotherapy patients: Improvements in hemoglobin and quality of life are similar to three-times-weekly dosing. J Clin Oncol 2001;19:2875-82.

8. Ford PA, Mastoris J. Strategies to optimize the use of erythropoietin and iron therapy in oncology patients. Transfusion 2004;44(Dec Suppl):15S 25S.

9. Aranesp (darbepoetin alfa) prescribing information. Thousand Oaks, CA: Amgen Inc., 2003. [Available at http://www.amgen.com/medpro/aranesp_pi.html (accessed August 6, 2007).]

10. Glaspy JA, Jadeja JS, Justice G, et al. Darbepoetin alfa given every 1 or 2 weeks alleviates anaemia associated with cancer chemotherapy. Br J Cancer 2002; 87:268-76.

11. Hesketh PJ, Arena F, Patel D, et al. A randomized controlled trial of darbepoetin alfa administered as a fixed or weight-based dose using a front-loading schedule in patients with anemia who have nonmyeloid malignancies. Cancer 2004;100:859-68.

12. Acs G, Acs P, Beckwith SM, et al. Erythropoietin and erythropoietin receptor expression in human cancer. Cancer Res 2001;61:3561-5.

13. Acs G, Xu X, Chu C, et al. Prognostic significance of erythropoietin expression in human endometrial carcinoma. Cancer 2004;100:2376-86.
14. Singh AK, Szczech L, Tang KL, et al. Correction of anemia with epoetin alfa in chronic kidney disease. N Engl J Med 2006; 355:2085-98.
15. Henke M, Laszig R, Rube C, et al. Erythropoietin to treat head and neck cancer patients with anemia undergoing radiotherapy: Randomized, double-blind, placebo-controlled trial. Lancet 2003;362:1255-60.
16. Leyland-Jones B, Semiglazov V, Pawlicki M, et al. Maintaining normal hemoglobin levels with epoetin alfa in mainly nonanemic patients with metastatic breast cancer receiving first-line chemotherapy: A survival study. J Clin Oncol 2005;23:5960-72.
17. Amgen Inc. Results from a phase 3, randomized, double-blind, placebo-controlled study of darbepoetin alfa for the treatment of anemia in patients with active cancer not receiving chemotherapy or radiotherapy. Clinical Study Results, 2008. [Available at http://www.clinicalstudyresults.org/documents/company-study_2157_0.pdf (accessed January 4, 2008).]
18. Wright JR, Ung YC, Julian JA, et al. Randomized, double-blind, placebo-controlled trial of erythropoietin in non-small-cell lung cancer with disease-related anemia. J Clin Oncol 2007;25:1027-32.
19. Food and Drug Administration. Package Insert. Aranesp (darbepoetin alfa). Amgen Inc. Rockville, MD: Center for Drug Evaluation and Research, 2003. [Available at http://www.fda.gov/cder/foi/label/2001/darbamg091701LB.htm (accessed January 4, 2008).]
20. Faich G, Strobos J. Sodium ferric gluconate complex in sucrose: Safer intravenous iron therapy than iron dextrans. Am J Kidney Dis 1999;33:464-70.
21. Michael B, Coyne DW, Fishbane S, et al. Sodium ferric gluconate complex in hemodialysis patients: Adverse reactions compared to placebo and iron dextran. Kidney Int 2002;61:1830-9.
22. Venofer (iron sucrose injection, USP) prescribing information. Shirley, NY: American Regent Inc., 2003. [Available at http://www.americanregent.com/PDF_For_Products/Venofer%20IN2340%20Rev%2002_07.pdf (accessed August 6, 2007).]
23. Kosch M, Bahner U, Bettger H, et al. A randomized, controlled parallel-group trial on efficacy and safety of iron sucrose (Venofer, American Regent Inc., Shirley, NY) vs iron gluconate (Ferrlecit, Watson Nephrology, Morristown, NJ) in haemodialysis patients treated with rHuEpo. Nephrol Dial Transplant 2001; 16:1239-44.
24. Patruta SI, Hörl WH. Iron and infection. Kidney Int 1999;69:S125-30.
25. Gaydos LA, Freireich EJ, Mantel N. The quantitative relation between platelet count and hemorrhage in patients with acute leukemia. N Engl J Med 1962; 266:905-9.
26. Schiffer CA, Anderson KC, Bennett CL, et al. Platelet transfusion for patients with cancer: Clinical practice guidelines of the American Society of Clinical Oncology. J Clin Oncol 2001;19:1519-38.
27. Slichter SJ. Relationship between platelet count and bleeding risk in thrombocytopenic patients. Transfus Med Rev 2004;18:153-67.
28. Ballen KK, Becker PS, Yeap BY, et al. Autologous stem-cell transplantation can be performed safely without the use of blood-product support. J Clin Oncol 2004;22:4087-94.

29. Bartholomew JR, Salgia R, Bell WR. Control of bleeding in patients with immune and nonimmune thrombocytopenia with aminocaproic acid. Arch Intern Med 1989;149:1959-61.
30. Vander Salm TJ, Kaur S, Lancey RA, et al. Reduction of bleeding after heart operations through the prophylactic use of epsilon-aminocaproic acid. J Thorac Cardiovasc Surg 1996;112:1098-107.
31. Bharucha MR. Progestogens in gynaecological practice. Indian Med Trib 1995;3:6-7.
32. Roberts HR. Thoughts on the mechanism of action of FVIIa. Second symposium on new aspects of hemophilia treatment. Copenhagen, Denmark: Medicom Europe, 1991:153-6.
33. Tepler I, Elias L, Smith JW, et al. A randomized placebo-controlled trial of recombinant human interleukin-11 in cancer patients with severe thrombocytopenia due to chemotherapy. Blood 1997;87:3607-14.

In: Waters JH, ed.
Blood Management: Options for Better Patient Care
Bethesda, MD: AABB Press, 2008

6

Pretransfusion Testing

MARK H. YAZER, MD, FRCP(C)

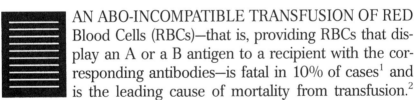 AN ABO-INCOMPATIBLE TRANSFUSION OF RED Blood Cells (RBCs)—that is, providing RBCs that display an A or a B antigen to a recipient with the corresponding antibodies—is fatal in 10% of cases[1] and is the leading cause of mortality from transfusion.[2] Errors leading to ABO-incompatible transfusions are nearly always clerical in origin and can occur at any phase of specimen collection, testing, or blood administration.[3] Fastidious adherence to proper patient identification and labeling procedures is

Mark H. Yazer, MD, FRCP(C), Medical Director, RBC Serology Reference Laboratory, The Institute for Transfusion Medicine, and Assistant Professor, Department of Pathology, University of Pittsburgh, Pittsburgh, Pennsylvania
(Parts of this chapter have been previously published as "The blood bank 'blackbox' debunked: Pretransfusion testing explained"—Reprinted from CMAJ 2006;174:29-32, by permission of the publisher. © 2006 Canadian Medical Association.)

required of all individuals involved in the transfusion process, as outlined in this chapter. Given the importance of ABO typing in ensuring a safe transfusion, this chapter will describe the testing performed by the blood bank when a "type and screen" is ordered.

Patient Identification

For a patient to receive a transfusion, it is important to establish the recipient's ABO and Rh(D) type. That process commences when an order for a type and screen (with or without an order for transfusion) is placed and when a nurse or phlebotomist is dispatched to collect a blood sample to be sent to the blood bank. Perioperative patients should have a type and screen performed in the days before surgery, if possible, to identify the small number of patients with a red cell antibody. Before a patient enters the operating room, it should be confirmed that the type and screen has been done and that crossmatched blood is available if indicated. A surgical blood ordering schedule is a list of all the surgical procedures offered at an institution; it delineates the extent of blood-bank testing and the number of crossmatched units that are typically required for each procedure. If such a schedule is available, it should be consulted before the patient's arrival in the operating room.

Whether it occurs on the ward or in the operating room, patient identification is of the utmost importance in ensuring a safe transfusion. The AABB mandates that, at a minimum, two unique patient identifiers must be present on both the blood sample and the accompanying paperwork (often an order form specifying the type and quantity of blood product required).[4] Typically, that requirement is met by using the patient's full name and medical record number, although other identifiers such as birthdate or social security number might also be acceptable, depending on hospital policy or government guidelines.

Sample Collection

The identification of the patient must occur at the bedside. This identification must also occur when a blood-bank sample is procured from a patient in the operating room. Hospital policy should dictate which members of the clinical staff can—and how many of them are required to—participate in the identification of the patient, although a nurse or a physician typically performs this vital task. It is important that the patient's identity information is actually attached to the patient through a hospital-issued bracelet or similar device. Verifying the patient's identification against the patient's chart outside his or her room or from a house staff member not physically located at the bedside increases the chances of drawing the wrong blood into the labeled tube ("wrong blood in tube"). Such errors are potentially serious because they can lead to ABO-incompatible transfusions; unfortunately, they are also quite common—estimated in a large multicenter study at 1:1986 samples collected.[5]

One possible exception to the rule that patient identification must be made by using the wristband attached to the patient is in the operating room. In that setting, the wristband might have been detached for venous access, or it might not be easily accessible because of the sterile environment. If the wristband is to be detached during the procedure, there must be a policy for identification of the patient during the time that he or she is unbanded. Ensuring that the wristband does not leave the operating room and is easily available for pretransfusion identity confirmation, such as by placing it in the patient's chart, will help reduce errors. The band should be reattached to the patient as soon as possible and definitely before the patient leaves the operating room. Otherwise, a new type and screen must be performed before crossmatch-compatible blood can be issued to that patient. The sample is linked to the patient by the wristband. If that wristband becomes lost or is not replaced after a surgical procedure, then the link to the blood-bank testing performed on that sample and on any crossmatched units is broken, and a new sample will have to be drawn.

After the patient has been properly identified, the phlebotomy can begin. At its conclusion, the sample must be labeled promptly, preferably while the tube and paperwork are still at the bedside or in the operating room. Hospital policies vary as to the suitability of preprinted stamps (eg, Addressograph) or of handwritten labels—but with any label, the two unique patient identifiers must be clearly legible and consistent between the sample and the paperwork.

A common error at this step is for the phlebotomist to put the unlabeled tube in his or her pocket and then search for a suitable label at the nursing station. There is less of a danger in an operating room, where the labels are likely to be in the same room as the patient, but the potential for applying the wrong identification to the tube of blood is unacceptably high in either scenario. Likewise, it is probably safer if the phlebotomist does not preapply the label to an empty tube of blood because the potential to accidentally draw blood into a tube labeled for a different patient also exists. In one British hospital, banning the use of preprinted patient identification labels resulted in an increased number of specimens rejected for mislabeling, but no wrong blood in tube errors were detected.[6]

Mislabeling of specimens occurs at a high rate, estimated at 1:165 samples in a large, multinational study.[5] Mislabeling errors can have dire consequences for the recipient ranging from a delay in providing blood while a new specimen is drawn to receiving an ABO-incompatibile transfusion. In fact, according to the British Serious Hazards of Transfusion (SHOT) database, the risk of death caused by "an incorrect blood component transfused" (ie, a case whereby a recipient inadvertently receives a blood component intended for another or whereby the component is transfused to the intended recipient but otherwise fails to be processed properly) is 1:1.5 million.[7] Efforts are being focused on using automated patient identification processes—such as barcodes that link the patient with his or her sample and the component—to reduce errors[8-11] or on requiring the ABO group to be verified on a second, separately collected blood sample in patients without a historical ABO group.[12] However, because errors can occur at any point in the specimen's travels from the patient, through the laboratory, and back to the patient, vigilance at each step is critical to ensuring a safe transfusion.[13,14]

Type and Screen

When the sample of the recipient's blood and the requisition or order arrive in the blood bank, the identifying information is compared to ensure that the information is consistent and complete, as discussed above. If there is any discrepancy or if information is missing, the specimen is rejected and the ward is then notified that a recollection is necessary. Even the most seemingly minor labeling error can be associated with an extremely high risk of recipient misidentification; hence such specimens are usually discarded.[15] (Interested readers should consult Dzik[16] for a detailed description of current and future practices to reduce such errors.)

If the specimen is acceptable for pretransfusion testing, the first step in ensuring serologic compatibility between the donor and the recipient is to perform a type and screen, which takes approximately 45 minutes (see Table 6-1). It consists of two distinct tests that are independent of each other. The "type," sometimes called a "group," is a test that determines which ABO antigens are present on the patient's red cells. It usually features a test for the D antigen. The type is divided into two parts. The first part uses commercially available monoclonal antibodies that will react with either the A or B antigens, if they are present, on the recipient's red cells and will cause them to agglutinate. That process is known as forward (cell) typing. The red cells from a group AB person will react with both anti-A and anti-B, whereas a group O person will not react with either. The D antigen is tested in the same manner; commercially available anti-D antibodies are mixed with the recipient's red cells and the mixture is inspected for hemagglutination (see Table 6-2).

In the second part of the type the recipient's plasma is reacted with commercially available A and B cells. That process is

---

Table 6-1. Estimated Turnaround Time for Pretransfusion Testing Phases[17]

Procedure	Estimated TAT* (min)	Risk of Acute Hemolysis (%)[†]
Emergency issue of uncross-matched RBCs	5	5
ABO and D type only	15	5
Type and screen	45	<0.1
Type and screen, and computer crossmatch[‡]	60	<0.1
Type and screen, and serologic crossmatch	>120[§]	<0.1

TAT = turnaround time; RBCs = Red Blood Cells.

*TATs will vary from institution to institution. The term refers to the time interval from receipt of the order in the blood bank until testing or issuing is complete.

[†]These figures estimate the probability of the RBC recipient suffering an acute hemolytic transfusion reaction if RBCs are administered after each phase of pretransfusion testing. Overall, approximately 5% of recipients will have an unexpected antibody; the risk of acute hemolysis is diminished only when antibody screening methods are performed.

[‡]These procedures can be performed when no unexpected antibodies are identified. The time represents the fastest time that crossmatched blood can be provided to a ward.

[§]Antibody identification can take several hours, depending on the nature of the antibody. Locating rare RBC units that lack a high-incidence antigen or combination of antigens can take days and may require consulting a rare donor registry or using frozen RBCs.

called reverse (serum) typing. Almost everyone has naturally occurring antibodies to the ABO antigens that they lack: group O individuals will have both anti-A and anti-B in their plasma but group AB individuals will have neither of the antibodies in their plasma. The two parts of the type test are complementary; used together, they establish the patient's ABO group. There are occasions when the results of the forward and reverse typings will

Table 6-2. Key Facts Regarding Red Cell Antigens[17]

Notes on the Rh blood group system:
- Next to the ABO system, Rh is the most clinically significant blood group system.
- Antibodies in the Rh system are generally IgG and will cause extravascular hemolysis of antigen-positive transfused red cells.
- There are more than 45 antigens in this system. The five main antigens are D, C, c, E, and e.
- The designation "Rh positive" indicates that the D antigen is present; "Rh negative" indicates the absence of the D antigen. Testing for the presence of other Rh antigens is not routinely performed.
- Unlike the ABO antibodies, anti-D is not naturally occurring. It is formed only after exposure to Rh-positive RBCs.
- The D antigen is the most immunogenic antigen. That is if a D-negative recipient or pregnant female is highly likely to produce an anti-D antibody if exposed to even small quantities of D-positive blood.
- This is why testing for the presence of the D antigen is routinely included in pretransfusion testing.

General notes on red cell antigens:
- There are more than 250 antigens on a typical red cell surface.
- Only a few antigens elicit the production of an antibody that would shorten the survival of an antigen-positive transfused red cell.
- These are known as clinically significant antibodies.
- Some clinically significant antigens are Kell (K), Duffy (Fy), Kidd (Jk), and Rh.
- Other antibodies are not usually considered clinically significant because they do not cause hemolysis of antigen-positive red cells at normal body temperature.
- Some of these insignificant antibodies are anti-Lewis (Le), -H, -I/i, and -M/N.

not coincide, and these situations are known as ABO discrepancies (see Table 6-3). Some discrepancies can be resolved by inquiring into the patient's medical history, but others require detailed laboratory investigation, which can delay the provision of crossmatched blood (see next for a discussion of the use of uncrossmatched blood).

Table 6-3. Causes of ABO Discrepancies*

Unexpected reactivity on forward typing:
- Stem cell transplant (transplantation can cause discrepancies if the native marrow is replaced by the donor marrow of a different ABO group)
- ABO subtype (weak reactivity on forward typing might conflict with an unexpected antibody on reverse typing)
- Rouleaux, Wharton's jelly
- Acquired B phenotype (in bacterial sepsis, the A antigen can be converted in rare cases into a B-like antigen that can be agglutinated by some anti-B reagents but is mostly of historical significance)

Unexpected absence of reactivity on forward typing:
- Stem cell transplant
- ABO subtype (weak reactivity might not be detected on forward typing)
- Old or young age
- Hematologic disease (loss of A and B antigens has been documented as disease progresses)
- Massive transfusion of group O blood to a non-group-O recipient

Unexpected reactivity on reverse typing:
- Transfusion of ABO-incompatible, non-group-AB platelets (anti-A and anti-B can be passively transfused in the plasma component of platelets)
- Cold agglutinin (if the thermal amplitude is reactive at room temperature)
- Administration of intravenous immunoglobulin
- ABO subtype

Unexpected lack of reactivity on reverse typing:
- Acquired or congential hypogammaglobulinemia
- Neonates[†]

---

*Preanalytical variables such as improper centrifugation speeds, dirty glassware, expired reagents, and wrong blood in tube are not included.
[†]In many blood banks, a reverse type is not performed on infants up to 4 months of age because of the immaturity of the infant's immune system and the unlikelihood of alloimmunization. Should an infant in this age group need transfusion, an antibody screen can be performed by using maternal plasma, with the assumption that any antibodies present in the infant's circulation were passively acquired from the mother. RBCs transfused would thus have to be compatible with the maternal serum. In the absence of a reverse type to confirm the findings on forward typing, many institutions transfuse only group O units to neonates.

The "screen" test is done to determine if the recipient has formed what are known as "unexpected" red cell antibodies. Approximately 3% to 10% of recipients who have been multiply transfused with RBCs will develop antibodies to non-ABO red cell antigens.[18,19] This phenomenon is in contrast to the regular, predictable occurrence of antibodies to the ABO antigens that the recipient lacks—hence the moniker "unexpected" (see Table 6-2). Alloimmunization is significantly higher in individuals with sickle cell issues, probably because of the different antigen frequencies between donors who are usually White, and Black patients.[20]

The antibody screen is performed by using either two or three commercially available group O cells that together express essentially all of the approximately 20 clinically significant red cell antigens. By incubating the recipient's plasma with those cells and then looking for agglutination of the red cells or for hemolysis caused by antigen-antibody interactions, the technologist can detect unexpected antibodies and can set the identification process in motion (the risk of overt hemolysis caused by abbreviated pretransfusion testing is estimated in Table 6-1). Patients with unexpected antibodies require additional testing. It sometimes takes several hours to identify the antibody specificity and to locate antigen-negative units for transfusion. A type and screen is valid for up to 3 days for hospitalized patients. A type and screen performed in the outpatient setting can remain valid for up to 30 days, provided the recipient has not been transfused or pregnant in the previous 3 months (see discussion that follows).

Crossmatch

A crossmatch is performed to ensure compatibility of the donor red cells selected for transfusion with the recipient's plasma. The crossmatch can be done serologically to ensure compatibility with both ABO and non-ABO antibodies or by computer as a check on ABO compatibility. If the recipient has a negative antibody screen (ie, has not formed unexpected antibodies), the computer can electronically match the ABO group of the recipient with a donor unit by using laser wands and bar code technology. The computer system must have the logic to recognize and allow a unit of RBCs to be issued if the ABO match between donor and recipient is compatible and to reject units that are incompatible. (The safety and use of the electronic crossmatch are reviewed in Judd[21] and Butch.[22])

If a recipient has formed an unexpected antibody, the blood bank cannot use the computer-crossmatching procedure. Instead, a serologic crossmatch is required. That method involves mixing the recipient's plasma with potential donor RBC units and inspecting for agglutination or hemolysis to ensure that the unit of RBCs—selected by further immunologic testing to be antigen negative—truly lacks the antigen corresponding to the patient's antibody. This crossmatching process adds 30 minutes to the pretransfusion testing (see Table 6-1). A compatible RBC unit would show no agglutination or hemolysis when it is mixed with recipient plasma. Figure 6-1 summarizes the process. In the absence of computer crossmatch technology, a serologic crossmatch is required to ensure ABO compatibility (see Fig 6-2).

Blood Administration

The final opportunity to recognize an error is just before the transfusion commences. The recipient's identification attached to the blood component must match exactly the identification on the intended recipient's wristband, and the ABO group and Rh type printed on the blood component must be compared to the compatibility tag. Recipient identity verification must be performed to confirm that the blood is being administered to the intended recipient. Although that sounds simple, a recent study[3] of more than 250 transfusion services in New York state found that administering a properly labeled unit of blood to someone other than the intended recipient was the most fre-

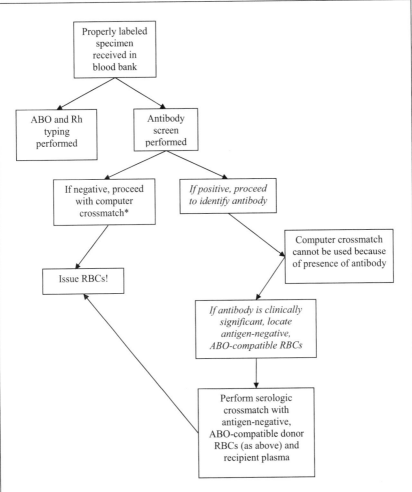

Figure 6-1. Steps before a crossmatch-compatible Red Blood Cell (RBC) unit is issued for transfusion. Steps in italics represent the major, time-consuming procedures in pretransfusion testing before RBC issue.
*If computer crossmatch is unavailable, a second verification of ABO compatibility between donor RBCs and recipient plasma is required (see Fig 6-2). Used with permission from Yazer.[17]

quent error associated with transfusion. That same study also found that the blood bank alone was responsible for 29% of all transfusion-associated errors. These data once again reinforce

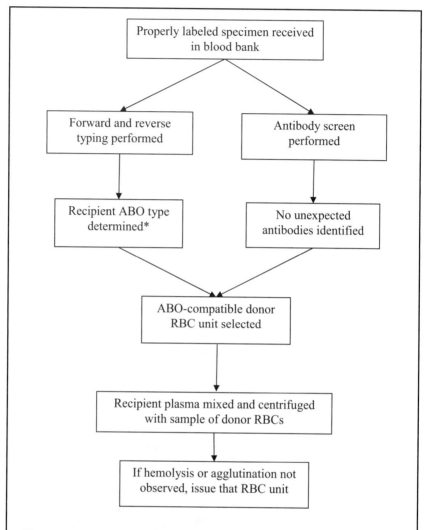

Figure 6-2. In the absence of a computer crossmatch system, a second ABO verification must occur before an RBC unit can be issued. After the type and screen are performed and no unexpected antibodies are detected, an ABO-compatible RBC unit is selected and mixed with the recipient's plasma. That mixture is briefly centrifuged and inspected for hemolysis or agglutination; if both are absent, ABO compatibility is verified and the RBC unit can be issued. This procedure must be repeated for each RBC unit issued. If unexpected antibodies are detected, a similar procedure is used to verify ABO compatibility, but the donor RBC units are also selected to be compatible with the recipient's antibody. Used with permission from Yazer.[17]

the need for rigorous attention to detail at each step in the transfusion process.

Uncrossmatched Blood

Uncrossmatched RBC units are group O (universal donor). Thus, they can be safely transfused to virtually any recipient in an emergency when the typically short delay caused by pre-transfusion testing to find ABO-matched units would jeopardize the patient's life. Usually, uncrossmatched blood is issued to unstable, hemorrhaging trauma victims on presentation to the emergency department, where RBCs are urgently required and the blood-bank testing has not been performed. However, uncrossmatched blood can be given to any patient who suddenly requires blood because of a deterioration in his or her clinical status related to bleeding and who does not have a valid type and screen. In such patients, the benefits of receiving uncrossmatched RBC transfusions during their resuscitation outweigh the small risks of alloimmunization or extravascular hemolytic reactions. Intravascular hemolysis mediated by the recipient's naturally occurring immunoglobulin M (IgM) anti-A or -B antibodies will not occur because these units will always be group O. There is a small risk of immunoglobulin G (IgG)-mediated extravascular hemolysis if the recipient has been exposed to foreign red cell antigens through pregnancy or previous transfusions and has become alloimmunized (ie, formed an unexpected antibody as described above). That type of hemolysis is usually much less severe than IgM-mediated intravascular hemolysis because the red cells are not lysed inside the vascular space. The risk of extravascular hemolysis in an uncrossmatched RBC recipient is directly proportionate to the recipient's a priori probability of having become alloimmunized.

An Australian study[23] stratified the risk of alloimmunization by recipient age and clinical condition and found the lowest rates of alloimmunization to clinically significant antigens (defined in the study as Kell, Kidd, Rh, Duffy, and MNS) among both males and females who were less than 30 years old. The incidence of alloimmunization to clinically significant antigens rose steadily with age. Most patients were alloimmunized to either Rh or Kell system antigens, although the specific antigens within these systems were not reported. The rates of alloimmunization in trauma and emergency department patients, that is, those who are most likely to receive uncrossmatched blood, were low and ranged from 0.5% of patients who were less than 30 years old to approximately 4% of patients who were more than 60 years old.[21]

In another study,[24] 581 uncrossmatched group O units were transfused to 161 trauma patients, and no acute transfusion reactions were noted. Of the 10 males who were subsequently found to be D negative, but who had received D-positive uncrossmatched blood during their resuscitation, only one became alloimmunized to the D antigen. That patient received only 1 D-positive unit and 11 crossmatch-compatible units in the first 24 hours of his admission.[24] These data indicate that the vast majority of trauma patients will not be at risk of clinically significant hemolysis from receiving uncrossmatched group O RBCs.

The decision to use D-positive or D-negative uncrossmatched units is complex and depends on the supply of group O-negative blood, the anticipated patient population requiring the uncrossmatched blood, and the anticipated frequency with which it will be used. For example, hospitals specializing in women's health or pediatrics might wish to use only D-negative uncrossmatched RBCs, whereas hospitals in smaller communities might use D-positive blood because of the limited supply of D-negative RBCs. D negative recipients are potentially at risk of forming D antibodies if they are exposed to D-positive blood components. Anti-D has been implicated in causing both acute hemolytic reactions and hemolytic disease of the fetus and newborn. Thus, preventing alloimmunization—especially in females of childbearing potential and in children—is important and is a driving factor for the use of D-negative uncrossmatched blood in hospitals that specialize in these patients.

Whenever uncrossmatched blood is used, it is essential that a properly labeled blood-bank specimen be procured from the recipient early in the transfusion course. That step is important in managing the blood-bank inventory because supplies of group O-negative RBCs are usually very limited and need to be maintained for those who need them, such as D-negative females of childbearing potential or individuals already sensitized to the D antigen.

Massive Transfusion

A massive transfusion is usually defined as the transfusion of one blood volume within 24 hours. For a typical 70-kg male, one blood volume is equal to approximately 10 units of RBCs. Massive transfusions often occur in the emergency department during the resuscitation of trauma patients. Surgical patients who receive uncrossmatched blood because of the acuity of their clinical situation frequently undergo a massive transfusion.

Aside from the patient's condition that necessitates a massive transfusion, another important consideration in managing such a patient is the development of a coagulopathy. Some factors contributing to the coagulopathy are listed in Table 6-4. By the time the patient has been transfused with two blood volumes of RBCs, his or her platelet count has likely dropped below the 50,000/μL threshold for surgical hemostasis.[25] There might also be functional platelet defects from the temperature and pH

Table 6-4. Some of the Factors Contributing to the Coagulopathy of Massive Transfusion

- Thrombocytopenia caused by dilution of platelets with crystalloid/colloid fluids and other blood components, and increased platelet consumption
- Dilution and consumption of soluble clotting factors
- Hypothermia
- Acidosis
- Disseminated intravascular coagulation
- Anemia

perturbations associated with conditions requiring massive transfusion. Given the quantitative and qualitative platelet problems associated with massive transfusion, the inability of a platelet count to accurately capture the patient's hemostatic potential, and the fact that RBC transfusion depresses platelet count to a greater extent than does colloid administration,[26] it is reasonable to maintain a platelet count of >50,000/μL during the resuscitation, with further platelet transfusions guided by the extent of bleeding.[27]

Quantitative and qualitative defects exist for soluble coagulation factors as well as for platelets. Although individual recipients vary in their ability to maintain a normal partial thromboplastin time (PTT) and prothrombin time (PT) in the setting of a massive transfusion, some data suggest that early intervention with Fresh Frozen Plasma (FFP) might be important. In a study of 39 patients[28] who received at least 10 units of allogeneic RBCs, recovered antologous units, or whole blood units in 24 hours, the PT and PTT became abnormal after the transfusion of 12 units of RBCs. However, the platelet count did not drop below 50,000/μL until almost 20 units of RBCs had been transfused (see also Ketchum[29] and Ho[30]). Those findings suggest that the FFP (see next section and Chapter 4) should be administered early in the course of the resuscitation, with a view to keeping the international normalized ratio (INR) <1.5 and PTT within 1.5 times the upper limit of the normal reference range.[27] Cryoprecipitate, which contains a minimum of 150 mg of fibrinogen per unit, can be used to maintain a fibrinogen level >100 mg/dL. It is important to keep in mind that both platelet and FFP units contain 2 to 4 mg/mL of fibrinogen; thus the amount of cryoprecipitate can be tempered by the number of platelet and FFP units infused.

Pretransfusion Testing and Same-Day Surgery

Hospitals that feature a significant number of same-day surgery admissions face two major issues: how to manage the workload associated with an influx of samples, typically early in the morning on the day of surgery, and how to manage patients with alloantibodies. One way to deal with the former problem is to extend the validity of the type and screen from 3 days to 30 days for qualified recipients. In the reported experience of one large tertiary care center, extending the validity of the type and screen to 30 days resulted in no surgical delays caused by lack of in-date type and screens.[31]

Qualified patients were those who in the preceding 3 months denied receiving a blood component, being pregnant or having an abortion, or having undergone surgery or general anesthesia and who were not scheduled to receive blood between the time the type and screen was drawn and the surgery date. If these criteria were met, then during the patient's preoperative consultation with the anesthesiologist <30 days before the surgery date, a sample for a type and screen was drawn, and the blood bank could conduct its investigations before the day of surgery. Patients who had unexpected antibodies on previous screens were excluded from the program.

The ability to order type and screens well before the surgery date keeps the blood bank from becoming inundated with a large volume of tests ordered on the actual day of surgery, thereby facilitating a more predictable and manageable laboratory workload. Under such a protocol, antibodies can be identified in advance of the surgery and crossmatch-compatible blood can be sought if necessary, thus reducing delays in providing blood.

The patients who are eligible for an extension of the type and screen validity period are those at the lowest risk of becoming alloimmunized. Managing patients who are already alloimmunized or whose antibodies are discovered at the time of admission for their same-day surgery can pose different challenges to both the blood bank and the surgical team. Antibody identification can take several hours (or longer, depending on the number and complexity of the antibodies); therefore, crossmatch-compatible blood might not be available at the patient's scheduled procedure time. Identifying antibodies before the day of surgery would ameliorate many of these delays. Note that the use of uncrossmatched blood in situations where an unexpected antibody is present but not yet identified is not recommended in nonemergency situations because serologic compatibility cannot be guaranteed.

Compatibility Requirements for Plasma, Platelets, and Cryoprecipitate

Plasma is transfused to correct the dilutional coagulopathy associated with massive transfusion of RBCs, to correct a complex coagulopathy (eg, liver failure), to immediately reverse the effects of oral anticoagulants, and to replace clotting factors for which a sterile concentrate is not available. It is not used for volume replacement. Because of ABO antibodies in units of plasma, only ABO-compatible units can be used (see Table 6-5). Thus, the patient's ABO type is needed for plasma transfusion. Because plasma from AB individuals does not contain ABO antibodies, any patient can receive AB plasma; it is used for emergency transfusion in patients with unknown blood types. Crossmatching of plasma is not required because there are no red cells in plasma products.

Platelets are transfused when a patient is thrombocytopenic. Such patients might be bleeding, might require prophylaxis from spontaneous bleeding, or might need to surpass a platelet-count threshold in advance of an invasive procedure. Non-thrombocytopenic patients might also require platelet transfusions because of platelet functional defects acquired as a result of medications or following cardiac bypass, for example. ABO compatibility for platelet transfusion is desirable but not required. The reason is that each unit contains approximately 60 mL of plasma, which is a substantial amount given that a standard dose of platelets is usually composed of 5 or 6 individual donor units.

Table 6-5. Selection of Blood Components[17]

Recipient ABO Group	Compatible Plasma	Compatible RBCs	Compatible Platelets First Choice	Compatible Platelets Second Choice
A	A, AB	A, O	A, AB	B, O
B	B, AB	B, O	B, AB	A, O
O	O, A, B, AB	O	O*	A, B, AB
AB	AB	O, A, B, AB	AB	A, B, O

RBC = Red Blood Cell.
*Although group O RBCs do not have A or B antigens, the recipient's plasma contains anti-A and anti-B, which could reduce the recovery of transfused platelets bearing A or B antigens.

However, because platelets have a short in-date (5 days) and ABO-matched pools may not be available for the recipient, most institutions will cross ABO boundaries when issuing platelets (eg, issuing A platelets to a B recipient). Typically, the only adverse event from crossing ABO lines is that the recipient might develop a positive direct antiglobulin test, but significant hemolysis is very uncommon. It is important to remember that platelets themselves have ABO antigens on their surface, and thus a donor-recipient ABO mismatch might result in a poor posttransfusion platelet increment.

Each unit of cryoprecipitate contains a small amount of plasma (15 mL/unit) and thus does not require ABO compatibility. This product contains at least 150 mg of fibrinogen and significant amounts of clotting Factor VIII and von Willebrand factor, although sterile preparations of those factors are recommended for the treatment of hemophilia A and von Willebrand's disease, respectively.

Conclusion

The steps in pretransfusion testing are relatively simple, but complete accuracy is required at each step. ABO compatibility between donor and recipient is of paramount importance. Understanding the relationship between the ABO antigens and their reciprocal antibodies and knowing exactly whose blood is being tested are the keys to a safe transfusion.

Acknowledgment

The author is grateful to Dr. Darrell Triulzi for thoughtful discussion and critical review of this chapter.

References

1. Mollison PL, Engelfriet CP, Contreras M. Blood transfusion in clinical practice. 10th ed. Oxford: Blackwell, 1997.
2. Sazama K. Reports of 355 transfusion-associated deaths: 1976 through 1985. Transfusion 1990;30:583-90.
3. Linden JV, Paul B, Dressler KP. A report of 104 transfusion errors in New York State. Transfusion 1992;32:601-6.
4. Silva MA, ed. Standards for blood banks and transfusion services. 24th ed. Bethesda, MD: AABB, 2006.
5. Dzik WH, Murphy MF, Andreu G, et al. An international study of the performance of sample collection from patients. Vox Sang 2003;85:40-7.
6. Cummins D, Sharp S, Vartanian M, et al. The BCSH guidelines on addressograph labels: Experience at a cardiothoracic unit and findings of a telephone survey. Transfus Med 2000;10:117-20.
7. Stainsby D, Russell J, Cohen H, et al. Reducing adverse events in blood transfusion. Br J Haematol 2005;131:8-12.
8. Davies A, Staves J, Kay J, et al. End-to-end electronic control of the hospital transfusion process to increase the safety of blood transfusion: Strengths and weaknesses. Transfusion 2006;46:352-64.
9. Sandler SG, Langeberg A, Dohnalek L, et al. Bar code technology improves positive patient identification and transfusion safety. Dev Biol (Basel) 2005; 120:19-24.
10. Turner CL, Casbard AC, Murphy MF. Barcode technology: Its role in increasing the safety of blood transfusion. Transfusion 2003;43:1200-9.

11. Lau FY, Wong R, Chui CH, et al. Improvement in transfusion safety using a specially designed transfusion wristband. Transfus Med 2000;10:121-4.

12. Figueroa PI, Ziman A, Wheeler C, et al. Nearly two decades using the check-type to prevent ABO incompatible transfusions: One institution's experience. Am J Clin Pathol 2006;126:422-6.

13. Callum JL, Kaplan HS, Merkley LL, et al. Reporting of near-miss events for transfusion medicine: Improving transfusion safety. Transfusion 2001;41:1204-11.

14. Sharma RR, Kumar S, Agnihotri SK, et al. Sources of preventable errors related to transfusion. Vox Sang 2001;81:37-41.

15. Lumadue JA, Boyd JS, Ness PM. Adherence to a strict specimen-labeling policy decreases the incidence of erroneous blood grouping of blood bank specimens. Transfusion 1997;37:1169-72.

16. Dzik WH. Emily Cooley Lecture 2002: Transfusion safety in the hospital. Transfusion 2003;43:1190-8.

17. Yazer MH. The blood bank "black box" debunked: Pretransfusion testing explained. CMAJ 2006;174:29-32.

18. Blumberg N, Ross K, Avila E, et al. Should chronic transfusions be matched for antigens other than ABO and Rho(D)? Vox Sang 1984;47:205-8.

19. Fluit CR, Kunst VA, Drenthe-Schonk AM. Incidence of red cell antibodies after multiple blood transfusions. Transfusion 1990;30:532-5.

20. Rosse WF, Gallagher D, Kinney TR, et al. Transfusion and alloimmunization in sickle cell disease. The Cooperative Study of Sickle Cell Disease. Blood 1990;76:1431-7.

21. Judd WJ. Requirements for the electronic crossmatch. Vox Sang 1998;74 (Suppl 2):409-17.

22. Butch SH for the Scientific Section Coordinating Committee. Guidelines for implementing the electronic crossmatch. Bethesda, MD: AABB, 2003.

23. Saverimuttu J, Greenfield T, Rotenko I, et al. Implications for urgent transfusion of uncrossmatched blood in the emergency department: The prevalence of clinically significant red cell antibodies within different patient groups. Emerg Med 2003;15:239-43.

24. Dutton RP, Shih D, Edelman BB, et al. Safety of uncrossmatched type-O red cells for resuscitation from hemorrhagic shock. J Trauma 2005;59:1445-9.

25. Hiippala S, Myllyla G, Vahtera E. Hemostatic factors and replacement of major blood loss with plasma-poor red cell concentrates. Anesth Analg 1995;81:360-5.

26. Noe DA, Graham SM, Luff R, et al. Platelet counts during rapid massive transfusion. Transfusion 1982;22:392-5.

27. Spence RK, Mintz PD. Transfusion in surgery, trauma and critical care. In: Mintz PD, ed. Transfusion therapy: Clinical principles and practice. 2nd ed. Bethesda, MD: AABB Press, 2005:203-41.

28. Leslie SD, Toy PT. Laboratory hemostatic abnormalities in massively transfused patients given red blood cells and crystalloid. Am J Clin Pathol 1991;96:770-3.

29. Ketchum L, Hess JR, Hiippala S. Indications for early Fresh Frozen Plasma, cryoprecipitate, and platelet transfusion in trauma. J Trauma 2006;60:S51-8.

30. Ho AM, Karmakar MK, Dion PW. Are we giving enough coagulation factors during major trauma resuscitation? Am J Surg 2005;190:479-84.
31. Narvios AB, Rozner M, Lichtiger B. Thirty-day typing and screening for patients undergoing elective surgery: Experience at a large cancer center. Transfusion 2006;46:348-51.

In: Waters JH, ed.
Blood Management: Options for Better Patient Care
Bethesda, MD: AABB Press, 2008

7

Preoperative Optimization

LAWRENCE TIM GOODNOUGH, MD, AND
DALE F. SZPISJAK, MD, MPH

IN THE PREOPERATIVE PERIOD, EVERY EFFORT should be made to optimize the patient's condition before the day of surgery. This can take place through optimizing hemoglobin and eliminating factors that make the patient more prone to bleeding. The value of optimizing hemoglobin concentration in surgical patients is evidenced by the many reports of the prevalence of preoperative anemia—5% to 75% of patients, depending upon the patient population.[1] As might be predicted, the largest risk factor for an intraoperative blood transfusion is this preexisting

Lawrence Tim Goodnough, MD, Professor of Pathology and Medicine, Stanford University, Stanford, California, and Dale F. Szpisjak, MD, MPH, Associate Professor of Anesthesiology, Uniformed Services University of the Health Sciences, Bethesda, Maryland anemia.[2,3] The following discussion describes how one might proceed in optimizing patient hemoglobin concentration. It will then transition into a discussion of factors that might interfere with coagulation function.

Optimizing Hemoglobin Concentration

Anemia is frequently discovered during routine preadmission testing in patients scheduled for elective surgery. Hospital medical committees are developing policies and procedures to address this issue.[4] Single-center reports indicate that approximately one-third of such patients (mostly female) will have iron-deficiency anemia.[3] The remaining patients will have anemia associated with inflammation or chronic disease.[5] Optimization of hemoglobin levels before surgery is an important strategy to reduce the need for allogeneic blood transfusion during surgery.[6]

Little is known about current use of erythropoietic therapeutic strategies to reduce allogeneic blood transfusion.[7] In a survey[8] sent to 1000 US hospitals in 1997, 43% of respondents stated that recombinant human erythropoietin (EPO) therapy (ie, epoetin alfa) was available, although only 11% stated that EPO was routinely (2%) or sometimes (9%) prescribed. The remainder stated that EPO was never used (57%) or almost never used (32%), despite approval of EPO therapy in 1996 for perisurgical use in the US.[9]

Erythropoiesis in Response to Blood Loss

In 2000, a review summarized the data about the relationships among EPO, iron, and erythropoiesis in patients undergoing preoperative autologous blood donation (PAD) (as a model for blood loss anemia), with or without EPO therapy.[10] Table 7-1 presents a summary of selected prospective controlled trials of patients undergoing PAD that are discussed in the review. In this setting, endogenous EPO-mediated erythropoiesis in re-

Table 7-1. Endogenous Erythropoietin-Mediated Erythropoiesis[7]

| | Blood Removed (Donated) | | | Blood Produced | | |
Patients (n)	Requested (donated units)	Red Cells (mL)	Baseline Red Cells (mL)	Red Cells (mL)	Expansion (%)	Iron Therapy
Standard phlebotomy						
108	3 (2.7)	522	1884	351	19	PO
22	3 (2.8)	590	1936	220	11	None
45	3 (2.9)	621	1991	331	17	PO
41	3 (2.9)	603	1918	315	16	PO + IV
Aggressive phlebotomy						
30	3 (3.0)	540	2075	397	19	None
30	3 (3.1)	558	2024	473	23	PO
30	3 (2.9)	522	2057	436	21	IV
24	6 (4.1)	683	2157	568	26	PO
23	6 (4.6)	757	2257	440	19	PO

Data are expressed as means.
PO = oral; IV = intravenous.

sponse to PAD under standard conditions of 1 blood unit donated weekly generates 397 to 568 mL of red cells, or the equivalent of 2 to 3 units of blood. Exogenous EPO therapy in patients undergoing PAD generates 358 to 1102 mL of red cells, or the equivalent of 2 to 5 units of blood (see Table 7-2). With enhanced erythropoiesis during exogenous EPO therapy, iron-restricted erythropoiesis occurs even in patients with measurable storage iron (see Fig 7-1). The superior erythropoietic response (1764 mL red cells) in a patient with hemochromatosis further suggests that iron-restricted erythropoiesis occurs in patients receiving EPO therapy (see Table 7-2), even with oral iron supplementation.

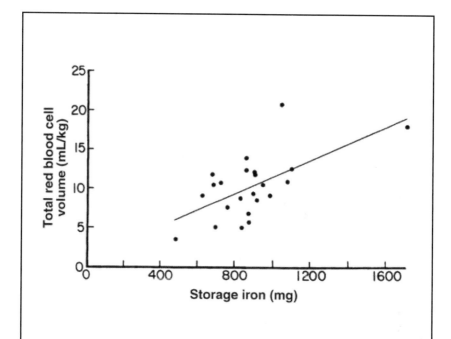

Figure 7-1. Relationship between initial storage iron (mg) and red cell volume expansion (mL/kg) in patients undergoing aggressive phlebotomy with epoetin alfa therapy. Linear regression analysis demonstrates a significant correlation (r = 0.6; p = 0.02). (Used with permission from Goodnough et al.[10])

Table 7-2. Erythropoiesis during Blood Loss and Epoetin Alfa Therapy[7]

Patients (n/gender)	Total EPO Dose (IU/kg)	Blood Removed		Baseline Red Cells (mL)	Blood Produced		Iron Therapy
		Units	Red Cells (mL)		Red Cells (mL)	Expansion (%)	
10/F	900 IV	3.4	435	1285	358	28	IV
24	900 IV	5.2	864	1949	621	32	PO
10/F	1800 IV	4.3	526	1293	474	37	IV
26	1800 IV	5.5	917	2032	644	32	PO
11/F	3600 IV	4.9	809	1796	701	39	PO
12/M	3600 IV	5.9	1097	2296	1102	48	PO
23	3600 IV	5.4	970	2049	911	45	PO
18	3600 IV	5.6	972	2019	856	42	PO
1/M	4200 SQ	8.0	1600	2241	1764	79	Hemochro-matosis

Data are expressed as means.
EPO = erythropoietin; F = female; M = male; SQ = subcutaneous; IV = intravenous; PO = oral.

Erythropoietin Therapy

An analysis of the relationship between EPO dose and the response in red cell production has demonstrated a good correlation (see Fig 7-2).[11] EPO-stimulated erythropoiesis is independent of age and gender,[12] and the variability in response among patients is in part the result of iron-restricted erythropoiesis.[13] There is no evidence that surgery or EPO therapy affects the endogenous EPO response to anemia or the erythropoietic response to EPO.[14]

Red cell expansion is seen with an increase in reticulocyte count by day 3 of treatment in iron-replete nonanemic patients

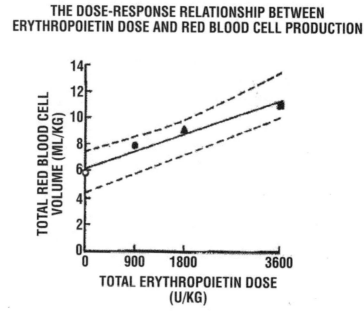

Figure 7-2. The dose-response relationship between total (cumulative) amount of epoetin alfa administered and the red cell volume increase during the preoperative interval for patients treated intravenously with placebo, 150 IU/kg, 300 IU/kg, and 600 IU/kg. Doses of epoetin alfa are given in total (cumulative) units per kilogram of body weight for all six treatments combined over a period of 3 weeks; increases in red cell volume are given in milliliters per kilogram of body weight. The dotted lines indicate the 95% confidence interval. (Used with permission from Goodnough et al.[11])

treated with EPO.[15] As illustrated in Fig 7-3, the equivalent of 1 blood unit is produced by day 7, and the equivalent of 5 blood units is produced over 28 days.[16] If 3 to 5 blood units are necessary in order to minimize allogeneic blood exposure in patients undergoing complex procedures such as orthopedic joint replacement surgery, the preoperative interval necessary for EPO-stimulated erythropoiesis can be estimated to be 3 to 4 weeks.

Normal individuals have been shown to have difficulty providing sufficient iron to support rates of erythropoiesis that are greater than three times the basal rate.[17] A 1998 study confirmed that the maximum erythropoietic response in the acute setting, which is seen in EPO-treated patients with measurable storage iron, is approximately four times basal marrow red cell

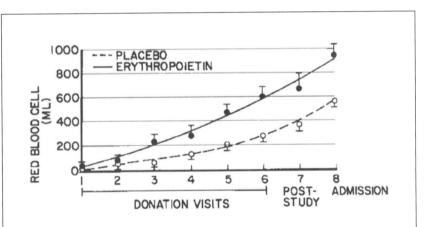

Figure 7-3. Red cell production during autologous blood donation in 23 placebo-treated (open circles) and 21 epoetin alfa-treated (closed circles) patients. Data points represent calculated red cell production (mL) at donation visits 1 through 6, the poststudy visit, and hospital admission. Red cell production is indicated by polynomial regression curve for each treatment group (n = 44 at each point). The rate of red cell production can be derived for any preoperative interval. The mean cumulative interval since donation visit 1 was 3.5 days to visit 2, 7.2 days to visit 3, 10.6 days to visit 4, 14.2 days to visit 5, 17.6 days to visit 6, 20.9 days to visit 7 (poststudy visit), and 26.3 days to visit 8 (hospital admission). (Used with permission from Goodnough et al.[16])

production.[13] Previous investigators have shown that conditions associated with enhanced plasma iron and transferrin saturation are necessary to produce a greater marrow response, such as in patients with hemochromatosis[18] or in patients supplemented with intravenous iron administration.[19]

In hemochromatosis, marrow response has been estimated to increase by six to eight times over baseline red cell production with aggressive phlebotomy.[18] The term "relative iron deficiency" has thus been shown by Finch[20] to describe occurrences in individuals when the iron stores are normal but the increased erythron iron requirements exceed the available supply of iron. Although iron supplementation with at least 100 mg of elemental iron per day taken with food can cover the increased iron needs from endogenous EPO in autologous blood donors, there is a significant positive relationship between storage iron and marrow response in patients receiving EPO therapy.[13] These results suggest that storage iron is important for maintaining sufficient plasma transferrin saturation for optimal erythropoiesis.

Iron Therapy

In circumstances with significant ongoing iron losses, oral iron does not provide enough iron to correct the iron-deficient erythropoiesis, and intravenous iron therapy should be considered. Patients undergoing renal dialysis have such blood losses, and the role of intravenous iron therapy has been best defined in clinical trials achieving target hematocrit levels in that setting. Addressing iron deficiency with intravenous iron therapy allows correction of anemia along with use of lower EPO dosage.[21] Another role for intravenous iron therapy is in the arena of bloodless medicine and bloodless surgery programs for patients who refuse blood transfusions because of religious beliefs. Common clinical settings in that arena include pregnant or postpartum females[22] and female patients who have dysfunctional uterine bleeding and are scheduled for hysterectomy.[23]

Intravenous iron therapy has been closely scrutinized for risks and adverse events.[24] Imferon (iron dextran BP; Fisons Ltd, Loughborough, Leicestershire, UK) is an iron preparation previously associated with a 0.6% risk of life-threatening anaphylactoid reactions and 1.7% risk of severe, delayed reactions that were serum-sickness-like and characterized by fever, arthragias, and myalgias. An increased incidence of delayed reactions of up to 30% and severe reactions of 5.3% was subsequently described. The product was eventually withdrawn from use.

INFeD (iron dextran USP; Schein Pharmaceutical, Florham Park, NJ) is currently approved for parenteral (intramuscular or intravenous) use, with widespread intravenous administration in renal dialysis patients. Clinical studies have shown that IN-FeD administered intravenously during the dialysis procedure was associated with clinically significant adverse reactions in 4.7% of patients, of which 0.7% were serious or life threatening, and another 1.75% were characterized as anaphylactoid reactions.[25] The prevalence of these reactions does not appear to differ among patients receiving low-dose (100 mg) or higher-dose (250-500 mg) infusions.[26] A 1999 review reported 196 allergy or anaphylaxis cases with the use of iron dextran in the United States between 1976 and 1996, of which 31 (15.8%) were fatal.[27]

Safety aspects of parenteral iron (iron dextran, ferric gluconate, and iron saccharate) in patients with end-stage renal disease have been scrutinized.[28] Iron saccharate is a preparation available in Europe but not in the United States. Although allergic reactions are very rare, possible adverse effects include a metallic taste, arthralgia, chest pain, and bronchospasm.[28-30] Ferric gluconate (Ferrlecit, Watson Nephrology, Morristown, NJ) was approved for use in the United States in February 1999 as an intravenous iron preparation in renal dialysis patients. Dosage of Ferrlecit is limited to 125 mg over a 1-hour infusion at each administration.[31] The rate of allergic reactions (3.3 episodes per million doses) appears lower than with iron dextran (8.7 episodes per million doses) and the safety profile of iron gluconate is substantially better. Among 74 adverse events from

1976 to 1996 that were reported as severe, there were no deaths.[27]

Adverse events associated with ferric gluconate that have been reported include hypotension, rash, and chest or abdominal pain, with an incidence of less than 5%.[32] Another potential adverse effect of intravenous iron therapy is a clinical syndrome of acute iron toxicity (nausea, facial reddening, and hypotension) that has been attributed to oversaturation (>100%) of transferrin. That effect has been described with rapid infusion of ferric gluconate (62.5-125 mg within 30 minutes) in a study of 20 dialysis patients.[33] However, a later report disputed the existence of the effect of oversaturation of transferrin by demonstrating that two laboratory assays for measurement of serum iron yield misleading results for transferrin saturation if performed within 24 hours after infusion.[34] One European study reported serious reactions, including one hypotensive event, in only 3 of 226 patients (1.3%) undergoing renal dialysis while being treated with ferric gluconate.[35]

Previous studies[36] have indicated that the increased erythropoietic effect (4.5 to 5.5 times basal rate) of intravenous iron dextran (with an estimated half-life of 60 hours) is transient and lasts from 7 to 10 days, after which time the iron is sequestered in the reticuloendothelial system and erythropoiesis returns to 2.5 to 3.5 times normal.[37] Intravenous iron therapy is therefore recommended to be administered at intervals of 1 to 2 weeks. A dose-response relationship of EPO and erythropoiesis that is affected favorably by intravenous iron, even in iron-replete individuals, has important implications for EPO dosage, especially if the cost of therapy is taken into account.[9] Intravenous iron may potentiate the erythropoietic response in the setting of EPO therapy by improving iron-restricted erythropoiesis induced by EPO therapy. The value of this approach has been best demonstrated in patients with chronic kidney disease undergoing dialysis. Clinical trials have been conducted to establish the value of parenteral iron supplementation in other clinical settings employing erythropoietin therapy.[38]

Maximizing Coagulation Function

If at all possible, drugs that could adversely affect clotting [aspirin, nonsteroidal anti-inflammatory drugs (NSAIDs), heparin, warfarin, and anti-platelet drugs] should be discontinued before surgery. In addition, attention should be paid to herbal and vitamin supplements.

Avoidance of Anticoagulants

Coagulation function can be affected by many factors, all of which should be taken into consideration before a patient undergoes surgery. For example, the avoidance of anticoagulants should include not only drugs and medications, but also herbal supplements. In addition, a thorough patient history may reveal genetic coagulation abnormalities that should be addressed.

Nonsteroidal Anti-Inflammatory Drugs

Platelet aggregation decreases with the inhibition of cyclooxygenase (COX_1), an enzyme located within the platelet. COX_1 inhibition prevents the conversion of arachidonic acid to thromboxane A_2. Because the latter is a potent stimulus of platelet aggregation, decreasing its production through COX_1 inhibition thereby decreases platelet adhesiveness.

Aspirin and NSAIDs both inhibit COX_1, although COX_2-specific NSAIDs are now available. (COX_2 is more commonly found in inflammatory cells; therefore, its inhibition should have little effect on platelet adhesiveness.[39]) The duration of the antiplatelet effect depends on the pharmacodynamic effects of aspirin and on the pharmacodynamic and pharmacokinetic effects of the NSAIDs. Aspirin inhibits COX irreversibly and thus decreases platelet adhesiveness for the 7- to 10-day life span of the platelet. The effects of most other non-aspirin NSAIDs are reversible after 48 hours, although exceptions include oxaprozin (12 days) and pirixicam (14 days).[40]

The perioperative use of NSAIDs has increased because of the new emphasis on multimodal pain therapies. Perioperative use of non-COX-specific NSAIDs does not appear to increase bleeding in children, but studies have produced inconsistent results.[41] Use of non-COX-specific NSAIDs in adults has been associated with increased blood loss in abdominal hysterectomy and plastic surgery.[42] Perioperative use of ketorolac is not associated with increased bleeding.[43] NSAIDs may reasonably be avoided in procedures in which hematoma formation would potentially compromise the surgical outcome.[39] Currently, no pharmacologic reversal agents are available for aspirin and NSAIDs.

Antiplatelet Drugs

Antiplatelet drugs are commonly used as prophylaxis against the cardiovascular risks of stroke and myocardial ischemia. Both oral and intravenous medications are in clinical use, and the mechanisms of action vary.

The thienopyridines ticlopidine and clopidogrel are orally administered. Although there is uncertainty about the mechanism of action, the effect of these drugs is likely the result of an irreversible blockade of adenosine diphosphate (ADP)-mediated platelet effects and the subsequent reduction of the responses to thromboxane A_2, platelet activating factor, collagen, and thrombin.[39,44] The thienopyridines should be discontinued between 7 and 10 days before surgery.[40] There are currently no pharmacologic reversal agents.

Dipyridamole is a phosphodiesterase inhibitor that increases cyclic adenosine monophosphate and cyclic guanosine monophosphate, thus inhibiting platelet activation.[39] Its use should be discontinued 2 days before surgery.[40]

The intravenous agents abciximab, eptifibatide, and tirofiban are used to inhibit platelets after coronary angioplasty and stent procedures. Abciximab is a monoclonal antibody fragment, while eptifibatide and tirofiban are low-molecular-weight compounds.[45] Their mechanism of action is blockade of the platelet's glycoprotein IIb/IIIa (GPIIb/IIIa) receptor, which inhibits fibrinogen binding.[39] These agents rapidly saturate the glycoprotein receptors and have rapid clearance from the plasma. Despite the short plasma half-life, abciximab has a GPIIb/IIIa receptor dissociation half-life of 4 hours,[45] and the receptors may remain bound for 2 weeks.[39] Thus, the effects of abciximab are longer lasting than the competitive inhibitors eptifibatide and tirofiban. Therapeutic effects require roughly 80% receptor blockade.[45] After discontinuation of an infusion, normal hemostatic function returns in approximately 72 hours with abciximab and in 4 hours with eptifibatide and tirofiban. Eptifibatide and tirofiban are renally excreted, and the risk of hemorrhage increases with renal insufficiency.[44] All three agents can induce thrombocytopenia in 1% to 5% of patients.[46]

Reversal of the effects of abciximab can be accelerated with platelet transfusion, which leads to redistribution of the drug, effectively "diluting" the bound receptors. The exact quantity of platelets required is not known.[41] Fibrinogen administration does not reverse abciximab.[47]

The effects of eptifibatide and tirofiban will reverse within 4 to 8 hours after discontinuing an infusion if patients have normal renal function. In contrast, fibrinogen [Fresh Frozen Plasma (FFP) or Cryoprecipitated AHF] with or without platelets will acutely reverse the effects of eptifibatide and tirofiban.[48] The reversal dose decreases as time from infusion discontinuation increases. The recommended dose of fibrinogen—extrapolated from laboratory, not clinical, data—is 2400 mg after acute discontinuation, but the dose is decreased to 1200 mg if the infusion has been stopped for 4 hours.[48]

Warfarin

Warfarin is an orally administered anticoagulant used in the treatment and prevention of thromboembolic complications.[49] Its mechanism of action is inhibition of vitamin K-dependent carboxylation of clotting Factors II, VII, IX, and X, which markedly decreases their clotting activity. Also included among the vitamin-K-dependent clotting factors are the anticoagulants protein C and protein S.[50]

The degree of anticoagulation is expressed in multiples of the international normalized ratio (INR), with the usual therapeutic range defined as an INR of 2.0 to 3.0.[50] The potential for hemorrhagic complications increases with warfarin therapy, especially with an INR >4.5.[51]

Reversal of warfarin anticoagulation is needed to decrease the hemorrhagic risk when the INR is supratherapeutic. A therapeutic INR may also need correction if the patient is actively bleeding or anticipating surgery. The prescribed reversal regimen should be based on the degree of INR elevation, the seriousness of bleeding, and the preoperative time available if surgery is planned.

Nonbleeding patients with supratherapeutic INRs rarely require transfusion therapy. They may be managed by simply holding warfarin therapy and adjusting the dose according to follow-up of the INR, although more rapid correction is obtained by adding oral vitamin K therapy.[50] Holding warfarin therapy is also an appropriate strategy when preparing an anticoagulated patient for elective surgery, although such a patient may need short-term preoperative prophylactic anticoagulation with standard- or low-molecular-weight heparin (LMWH).

Bleeding patients and those scheduled for urgent or emergent surgery require a more aggressive approach. The following recommendations are based on the reviews by Warkentin and Crowther[50] and by Goodnough et al.[52] Nonbleeding patients who have therapeutic INRs and who are about to undergo urgent surgery (ie, within 18-24 hours) can be managed by holding warfarin, administering 2 to 5 mg of intravenous vitamin K, and rechecking for correction of the INR. Nonbleeding patients requiring emergent surgery should also have warfarin held and should receive 2 to 5 mg of intravenous vitamin K, as well as transfusion of either FFP or recombinant activated Factor VII (rFVIIa). (See the following paragraph.) The dose of FFP varies with the INR. Patients with therapeutic INRs may correct with a

5 to 8 mL/kg dose of FFP, whereas the dose for patients with supratherapeutic INRs is 15 mL/kg. Patients with major or life-threatening bleeding should have warfarin held and should receive up to 10 mg of intravenous vitamin K, as well as FFP or rFVIIa. The effectiveness of these measures should always be verified by rechecking the INR.

A special note is required regarding the use of rFVIIa, whose labeled indication is the treatment of hemophilia in patients with inhibitors. An uncontrolled case series used the preparation to acutely reverse the effects of warfarin with doses that ranged from 15 to 90 µg/kg.[49] (The editors of the journal that published the study advised controlled studies before changing treatment policies.) Such therapy may be helpful in patients who cannot tolerate the fluid load associated with FFP or the time required to obtain it. Another potential benefit is that rFVIIa has been rarely associated with the thrombotic complications attributed to prothrombin complex concentrates (PCCs), which have also been used to reverse warfarin therapy.[49,50] Goodnough et al[52] recommend that patients treated with rFVIIa to acutely reverse warfarin therapy should also receive FFP to increase levels of functional Factors II, IX, and X.[52] They further recommend a transfusion medicine consultation to assist with additional dosing of this expensive new therapy.

Heparin

Heparin inhibits coagulation by enhancing the effects of the physiologic clotting inhibitor, antithrombin (AT). AT inhibits circulating factors, including Factors IIa, IXa, Xa, XIa, and the tissue factor-Factor VIIa complex, although it does not inhibit thrombin already bound to a clot or Factor Xa already bound to platelets.[50] There are two main types of heparin: unfractionated heparin (UFH) and LMWH.

UFH is effectively reversed by protamine. The dose is based on the amount of UFH administered in the previous 4 hours, and it is calculated as 1 mg of protamine per 100 units of UFH. The serum half-life of UFH is 90 minutes and should be considered when calculating the dose of protamine.[50] Slow intravenous drip is the safest route of administration. Because the half-life of UFH exceeds that of protamine, redosing may be needed.

In contrast, protamine reverses only about 60% of the anticoagulant effect of LMWH.[50] The dose is calculated on a mg-per-mg basis, and again the half-life of LMWH (3-4 hours) should be taken into account when considering either the initial protamine dose or the need for redosing.

Herbal Supplements

The use of herbal or other complementary, alternative medical therapies is prevalent, with estimates ranging from 6.8%[53] to 32%[54] among perioperative patients. Especially concerning is that 70% of such patients may not reveal this information during preoperative interviews.[54,55] These substances are considered dietary supplements by the Food and Drug Administration and are exempt from the testing required of scientific medications.[55,56] Nevertheless, many of those substances have been associated with coagulation problems.

Garlic is used by 15% of patients who consume herbals.[56] Garlic decreases thromboxane synthesis and alters arachidonic acid metabolism, causing antiplatelet effects.[55] These effects may be mediated by a component, ajoene, and they may be irreversible.[57] Reports of bleeding problems associated with garlic are anecdotal.[58,59] Garlic may also potentiate the effects of warfarin.[55] The most conservative recommendation, because of the potential for irreversible platelet effects, is to discontinue use of garlic 7 days before surgery.[57]

Ginkgo is used by 18% of patients who consume herbals.[56] It inhibits platelet activating factor[60] and has been associated with anecdotal reports of spontaneous[61-65] and surgical[66] bleeding. Use of ginkgo should be discontinued at least 36 hours before surgery.[57]

Ginseng is used by 15% of patients who consume herbals.[56] Because ginseng inhibits platelets irreversibly in humans,[67] it should be discontinued 7 days before surgery.

Ginger decreases platelet aggregation through COX_1 inhibition,[68] and it potentiates warfarin.[69] The most conservative recommendation is to discontinue ginger consumption 7 days before surgery, although no adverse bleeding attributed solely to ginger has been reported.[55]

St. John's wort is used by 15% of patients who consume herbals.[56] It may accelerate the metabolism of warfarin,[57] in contrast to the other agents described above.

Danshen potentiates the effects of warfarin, inhibits platelet aggregation, and has AT-like effects.[55]

Dong quai is a naturally occurring vitamin K antagonist and may potentiate the effects of warfarin.

Genetic Coagulation Abnormalities

Platelet Disorders

Bernard-Soulier disease (also known as giant platelet syndrome) is a rare, autosomal-recessive platelet disorder caused by a deficiency of platelet membrane proteins Ib, IX, and V.[70-72] The pathophysiology is reduced von Willebrand factor (vWF)-dependent platelet adhesion. Clinical signs and symptoms include giant platelets, prolonged bleeding time, spontaneous bleeding, and thrombocytopenia. The administration of 1-deamino-8-D-arginine vasopressin [DDAVP (Ferring Pharmaceuticals, Parsippany, NJ] may be helpful,[73] but platelet transfusion may still be needed.

Fanconi anemia is a rare, autosomal-recessive disorder associated with pancytopenia and high risk for acute myeloid leukemia, in addition to other nonhematologic abnormalities.[74,75] The disease presents in childhood. Patients may require erythrocyte or platelet transfusion, or both.

Glanzmann's thrombasthenia is an autosomal recessive disease characterized by severely reduced or absent platelet aggregation. The pathophysiology is defective synthesis of GPIIb and IIIa. Patients can present with mild to severe bleeding and may require platelet transfusion.[72]

Immune thrombocytopenic purpura (ITP) is an autoimmune (not genetic) disease associated with platelet antibodies directed at GPIIb and IIIa. It has an incidence of 6:100,000. The pathophysiology is autoimmune destruction of platelets in the spleen, leading to thrombocytopenia. Clinical signs and symptoms include petechiae, easy bruising, epistaxis, and thrombocytopenia. Bleeding does not usually occur with platelet counts above 50,000/μL, although patients with ITP often tolerate lower levels. Patients may respond to steroids, intravenous immune globulin, anti-D immunoglobulin, chemotherapeutic agents, and plasmapheresis, although splenectomy may be required in refractory cases.[76] Patients may require platelet transfusion, although the transfused platelets may be destroyed by the same pathophysiologic mechanism. If platelets are to be transfused, they should be typed and crossed and leukocyte reduced to help prevent alloimmunization.

Storage pool disease and gray platelet syndrome are hereditary platelet disorders associated with decreased alpha granules, delta granules, or both, in platelets. Alpha granules contain vWF and platelet factor 4, among others. Delta granules contain ADP, which is essential in normal platelet aggregation. Patients with storage pool disease have the usual bleeding problems associated with defective platelets. Patients with delta storage pool disease may respond to DDAVP, although platelet transfusion may be required for all patients with the disorder.[70] Platelets should be typed and crossed and leukocyte reduced to help prevent alloimmunization.

Sea-blue histiocyte syndrome is a very rare autosomal recessive disease associated with thrombocytopenia, hepatosplenomegaly, occasional neurologic abnormalities, and a predisposition to parasitic infections.[77,78] The exact pathophysiology is unknown. Patients with albinism who have normal platelet counts may have elevated bleeding times.[78] Patients may need platelet transfusion, although it is rarely necessary in individuals with platelet counts >50,000/μL.

von Willebrand disease (vWD) is the most common inherited bleeding disorder in humans, with a prevalence of approximately 1%.[72] There are several subtypes of vWD, and treatment depends on proper diagnosis. The most common subtype is Type I (70%). It is characterized by a partial quantitative defect of normal vWF. Inheritance is autosomal dominant, with incomplete penetrance.[79]

Most of the remaining cases (20%-30%) are Type II, and they are characterized by both qualitative and quantitative defects of vWF. Type II has three variants of approximately equal prevalence.[72] Type IIA has autosomal dominant inheritance, and patients lack high-molecular-weight vWF multimers. Type IIB is also an autosomal dominant disease and is associated with both thrombocytopenia and loss of high-molecular-weight multimers.[79] Thrombocytopenia is secondary to accelerated clearance of platelets caused by increased binding of the abnormal vWF to platelet GPIb.[70,72,79] Type IIN is an X-linked recessive disorder associated with decreased binding of Factor VIII to vWF. That decreased binding leads to a rapid clearance of Factor VIII from the plasma, resembling hemophilia A.[70,72,79,80] A much rarer form, Type IIM, is associated with decreased vWF binding to platelet GPIb.[79]

Approximately 5% of patients with vWD have the Type III variant. It is autosomal recessive and associated with little to no production of vWF.[72,79]

In addition to the inherited forms of vWD, an acquired form exists. It is most commonly associated with lymphoproliferative disorders, cardiac disease, and cancer.[72,79] (See Table 7-3 for a list of laboratory diagnostic criteria for each subtype.)

Treatment of vWD depends on the subtype. Approximately 75% of patients with Types I, IIA, and IIM will respond to DDAVP, which releases vWF and Factor VIII from endothelial cells.[79] The dose is 0.3 μg/kg (maximum 20 μg) by intravenous infusion administered over approximately 30 minutes.[79] vWF levels double to triple within an hour and stay elevated for approximately 6 hours. When a patient is being prepared for elective surgery, a DDAVP challenge followed by verification of an increase in vWF levels is useful. The addition of an antifibrin-

Table 7-3. Diagnostic Tests in von Willebrand Disease*

Test	PTT	Plt Count	vWF:Ag	FVIII:c	vWF Multimer Pattern	vWF:RCof	RIPA
Type 1	⇑ /⇕	⇕	⇓⇓⇓	⇓/⇕	⇕	⇓	L none M ⇓/⇕ H ⇓/⇕
Type 2A	⇑ /⇕	⇕	⇓/⇕	⇓/⇕	⇓ HMW multimers	⇓	L none M ⇓ H ⇓/⇕
Type 2B	⇑ /⇕	⇓/⇕	⇓/⇕	⇓/⇕	⇓ HMW multimers	⇓	L + M ⇕ H ⇕
Type 2M	⇑ /⇕	⇕	⇓/⇕	⇓/⇕	⇕	⇓	L none M ⇓/⇕ H ⇓/⇕
Type 2N	⇑ /⇕	⇕	⇓/⇕	⇓/⇕	⇕	⇓/ ⇕	L none M ⇕ H ⇕
Type 3	⇑	⇕	⇓⇓⇓	⇓⇓⇓	Absent	⇓⇓⇓	L none M none H none

*Data from multiple sources.[70,72,79,80]

Plt = platelet; PTT = partial thromboplastin time; vWF = von Willebrand factor; Ag = antigen; FVIII = Factor VIII; RCof = ristocetin cofactor; HMW = high molecular weight; RIPA = ristocetin-induced platelet aggregation; ⇕ = normal; ⇑ = increased; ⇓ = decreased; L = low dose ristocetin (0.5 mg/mL); M = medium dose ristocetin (1.0 mg/mL); H = high dose ristocetin (1.5 mg/mL); + = positive.

olytic also improves clot stability.[79] DDAVP is contraindicated in Type IIB vWD because it may worsen thrombocytopenia. Also, because DDAVP may cause hyponatremia, electrolytes should be monitored with repeated dosing.

Patients who do not respond favorably to DDAVP will need exogenous vWF. Although vWF is present in Cryoprecipitated AHF, use of that product carries the risks of viral disease transmission. Purified plasma concentrates are now available. Expert consultation is recommended to assist with dosing. For surgery, patients should receive approximately 60 to 80 ristocetin cofactor activity units/kg every 8 to 12 hours, and this regimen should continue for 7 to 10 days after major surgery and for 3 to 5 days after minor surgery.[79]

Factor Deficiencies

Factor II deficiency is a rare autosomal recessive disorder characterized by either low or dysfunctional prothrombin.[79,81] Prothrombin levels may vary from <1% to 75%,[81] although levels from 5% to 50% are usually well tolerated except when challenged by trauma or surgery.[79] It is important to rule out vitamin K deficiency when diagnosing this disease. Prothrombin complex concentrates can be used to treat vitamin K deficiency. Prothrombin has a long serum half-life of about 60 hours, which simplifies maintenance therapy. The loading dose is 20 units/kg, with a maintenance dose of 5 units/kg/24 hours. FFP is an alternative, although it has increased risks of viral disease transmission[82] and fluid overload.[79] The loading dose of FFP is 20 mL/kg with maintenance doses of 5 mL/kg/24 hours.[81]

Factor V deficiency is an extremely rare, autosomal recessive disorder with approximately 200 reported cases.[83] Signs and symptoms include ecchymosis, epistaxis, gingival bleeding, menorrhagia, and excess bleeding associated with surgery or trauma.[79] Factor V is synthesized by the liver and has a serum half-life of 12 to 36 hours.[84] Surgical hemostasis is achieved when levels are approximately 30% of normal. Replacement therapy is FFP, 20 mL/kg, with maintenance doses of 5 to 10 mL/kg daily for 7 days.

Factor VII deficiency is an autosomal recessive disorder and the only hereditary clotting factor deficiency with a prolonged prothrombin time (PT) and normal partial thromboplastin time (PTT). Diagnosis requires a specific Factor VII assay. Heterozygotes are usually asymptomatic, but the bleeding in homozygotes does not always correlate with Factor VII levels. Replacement therapies have included PCCs and FFP; however, rFVIIa has advantages because it removes the risks of both viral disease transmission and fluid overload. Dosing regimens are still anecdotal. Surgical hemostasis may be achieved with Factor VII levels approximately 25% of normal, but this percentage is not certain.[81] A higher Factor VII level may be required when small amounts of bleeding would be poorly tolerated. For example, in neurosurgery, a loading dose of 50 units/kg followed by 20 units/kg every 12 hours has been successful.[85] Frequent dosing or continuous infusion may be required perioperatively because of Factor VII's short half-life of about 5 hours.[84] A patient with Factor VII deficiency (native level 5% of normal) underwent cesarean section without excess hemorrhage after 13.3 µg/kg bolus followed by 96 hours of continuous infusion (48 hours at 3.33 µg/kg/hour followed by 1.66 µg/kg/hour for an additional 48 hours).[86] Expert hematology consultation is recommended when using this expensive therapy.

Hemophilia A (Factor VIII deficiency) is an X-linked recessive disorder caused by a deficiency of Factor VIII. This defect occurs in approximately 1:10,000 males and is definitively diagnosed with a Factor VIII assay. Carriers have Factor VIII levels >50% of normal and are usually asymptomatic. Symptomatic patients are classified as mild, moderate, or severe.[79] Mildly affected patients (Factor VIII levels 6%-30% of normal) rarely suffer spontaneous hemorrhaging, although surgery or trauma may lead to excess bleeding. Moderately affected patients (Factor VIII levels 1%-5% of normal) have occasional spontaneous hemorrhages. Severely afflicted patients (Factor VIII <1% of normal) experience frequent, spontaneous hemorrhages from early infancy.[79]

Treatment varies with disease severity and should be coordinated through the patient's hematologist. Mildly affected patients may respond to DDAVP (either 0.3 µg/kg intravenously or 300 µg intranasally) and antifibrinolytic therapy with ε-aminocaproic acid[79] or tranexamic acid.[87] Despite such therapy, patients may still require Factor VIII replacement. Although both FFP and Cryoprecipitated AHF have been used, they are no longer considered first-line therapy because of the risks of viral disease transmission, uncertain Factor VIII content, and fluid overload (with FFP). PCCs have also fallen out of favor because of potential thromboembolic complications.[88]

The preferred agent is recombinant Factor VIII [Kogenate FS (Bayer Corp, Elkhart, IN)]. Although patients who experience moderate hemorrhages or who are undergoing minor surgical procedures may respond adequately when Factor VIII activity is increased to 30% to 60%, patients who have life-threatening hemorrhages or who are undergoing major surgery will need 100% of normal Factor VIII activity. Dosing is based on the assumption that 1 unit/kg will increase Factor VIII activity by 2%. The initial preoperative dose is 50 units/kg, and verification of 100% activity is needed to document benefit. This dose will need to be repeated every 6 to 12 hours because Factor VIII has a half-life of 13 hours. Maintenance of 100% Factor VIII activity will be required for 10 to 14 days or until healing is complete.[89]

Despite the advantages of recombinant Factor VIII therapy, the incidence of inhibitor formation to Factor VIII is approximately 30%,[90] and most are in the "severely afflicted" category.[79] Patients with inhibitors are classified as "high responders" (high inhibitor titers) or "low responders" (low inhibitor titers). Patients with low antibody titers may respond favorably to high doses of Factor VIII concentrates or porcine Factor VIII concentrates. Patients with high antibody titers generally do not respond favorably to Factor VIII concentrates and should be treated with rFVIIa. Before major surgery, the dose of rFVIIa is 90 µg/kg intravenously, with repeat dosing every 2 to 3 hours to maintain hemostasis.[52]

Hemophilia B (Factor IX deficiency) is an X-linked recessive disorder with an incidence of 1:25,000 males; it is clinically identical to hemophilia A. Similarly, mildly affected patients have Factor IX levels 5% to 40% of normal, moderately affected patients have levels in the 1% to 5% range, and severely afflicted patients have levels <1%. Definitive diagnosis is based on measuring Factor IX levels. Although PCCs have been used in the past, they are no longer the first-line therapy because of the risks of thromboembolic complications, as mentioned earlier in the discussion of hemophilia A. The preferred agent is recombinant Factor IX. Dosing is based on the assumption that 1 unit/kg will increase Factor IX activity by 1%. Recombinant Factor IX has a half-life of 18 hours, and maintenance doses should be repeated at intervals of 12 to 18 hours until healing occurs or has occurred. Therapy should be guided by measuring Factor IX levels.[79]

In contrast to patients with hemophilia A, only about 3% of hemophilia B patients will develop inhibitors to Factor IX.[91] Another difference is that hemophilia B patients with inhibitors have developed anaphylaxis and nephrotic syndrome on exposure to Factor IX.[92] In patients with Factor IX inhibitors, rFVIIa can be used and is dosed as described for hemophilia A patients with inhibitors.

Once again, it is important to coordinate therapy with the patient's hematologist.

Factor XI deficiency is a rare autosomal recessive disorder that occurs with a frequency of 1:450 among Ashkenazi Jews,[79] but with a frequency of about 1:1,000,000 outside that population.[93] Spontaneous bleeding is rare, but hemorrhaging often occurs with surgery or trauma.[79,93] Bleeding does not always correlate with Factor XI levels, and it can be associated with vWD.[94] Treatment with antifibrinolytics is often sufficient, especially for dental surgery[79,95]; fibrin sealant has also been used successfully.[96]

The preferred Factor XI therapy is FFP or Factor XI concentrate, but the former is associated with fluid overload and viral disease transmission while the latter is not available in the United States.[93] rFVIIa (major surgery: 90 µg/kg every 2 hours for 24 hours, followed by 90 µg/kg every 4 hours for 24 hours) in combination with tranexamic acid (15 mg/kg by mouth every 6 hours for 7 days) was used successfully in a pilot study with 14 patients, although one patient suffered a fatal cerebrovascular accident.[93]

Hageman factor (Factor XII) deficiency is a rare, autosomal recessive disorder that is not associated with a bleeding diathesis despite an elevated PTT. Paradoxically, the disorder has been associated with thromboembolic complications, although it is uncertain if such complications are related to Factor XII levels or to some other abnormality, such as antiphospholipid antibody syndrome or lupus anticoagulant.[97]

Factor XIII deficiency is a rare, autosomal recessive disorder often occurring with consanguinity.[98] It is characterized by a severe bleeding diathesis that often presents early in life. PT and PTT tests are normal, despite severe bleeding. Umbilical stump bleeding in the neonatal period is almost considered pathognomonic.[99,100] The most severe complication is intracranial bleeding, which occurs in 25% of patients.[99] Factor XIII has a half-life of 9 to 12 days[84] and has been successfully treated with replacement therapy (FFP, 5 mL/kg each month). Factor XIII concentrates have also been used,[101] but they are not available in the United States. Recombinant Factor XIII exists but is not yet marketed in the United States.[102]

Conclusion

Optimization of presurgical patients can be a complex process. For many surgeons and anesthesiologists, allogeneic transfusion is a simpler solution to any preexisting anemia or coagulation dysfunction. However, given the choice for themselves or one of their family members, many surgeons or anesthesiologists would likely choose the route of optimization. Although many conscientious surgeons would spend the time to minimize patient risk through optimization, it is important to have structures in place that aid all surgeons in this process and protect patients from unnecessary transfusion risk. In many hospitals, such a structure can take the form of an internal medicine preoperative clearance and treatment center, where an internist sees preoperative patients and optimizes their conditions before surgery. In other hospitals, this can take place through a preoperative anesthesia clinic. Critical to the success of both is adequate time for the internist or anesthesiologist to influence anemia or coagulation dysfunction.

References

1. Shander A, Knight K, Thurer R, et al. Prevalence and outcomes of anemia in surgery: A systematic review of the literature. Am J Med 2004;116(Suppl 7A): 58S-69S.
2. Madbouly KM, Senagore AJ, Remzi RH, et al. Perioperative blood transfusions increase infectious complications after ileoanal pouch procedures (IPAA). Int J Colorec Dis 2006;21:807-13.
3. Goodnough LT, Vizmeg K, Sobecks R, et al. Prevalence and classification of anemia in elective orthopedic surgery patients: Implications for blood conservation programs. Vox Sang 1992;63:90-5.
4. Waters J. The transfusion committee's role in blood management. In: Saxena S, Shulman I, eds. The transfusion committee: Putting patient safety first. Bethesda, MD: AABB Press, 2006:99.
5. Weiss G, Goodnough LT. Anemia of chronic disease. N Engl J Med 2005; 352: 1011-23.
6. Goodnough LT, Spence R, Shander A. Bloodless medicine: Clinical care without allogeneic blood transfusion. Transfusion 2003;43:668-76.
7. Goodnough LT, Brecher ME, Kanter MH, AuBuchon JP. Transfusion medicine, part II: Blood conservation. N Engl J Med 1999;340:525-33.
8. Hutchinson AB, Fergusson D, Graham ID, et al. Utilization of technologies to reduce allogeneic blood transfusion in the United States. Transfus Med 2001; 11:79-85.
9. Goodnough LT, Monk TG, Andriole GL. Erythropoietin therapy. N Engl J Med 1997;336:933-8.
10. Goodnough LT, Skikne B, Brugnara C. Erythropoietin, iron, and erythropoiesis. Blood 2000;96:823-33.
11. Goodnough LT, Verbrugge D, Marcus RE, Goldberg V. The effect of patient size and dose of recombinant human erythropoietin therapy on red blood cell expansion. J Am Coll Surg 1994;179:171-6.
12. Goodnough LT, Price TH, Parvin CA. The endogenous erythropoietin response and the erythropoietic response to blood loss anemia: The effects of age and gender. J Lab Clin Med 1995;126:57-64.

13. Goodnough LT, Marcus RE. Erythropoiesis in patients stimulated with erythropoietin: The relevance of storage iron. Vox Sang 1998;75:128-33.

14. Goodnough LT, Price TH, Parvin CA, et al. Erythropoietin response to anaemia is not altered by surgery or recombinant human erythropoietin therapy. Br J Haematol 1994;87:695-9.

15. Goodnough LT, Brittenham G. Limitations of the erythropoietic response to serial phlebotomy: Implications for autologous blood donor programs. J Lab Clin Med 1990;115:28-35.

16. Goodnough LT, Price TH, Rudnick S, Soegiarso RW. Preoperative red blood cell production in patients undergoing aggressive autologous blood phlebotomy with and without erythropoietin therapy. Transfusion 1992;32:441-5.

17. Coleman PH, Stevens AR, Dodge HT, Finch CA. Rate of blood regeneration after blood loss. Arch Intern Med 1953;92:341-8.

18. Crosby WH. Treatment of hemochromatosis by energetic phlebotomy. One patient's response to getting 55 liters of blood in 11 months. Br J Haematol 1958;4:82-8.

19. Goodnough LT, Merkel K. The use of parenteral iron and recombinant human erythropoietin therapy to stimulate erythropoiesis in patients undergoing repair of hip fracture. Int J Hematol 1996;1:163-6.

20. Finch CA. Erythropoiesis, erythropoietin, and iron. Blood 1982;60:1241-6.

21. Muirhead M, Bargman J, Burgess E, et al. Evidence-based recommendations for the clinical use of recombinant human erythropoietin. Am J Kidney Dis 1995;26:S1.

22. Kaisi M, Ngwalle EWK, Runyoro DE, Rogers J. Evaluation and tolerance of response to iron dextran (Imferon) administered by total dose infusion to pregnant women with iron deficiency anemia. Int J Gynaecol Obstet 1988;26:235-43.

23. Mays T, Mays T. Intravenous iron dextran therapy in the treatment of anemia occurring in surgical, gynecologic, and obstetric patients. Surg Gynecol Obstet 1976;143:381-4.

24. Auerbach M, Ballard H, Glaspy J. Clinical update: Intravenous iron for anaemia. Lancet 2007;369:1502-4.

25. Fishbane S, Ungureanu VD, Maeska JK, et al. The safety of intravenous iron dextran in hemodialysis patients. Am J Kidney Dis 1996;28:529-34.

26. Auerbach M, Winchester J, Wahab A, et al. A randomized trial of three iron dextran infusion methods for anemia in EPO-treated dialysis patients. Am J Kidney Dis 1998;31:81-6.

27. Faich G, Strobos J. Sodium ferric gluconate complex in sucrose: safer intravenous iron therapy than iron dextran. Am J Kidney Dis 1999;33:464-7.

28. Sunder-Plassmann G, Horl WH. Safety aspects of parenteral iron in patients with end stage renal disease. Drug Saf 1997;17:241-50.

29. Silverberg DS, Blum M, Peer G, et al. Intravenous ferric saccharate as an iron supplementation in dialysis patients. Nephron 1996;72:413-17.

30. Sunder-Plassmann G, Horl WH. Importance of iron supply for erythropoietin therapy. Nephrol Dial Transplant 1995;10:2070-6.

31. Nissenson AR, Lindsay RM, Swan S, et al. Sodium ferric gluconate complex in sucrose is safe and effective in hemodialysis patients: North American Trial. Am J Kidney Dis 1999;33:471-82.

32. Calvar C, Mata D, Alonso C, et al. Intravenous administration of iron gluconate during haemodialysis. Nephrol Dial Transplant 1997;12:574-5.

33. Zanen AL, Adriaansen HJ, Van Bommel EFH, et al. "Oversaturation" of transferrin after intravenous ferric gluconate (Ferrlecit) in haemodialysis patients. Nephrol Dial Transplant 1996;11:820-4.

34. Seligman PA, Schleicher RB. Comparison of methods used to measure serum iron in the presence of iron gluconate or iron dextran. Clin Chem 1999;45:898-901.

35. Pascual J, Teruel JL, Liano F, et al. Serious adverse reactions after intravenous ferric gluconate. Nephrol Dial Transplant 1992;7:271-2.

36. Hillman RS, Henderson PA. Control of marrow production by the level of iron supply. J Clin Invest 1969;48:454-60.

37. Henderson PA, Hillman RS. Characteristics of iron dextran utilization in man. Blood 1969;34:357-75.

38. Auerbach M, Picard M, Goodnough LT, Manaitas A. The role of intravenous iron in anemia management and transfusion avoidance. Transfusion 2008 (in press).

39. Russell MW, Jobes D. What should we do with aspirin, NSAIDs, and glycoprotein-receptor inhibitors? Int Anesthesiol Clin 2002;40:63-76.

40. Volkman J, Moore J, Schupp K, Ross M. Guidelines for perioperative use of "blood thinners." P&T News, February/March 2002. [Available at http://www.healthcare.uiowa.edu/pharmacy/PTNews/2002/0203PTNews.html (accessed December 16, 2007).]

41. Romsing J, Walther-Larsen S. Peri-operative use of nonsteroidal anti-inflammatory drugs in children: Analgesic efficacy and bleeding. Anaesthesia 1997;52:673-83.

42. Souter AJ, Fredman B, White PF. Controversies in the perioperative use of nonsteroidal antiinflammatory drugs. Anesth Analg 1994;79:1178-90.

43. Strom BL, Berlin JA, Kinman JL, et al. Parenteral ketorolac and risk of gastrointestinal and operative site bleeding. A postmarketing surveillance study. JAMA 1996;275:376-82.

44. Schroeder WS, Gandhi PJ. Emergency management of hemorrhagic complications in the era of glycoprotein IIb/IIIa receptor antagonists, clopidogrel, low molecular weight heparin, and third-generation fibrinolytic agents. Curr Cardiol Rep 2003;5:310-17.

45. Schror K, Weber AA. Comparative pharmacology of GP IIb/IIIa antagonists. J Thromb Thrombolysis 2003;15:71-80.

46. Abrams CS, Cines DB. Thrombocytopenia after treatment with platelet glycoprotein IIb/IIIa inhibitors. Curr Hematol Rep 2004;3:143-7.

47. Renda G, Rocca B, Crocchiolo R, et al. Effect of fibrinogen concentration and platelet count on the inhibitory effect of abciximab and tirofiban. Thromb Haemost 2003;89:348-54.

48. Li YF, Spencer FA, Becker RC. Comparative efficacy of fibrinogen and platelet supplementation on the in vitro reversibility of competitive glycoprotein IIb/IIIa receptor-directed platelet inhibition. Am Heart J 2002;143:725-32.

49. Deveras RA, Kessler CM. Reversal of warfarin-induced excessive anticoagulation with recombinant human factor VIIa concentrate. Ann Intern Med 2002;137:884-8.

50. Warkentin TE, Crowther MA. Reversing anticoagulants both old and new. Can J Anaesth 2002;49:S11-25.

51. Palareti G, Leali N, Coccheri S, et al. Bleeding complications of oral anticoagulant treatment: An inception-cohort, prospective collaborative study (ISCOAT). Italian Study on Complications of Oral Anticoagulant Therapy. Lancet 1996; 348:423-8.

52. Goodnough LT, Lublin DM, Zhang L, et al. Transfusion medicine service policies for recombinant factor VIIa administration. Transfusion 2004;44:1325-31.

53. Wang SM, Caldwell-Andrews AA, Kain ZN. The use of complementary and alternative medicines by surgical patients: A follow-up survey study. Anesth Analg 2003;97:1010-15, table of contents.

54. Kaye AD, Clarke RC, Sabar R, et al. Herbal medicines: Current trends in anesthesiology practice—a hospital survey. J Clin Anesth 2000;12:468-71.

55. Cheng B, Hung CT, Chiu W. Herbal medicine and anaesthesia. Hong Kong Med J 2002;8:123-30.

56. Tsen LC, Segal S, Pothier M, Bader AM. Alternative medicine use in presurgical patients. Anesthesiology 2000;93:148-51.

57. Ang-Lee MK, Moss J, Yuan CS. Herbal medicines and perioperative care. JAMA 2001;286:208-16.

58. German K, Kumar U, Blackford HN. Garlic and the risk of TURP bleeding. Br J Urol 1995;76:518.

59. Rose KD, Croissant PD, Parliament CF, Levin MB. Spontaneous spinal epidural hematoma with associated platelet dysfunction from excessive garlic ingestion: A case report. Neurosurgery 1990;26:880-2.

60. Chung KF, Dent G, McCusker M, et al. Effect of a ginkgolide mixture (BN 52063) in antagonising skin and platelet responses to platelet activating factor in man. Lancet 1987;i:248-51.

61. Rowin J, Lewis SL. Spontaneous bilateral subdural hematomas associated with chronic Ginkgo biloba ingestion. Neurology 1996;46:1775-6.

62. Vale S. Subarachnoid haemorrhage associated with Ginkgo bilobale (letter). Lancet 1998;352:36.

63. Gilbert GJ. Ginkgo biloba (letter). Neurology 1997;48:1137.

64. Matthews MK Jr. Association of Ginkgo biloba with intracerebral hemorrhage. Neurology 1998;50:1933-4.

65. Rosenblatt M, Mindel J. Spontaneous hyphema associated with ingestion of Ginkgo biloba extract (letter). N Engl J Med 1997;336:1108.

66. Fessenden JM, Wittenborn W, Clarke L. Ginkgo biloba: A case report of herbal medicine and bleeding postoperatively from a laparoscopic cholecystectomy. Am Surg 2001;67:33-5.

67. Teng CM, Kuo SC, Ko FN, et al. Antiplatelet actions of panaxynol and ginsenosides isolated from ginseng. Biochim Biophys Acta 1989;990:315-20.

68. Nurtjahja-Tjendraputra E, Ammit AJ, Roufogalis BD, et al. Effective anti-platelet and COX-1 enzyme inhibitors from pungent constituents of ginger. Thromb Res 2003;111:259-65.

69. Kruth P, Brosi E, Fux R, et al. Ginger-associated overanticoagulation by phenprocoumon. Ann Pharmacother 2004;38:257-60.

70. Fausett B, Silver RM. Congenital disorders of platelet function. Clin Obstet Gynecol 1999;42:390-405.

71. Finch CN, Miller JL, Lyle VA, Handin RI. Evidence that an abnormality in the glycoprotein Ib alpha gene is not the cause of abnormal platelet function in a family with classic Bernard-Soulier disease. Blood 1990;75:2357-62.

72. Ramasamy I. Inherited bleeding disorders: Disorders of platelet adhesion and aggregation. Crit Rev Oncol Hematol 2004;49:1-35.

73. Greinacher A, Potzsch B, Kiefel V, et al. Evidence that DDAVP transiently improves hemostasis in Bernard-Soulier syndrome independent of von Willebrand-factor. Ann Hematol 1993;67:149-50.

74. Giampietro PF, Adler-Brecher B, Verlander PC, et al. The need for more accurate and timely diagnosis in Fanconi anemia: A report from the International Fanconi Anemia Registry. Pediatrics 1993;91:1116-20.

75. Tischkowitz M, Dokal I. Fanconi anaemia and leukaemia—clinical and molecular aspects. Br J Haematol 2004;126:176-91.

76. Medeiros D, Buchanan GR. Current controversies in the management of idiopathic thrombocytopenic purpura during childhood. Pediatr Clin North Am 1996;43:757-72.

77. Hirayama Y, Kohda K, Andoh M, et al. Syndrome of the sea-blue histiocyte. Intern Med 1996;35:419-21.

78. Sawitsky A, Rosner F, Chodsky S. The sea-blue histiocyte syndrome, a review: Genetic and biochemical studies. Semin Hematol 1972;9:285-97.

79. Lee JW. von Willebrand disease, hemophilia A and B, and other factor deficiencies. Int Anesthesiol Clin 2004;42:59-76.

80. Nichols WC, Ginsburg D. von Willebrand disease. Medicine (Baltimore) 1997; 76:1-20.

81. Lechler E. Use of prothrombin complex concentrates for prophylaxis and treatment of bleeding episodes in patients with hereditary deficiency of prothrombin, Factor VII, Factor X, protein C, protein S, or protein Z. Thromb Res 1999;95(Suppl):S39-50.

82. Preiss DU, Eberspacher B, Abdullah D, Rosner I. Safety of vapour heated prothrombin complex concentrate (PCC) Prothromplex S-TIM 4. Thromb Res 1991;63:651-9.

83. Girolami A, Simioni P, Scarano L, et al. Hemorrhagic and thrombotic disorders due to factor V deficiencies and abnormalities: An updated classification. Blood Rev 1998;12:45-51.

84. VanCott EM, Laposata M. Coagulation. In: Jacobs D, ed. The laboratory test handbook. 5th ed. Cleveland: Lexi-Comp, 2001:327-58.

85. Cohen LJ, McWilliams NB, Neuberg R, et al. Prophylaxis and therapy with factor VII concentrate (human) immuno, vapor heated in patients with congenital factor VII deficiency: A summary of case reports. Am J Hematol 1995;50: 269-76.

86. Jimenez-Yuste V, Villar A, Morado M, et al. Continuous infusion of recombinant activated factor VII during caesarean section delivery in a patient with congenital factor VII deficiency. Haemophilia 2000;6:588-90.

87. Zanon E, Martinelli F, Bacci C, et al. Proposal of a standard approach to dental extraction in haemophilia patients: A case-control study with good results. Haemophilia 2000;6:533-6.

88. Kohler M. Thrombogenicity of prothrombin complex concentrates. Thromb Res 1999;95:S13-7.
89. Kogenate FS antihemophilic factor (recombinant) (package insert). Elkhart, IN: Bayer Health Care, 2002.
90. Scharrer I, Bray GL, Neutzling O. Incidence of inhibitors in haemophilia A patients—a review of recent studies of recombinant and plasma-derived factor VIII concentrates. Haemophilia 1999;5:145-54.
91. Shapiro AD, Di Paola J, Cohen A, et al. The safety and efficacy of recombinant human blood coagulation factor IX in previously untreated patients with severe or moderately severe hemophilia B. Blood 2005;105:518-25.
92. Warrier I, Ewenstein BM, Koerper MA, et al. Factor IX inhibitors and anaphylaxis in hemophilia B. J Pediatr Hematol Oncol 1997;19:23-7.
93. O'Connell NM. Factor XI deficiency. Semin Hematol 2004;41:76-81.
94. Tavori S, Brenner B, Tatarsky I. The effect of combined factor XI deficiency with von Willebrand factor abnormalities on haemorrhagic diathesis. Thromb Haemost 1990;63:36-8.
95. Berliner S, Horowitz I, Martinowitz U, et al. Dental surgery in patients with severe factor XI deficiency without plasma replacement. Blood Coagul Fibrinolysis 1992;3:465-8.
96. Rakocz M, Mazar A, Varon D, et al. Dental extractions in patients with bleeding disorders. The use of fibrin glue. Oral Surg Oral Med Oral Pathol 1993;75: 280-2.
97. Kitchens CS. The contact system. Arch Pathol Lab Med 2002;126:1382-6.
98. Ratnoff OD, Steinberg AG. Inheritance of fibrin-stabilising-factor deficiency. Lancet 1968;i:25-6.
99. Andreae MC, Amanullah A, Jamil S, Main C. Congenital factor XIII deficiency: A patient report and review of the literature. Clin Pediatr (Philadelphia) 1997; 36:53-5.
100. Anwar R, Miloszewski KJ. Factor XIII deficiency. Br J Haematol 1999;107: 468-84.
101. Lim W, Moffat K, Hayward CP. Prophylactic and perioperative replacement therapy for acquired factor XIII deficiency. J Thromb Haemost 2004;2:1017-19.
102. Lovejoy AE, Reynolds TC, Visich JE, et al. Safety and pharmacokinetics of recombinant Factor XIII-A2 administration in patients with congenital Factor XIII deficiency. Blood 2006;108:57-62.

In: Waters JH, ed.
Blood Management: Options for Better Patient Care
Bethesda, MD: AABB Press, 2008

8

Perioperative Blood Sequestration

JONATHAN H. WATERS, MD

TWO METHODS THAT ARE USED AT THE TIME of surgery for the purpose of avoiding allogeneic transfusion are acute normovolemic hemodilution (ANH) and component sequestration. At the beginning of a surgical procedure, whole blood can be removed from a patient, with the volume loss being replenished with crystalloid or colloid fluids.[1,2] The goal of this blood removal is to create a relative anemia in the patient so that blood shed during the operative procedure effectively has a reduced number of red cells in it. Once the threat of blood loss is diminished, the harvested cells are returned to the patient, thus minimizing the loss of blood during the operative procedure. This

Jonathan H. Waters, MD, Chief and Visiting Associate Professor, Department of Anesthesiology, Magee-Womens Hospital, University of Pittsburgh Medical Center, Pittsburgh, Pennsylvania whole blood sequestration is typically termed ANH; it is also termed autologous normovolemic hemodilution or isovolemic hemodilution. Component sequestration also involves the removal of whole blood, but the whole blood is immediately separated into its components so that individual components are selectively readministered as needed.

Acute Normovolemic Hemodilution

Figures 8-1 and 8-2 illustrate how ANH works and its theoretical benefits. The blood savings can be illustrated by a simplified

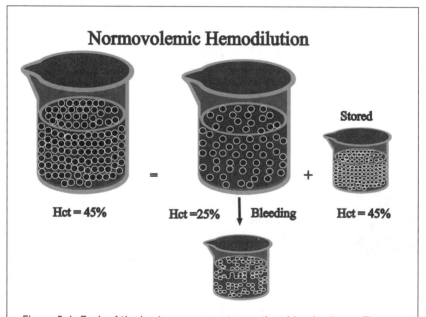

Figure 8-1. Each of the beakers represents a patient blood volume. The circles represent red cells in plasma. The beaker on the far left represents a patient with a concentrated hematocrit of 45%. The middle beaker shows the blood concentration after hemodilution, with the sequestered blood represented by the small beaker to the far right. Blood shed during a surgical procedure is lost at the concentration level of the middle beaker, so that the absolute number of red cells lost is smaller than it would have been without hemodilution. Hct = hematocrit.

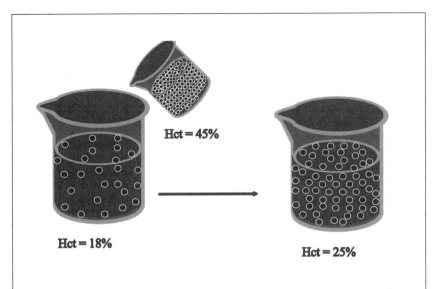

Figure 8-2. At the end of the surgical procedure, the patient has a low hematocrit and is given back the sequestered blood. By doing so, the patient's hematocrit is restored to a satisfactory level.

example. Hypothetically, if a patient were to lose 1000 mL of blood with a hemoglobin (Hb) level of 15 g/dL during a surgical procedure, this would amount to the loss of 150 g of Hb. If the patient were hemodiluted to 8 g/dL of Hb, the same 1000 mL of blood loss would result in 80 g of lost Hb. Thus, a savings of 70 g of Hb is achieved. One must realize that this scenario is idealized because a real patient's Hb will fall with the blood loss and not stay constant, so the actual blood-saving effect is much less than this example.

Physiology

During the hemodilution process, a number of physiologic mechanisms compensate for the drop in circulating red cells. Because this is one of the few areas of medicine where accurate mathematical models are in place, it is useful to discuss the mathematics in conjunction with the compensatory changes that occur during hemodilution.

The decreased number of red cells will decrease oxygen delivery to the various tissue beds. Oxygen delivery (O_2Del) is dependent upon cardiac output (CO) and blood oxygen content (C_aO_2) and may be defined by the following equation:

$$O_2Del = CO \times C_aO_2$$

C_aO_2 is a function of the oxygen saturation (S_aO_2), the hemoglobin concentration (Hb), and the partial pressure of oxygen (pO_2) dissolved in the plasma. It is defined as follows:

$$C_aO_2 = (1.34 \times Hb \times S_aO_2) + 0.003pO_2$$

The factor 1.34 relates to the volume of oxygen that is carried by every gram of Hb. The 0.003 factor is the solubility constant for oxygen in blood at 37 C. From these two equations, it can be seen that a fall in Hb will decrease oxygen content and, in turn, decrease oxygen delivery.

For most individuals, significant physiologic reserve exists to compensate for the declining Hb concentration. This compensation takes place through two primary mechanisms. First, cardiac output increases in order to maintain O_2 delivery. Cardiac output is dependent on heart rate, preload, afterload, and contractility. Increases in cardiac output take place through increases in heart rate[3] and contractility.[4] In addition, blood viscosity is reduced. This lowered viscosity reduces cardiac afterload by decreasing the pressure necessary to drive blood into the circulation. In turn, preload is enhanced by better venous return to the heart.[5] Consequently, hemodilution results in multiple enhancements in cardiac output to maintain oxygen delivery.

The second compensatory mechanism is the effect of enhanced oxygen extraction. Under normal circumstances, the amount of oxygen used at the tissue level is significantly smaller than the oxygen content of the blood being delivered to it. This physiologic reserve is narrowed during hemodilution, and oxygen extraction is enhanced to maintain tissue oxygen needs. As a result, the venous blood exiting the tissue bed has lower oxygen content than it would under normal circumstances.

The oxygen content equation shows that enhanced oxygen delivery can be achieved by increasing the concentration of oxygen being administered to the patient. This results in a larger pO_2 and enhances the contribution that dissolved oxygen makes to the overall content of the blood. (See section on hyperbaric medicine in Chapter 14.)

Increasing heart rate and contractility has the negative consequence of increasing myocardial oxygen utilization. Because the heart has higher oxygen needs than other tissue beds, the reserve for enhanced oxygen extraction is smaller for this organ.[6] The heart is primarily reliant on enhanced coronary blood flow from viscosity change to maintain oxygen delivery. In a patient with normal coronary arteries, the physiologic limit of hemodilution occurs at a Hb level of approximately 4 g/dL.[7] At this point, enhanced blood flow cannot keep up with oxygen needs, and the heart becomes ischemic. For a patient with coronary stenosis, enhanced coronary blood flow can be impeded, resulting in ischemia at higher Hb levels.

Advantages and Disadvantages

The advantages of ANH are as follows: 1) it may reduce the need for allogeneic blood during surgery, 2) no storage injury occurs to the blood, 3) the blood contains viable clotting factors, 4) minimal cost is incurred, and 5) the circuit used for the procedure can be kept in constant contact with the patient, thus making it a viable option for many Jehovah's Witness patients. The most significant disadvantage of ANH is that it is not very effective. It is estimated that the blood savings attributable to ANH amount to 100 to 200 mL, which is hardly enough to significantly reduce allogeneic exposure.[8]

The main value of ANH relates to plasma and platelets. If adequate amounts of whole blood are withdrawn (typically 1 L in an adult), the need for plasma and platelet transfusion during surgery with major blood loss can be significantly reduced.[9,10] The technique also offers some benefits when combined with blood recovery.[11] ANH reduces blood viscosity so that less shear stress is placed on the remaining red cells during the blood recovery suctioning and processing. This reduction may lead to higher blood recovery efficiency rates.

Inclusion and Exclusion Criteria[12]

In general, all patients undergoing surgery when significant (1000 mL) blood loss is anticipated should be considered for ANH. Contraindications to ANH include active ischemic heart disease, hemoglobinopathy, hemorrhagic or septic shock, and known coagulopathy associated with active bleeding or any other circumstance where the blood removal might put the patient at risk.

Calculation of Sequestered Volume

ANH involves a conceptually simple technique. Application of the technique can be marred by technical failures, however. Such failures arise primarily during the blood-drawing process. An inadequate harvest site, poor blood flow, or a failure to adequately anticoagulate the blood can turn this good idea into a bad one.

The first step in the process is to determine how much blood can be safely withdrawn from the patient. The following formula is frequently used:

$$V = EBV \times (H_i - H_f)/H_{av}$$

where
V = volume of blood to be withdrawn.
EBV = patient's estimated blood volume, which is typically 70 mL/kg × patient body weight in kg.
H_i = initial hematocrit before the start of the procedure.

H_f = final hematocrit after hemodilution.

H_{av} = hematocrit average during the hemodilution process.

For example, a 70-kg patient's blood volume would be estimated to be 4900 mL. If the patient had a starting hematocrit of 45% and the target hematocrit is 25%, the average hematocrit during the dilution process is 35% (45% + 25%, divided by two). The equation above may be applied as follows:

$$V = 4900 \text{ mL} \times (45\% - 25\%)/35\% = 2800 \text{ mL}$$

The formula would suggest that a sizeable amount of blood may need to be withdrawn in order to achieve the targeted Hb. Because the formula produces an estimation, it is sound practice to check the hematocrit between each unit collection. For instructions in how to perform ANH, see Appendix 8-1.

Readministration

Readministration of harvested units typically occurs in reverse order, compared with the draw. For instance, if 3 units are harvested, the third unit is given first and the first unit is readministered last. If blood recovery is being used in conjunction with ANH, the blood recovery components should be given first, with the ANH units being given as close to the end of surgery as possible so that clotting factors and platelets are restored when clotting is desired most.

Component Sequestration

The incidence of patients presenting to the operating room with preexisting anemia is high, ranging from 5% to 75% of elective surgical patients.[13,14] Anemia can be a significant obstacle to successful ANH. A small blood volume can also significantly limit the success of this technique. In such situations, the whole blood that is removed can be fractionated using a blood recovery machine. By changing centrifuge speeds on a standard blood recovery machine, high and low centrifugal forces separate the principal blood components (essentially the same process used by the blood bank to fractionate whole blood).

Technique

Component sequestration can take place through a "direct" or "indirect" draw technique. In the indirect technique, units of blood are removed in the same fashion as ANH. Here the blood removal is typically slow and methodical, allowing for adequate maintenance of the circulating blood volume. In a direct draw technique, the blood recovery machine is directly connected to a large-bore intravenous catheter, typically placed in the internal jugular vein. The draw speed can be varied but typically occurs at 100 mL/min. At this speed, significant hypovolemia can occur rapidly; thus careful hemodynamic monitoring is required. In addition, close observation of anticoagulation is imperative during the blood removal.

With component sequestration, varying amounts of red cells and plasma may be withheld or immediately reinfused in order to maintain blood volume or Hb level.[15] For an individual with a normal hematocrit and platelet count, fractionation will allow for generation of 3 to 4 units of red cells, 6 units of fresh plasma, and 4 to 6 units of concentrated platelets. To produce these components requires approximately 45 minutes; however, this processing can take place during the initial stages of the surgical procedure. With the generation of components instead of whole blood, specific patient needs can be addressed without sacrificing other components. If the patient is anemic, red cells are given. If the patient is not clotting, plasma and platelets are given.

Despite the logic of component sequestration, debate has arisen around the efficacy of the technique. Literature review shows variable success with the technique. However if evaluated closely, the studies that show minimal patient benefit are flawed by low yields of platelets and plasma. Yields for sequestered platelets and plasma must reach minimum therapeutic quantities recommended for any coagulopathy. Table 8-1 summarizes these studies of component sequestration. These studies show that a minimum of 0.5 units/kg of platelets and 10 mL/kg of plasma need to be harvested to avoid allogeneic transfusion. The standard recommendation for dosing of allogeneic platelets or plasma to correct a coagulation problem is 1 unit per 10 kg of platelets and 15 mL/kg of plasma. Therefore, it would seem logical that, when sequestering components, sim-

Table 8-1. Studies Comparing Yields from Plasmapheresis

| | | Platelet Yield | |
| | | | |
Author	Outcome	Units	Kg/Unit
Noon[16]	+	9.8	7
Davies[17]	+	7.0	11
Harke[18]	+	5.0	13
Jones[19]	+	5.0	14
Boldt[20]	+	4.8	16
Boldt[21]	+	3.9	20
Tobe[22]	−	3.6	29
Giordano[23,24]	+	3.0	23
Ferrari[25]	+ / −	2.9	28
Triulzi[26]	−	2.8	30
Ereth[27]	−	2.7	29
Wong[28]	−	2.5	33

+ = the study found that significant allogeneic avoidance occurred; − = the study found that no significant allogeneic avoidance occurred.

ilar amounts of autologous blood should be retained for clotting restoration.

Advantages and Disadvantages

The primary advantage of component sequestration is that the process can take place in patients who have a small body habitus or who present with an anemia where whole blood sequestration would be limited.

Disadvantages of component sequestration are that processing is time consuming and requires a technician with a high level of understanding of blood recovery equipment. The complexity of component sequestration is significantly greater than ANH or blood recovery. If a direct draw technique is being used, anticoagulation needs to be closely monitored. At high rates of blood removal, small errors in administration of anticoagulant can have significant patient consequences resulting from clotted, sequestered blood. In addition, monitoring of the processing requires considerable vigilance to manage the direction of blood flow. The processing bowl can explode if the clamps directing fluid flow are misdirected. Because of this complexity, the personnel involved should be experienced and familiar with their equipment.

Inclusion and Exclusion Criteria

Component sequestration may not be cost-effective unless appropriate patients are selected. Multilevel spine fusion and instrumentation, liver transplantation, open thoracoabdominal aneurysm repair, renal tumors enveloping the major vessels, and pediatric heart transplants are some of the cases where this technique might be useful. In Jehovah's Witnesses where blood loss is expected but no margin for error exists, consideration should be given to component sequestration. Because of the large volume shifts that occur during this process, hemodynamically unstable patients should be excluded from this process.

Readministration

When harvesting platelets, it is important to understand that the platelets should be reserved until the end of the surgical dissection. In heparinized patients, it is imperative that the platelets not be administered until protamine administration is complete and neutralization of heparin is confirmed. Protamine is a potent platelet antagonist, and exposure of the carefully preserved platelets to either heparin or protamine should not occur.

References

1. Ereth M, Oliver W, Santrach P. Subspecialty clinics: Perioperative interventions to decrease transfusion of allogeneic blood products. Mayo Clin Proc 1994; 69:575-86.
2. Olsfanger D, Fredman B, Goldstein B, et al. Acute normovolemic hemodilution decreases postoperative allogeneic blood transfusion after total knee replacement. Br J Anaesth 1997;79:317-21.
3. Weiskopf RB, Feiner J, Hopf H, et al. Heart rate increases linearly in response to acute isovolemic anemia. Transfusion 2003;43:235-40.
4. Habler OP, Kleen MS, Podtschaske AH, et al. The effect of acute normovolemic hemodilution (ANH) on myocardial contractility in anesthetized dogs. Anesth Analg 1996;83:451-8.
5. Monk TG. Acute normovolemic hemodilution. Anesthesiol Clin North America 2005;23:271-81.
6. Jan KM, Chien S. Effect of hematocrit variations on coronary hemodynamics and oxygen utilization. Am J Physiol 1977;233:H106-13.
7. Van der Linden P, De Hert S. Normovolemic hemodilution and the heart. Can J Anaesth 2005;52:130-2.
8. Goodnough LT, Grishaber JE, Monk TG, Catalona WJ. Acute preoperative hemodilution in patients undergoing radical prostatectomy: A case study analysis of efficacy. Anesth Analg 1994;78:932-7.
9. Friesen RH, Perryman KM, Weigers KR, et al. A trial of fresh autologous whole blood to treat dilutional coagulopathy following cardiopulmonary bypass in infants. Paediatr Anaesth 2006;16:429-35.
10. Milam JD, Austin SF, Nihill MR, et al. Use of sufficient hemodilution to prevent coagulopathies following surgical correction of cyanotic heart disease. J Thorac Cardiovasc Surg 1985;89:623-9.
11. Waters JH, Shin Jung Lee J, Karafa MT. A mathematical model of cell salvage compared and combined with normovolemic hemodilution. Transfusion 2004; 44:1412-16.
12. Shander A, Rijhwani TS. Acute normovolemic hemodilution. Transfusion 2004; 44(Dec Suppl):26S-34S.

13. Shander A, Knight K, Thurer R, et al. Prevalence and outcomes of anemia in surgery: A systematic review of the literature. Am J Med 2004;116(Suppl 7A): 58S-69S.

14. Bierbaum BE, Callaghan JJ, Galante JO, et al. An analysis of blood management in patients having a total hip or knee arthroplasty. J Bone Joint Surg Am 1999;81:2-10.

15. Christenson JT, Relise J, Badel P, et al. Platelet pheresis before redo CABG diminishes excessive blood transfusion. Ann Thorac Surg 1996;62:1373-9.

16. Noon GP, Jones J, Fehir, Yawn DH. Use of pre-operatively obtained platelets and plasma in patients undergoing cardiopulmonary bypass. J Clin Apher 1990;5:91-6.

17. Davies GG, Wells DG, Mabee TM, et al. Platelet-leukocyte plasmapheresis attenuates the deleterious effects of cardiopulmonary bypass. Ann Thorac Surg 1992;53:274-7.

18. Harke H, Tanger D, Furst-Denzer S, et al. [Effect of a preoperative separation of platelets on the postoperative blood loss subsequent to extracorporeal circulation in open heart surgery] (author's translation; article in German). Anaesthesist 1977;26:64-71.

19. Jones JW, McCoy TA, Rawitscher RE. Lindsley DA. Effects of intraoperative plasmapheresis on blood loss in cardiac surgery. Ann Thorac Surg 1990;49: 585-9.

20. Boldt J, von Bormann B, Kling D, et al. Preoperative plasmapheresis in patients undergoing cardiac surgery procedures. Anesthesiol 1990;72:282-8.

21. Boldt J, Zickmann B, Ballesteros M, et al. Influence of acute preoperative plasmapheresis on platelet function in cardiac surgery. J Cardiothorac Vasc Anesth 1993;7:4-9.

22. Tobe CE, Vocelka C, Sepulvada R, et al. Infusion of autologous platelet rich plasma does not reduce blood loss and product use after coronary artery bypass: A prospective, randomized, blinded study. J Thorac Cardiovasc Surg 1993; 105:1007-13.

23. Giordano GF Sr, Giordano GF Jr, Rivers SL, et al. Determinants of homologous blood usage utilizing autologous platelet-rich plasma in cardiac operations. Ann Thorac Surg 1989;47:897-902.

24. Giordano GF, Rivers SL, Chung GK, et al. Autologous platelet-rich plasma in cardiac surgery: Effect on intraoperative and postoperative transfusion requirements. Ann Thorac Surg 1988;46:416-19.

25. Ferrari M, Zia S, Valbonesi M, et al. A new technique for hemodilution, preparation of autologous platelet-rich plasma and intraoperative blood salvage in cardiac surgery. Int J Artif Organs 1987;10:47-50.

26. Triulzi DJ, Gilmor GD, Ness PM, et al. Efficacy of autologous fresh whole blood or platelet-rich plasma in adult cardiac surgery. Transfusion 1995;35:627-34.

27. Ereth MH, Oliver WC Jr, Beynen FM, et al. Autologous platelet-rich plasma does not reduce transfusion of homologous blood products in patients undergoing repeat valvular surgery. Anesthesiology 1993;79:540-7.

28. Wong CA, Franklin ML, Wade LD. Coagulation tests, blood loss, and transfusion requirements in platelet-rich plasmapheresed versus nonpheresed cardiac surgery patients. Anesth Analg 1994;78:29-36.

Appendix 8-1. How to Perform ANH

In general, 2 to 4 units of autologous whole blood are collected. Single-draw citrate-phosphate-dextrose-adenine-1 (CPDA-1) blood bags are used, and collection procedures follow the AABB and Food and Drug Administration guidelines for sterility and transfusion.[1-3] Under most circumstances, phlebotomy is the responsibility of the anesthesia personnel. Optimally, phlebotomy should proceed through a peripheral vein. However, in the presence of central venous or peripheral arterial access, blood may be removed through these routes as long as sterility is maintained. In general, flow through a multilumen central-line catheter will be inadequate, but a large-bore, single-lumen catheter will provide optimal phlebotomy conditions. Likewise, arterial line use will be optimal when the harvest site is at the end of the arterial catheter. If the connection is placed at the end of the arterial-line-monitoring tubing, inadequate flow will frequently result. Also, long, small-diameter tubing will impede successful blood harvesting.

When a peripheral vein is used, it is important to select a large, firmly attached vein in an area free of skin lesions. If multiple units of blood are to be withdrawn from a peripheral vein, a large-bore (14-16 gauge) intravenous line can be placed with a heplock for repeated access. A blood pressure cuff is used to make the veins more prominent. For best results, it should be inflated to 50 to 60 mm Hg, which is a level adequate to obstruct venous return but not high enough to impede arterial flow. Following is a list of general instructions for performing ANH:

1. Before phlebotomy, label the blood bag with a biohazard label, patient name, patient identification number, date and time of phlebotomy, 8-hour expiration time (24 hours if stored within 8 hours of collection at 1-6 C), and order of draw (if more than 1 unit is involved).
2. Prepare a sterile area at least 1½ inches in all directions from the intended site of venipuncture.
3. When phlebotomy is through a central venous or arterial line, apply the standard prep method to the heplock adapter.

4. Position the CPDA-1 bag on a scale. Tare the scale to zero with an empty blood bag before use.

5. Clamp the donor tubing just above the needle with a hemostat. Uncover the sterile needle, immediately perform the venipuncture, and release the hemostat. Make sure that the tubing is full of the anticoagulant so that blood clotting is inhibited at an early stage of harvesting. Tape the needle hub and tubing to hold the needle in place. Cover the site with a sterile gauze pad.

6. Check the blood flow periodically to ensure a 30 mL/minute flow rate. If this flow rate cannot be attained or if less than 300 mL of whole blood is collected, the unit should be discarded or transferred to a blood recovery reservoir. Slower flow rates will lead to blood clotting.

7. Stop the blood flow when approximately 450 mL of blood has been collected. A standard collection bag has a prescribed volume of anticoagulant calculated to anticoagulate 450 mL of blood (acceptable range = 415-508 g anticoagulant).

8. Deflate and remove the blood pressure cuff. Remove the needle from the arm. Apply pressure. Seal the tubing 4 to 5 inches from the needle by using a metal clip.

When multiple units of blood are drawn, it is important that the anesthesia personnel administer hetastarch or other volume expanders to the patient following removal of each unit in a volume equal to the volume of blood removed. Multiple units may be drawn until the patient's hematocrit is approximately 28% or until the anesthesia staff orders the procedure to be discontinued. The cutoff of 28% is a point of controversy, but decisions about cutoffs should depend on patient factors such as age and coexisting disease, including coronary artery disease and chronic obstructive pulmonary disease.

References

1. Brecher ME, ed. Technical manual. 15th ed. Bethesda, MD: AABB, 2005:126-30.

2. Price TH. Standards for blood banks and transfusion services. 25th ed. Bethesda, MD: AABB, 2008:22.
3. Ilstrup S, ed. Standards for perioperative autologous blood collection and administration. 3rd ed. Bethesda, MD: AABB, 2007:14-15.

In: Waters JH, ed.
Blood Management: Options for Better Patient Care
Bethesda, MD: AABB Press, 2008

9

Intraoperative Blood Recovery

GARY D. REEDER, CP, AND
JONATHAN H. WATERS, MD

THE PROCESS OF COLLECTING SHED BLOOD and readministering it is termed blood recovery (or cell salvage). This chapter addresses the process of intraoperative recovery of washed blood. If the technique is used appropriately, several blood volumes of red cells can be recovered and readministered. To properly perform intraoperative blood recovery and return a safe product to the patient, professionals need a sound understanding of the components of the system and how they work.

Gary D. Reeder, CP, President, Hema Rx Corporation, Broomfield, Colorado, and Jonathan H. Waters, MD, Chief and Visiting Associate Professor, Department of Anesthesiology, Magee-Womens Hospital, University of Pittsburgh Medical Center, Pittsburgh, Pennsylvania
Work performed at the Department of Anesthesiology, University of Pittsburgh Medical Center, and at Hema Rx Corporation.

Collection System

The blood recovery system can generally be broken into a collection component and a processing component (see Figs 9-1 and 9-2). Four subcomponents make up the collection system: suction, an anticoagulant, a suction line and suction tip, and the collection reservoir. Recovery of erythrocytes begins with aspiration of blood from the surgical wound or a surgical drain. Suction takes place through a suction tip into a double-lumen suction line (see Fig 9-2). At the suction tip, shed cells are mixed with an anticoagulant. The cells are then stored in a collection reservoir to await processing.

Suction

How the suction pressure is applied changes the shear forces applied to the red cells. In general, turbulence destroys red cells. Shear forces occur anytime a fluid moves in contact with a solid surface.[1] Shear-induced hemolysis can be produced with high-suction pressures. Therefore, the lowest-tolerable suction pressure should be applied when blood is sucked from the surgical field.

In addition to shear-induced hemolysis, subhemolytic trauma can occur, significantly shortening a red cell's life span following reinfusion. To avoid hemolytic and subhemolytic stress, vacuum pressure should be regulated to 80 to 120 torr, which is adequate for most surgical procedures.[2,3] The vacuum level can be temporarily raised to clear the field in the event of massive blood loss, then reduced to a lower level. It is important to remember that if multiple suction lines are attached to a collection reservoir, both lines need to be used simultaneously. Otherwise, when one suction line is placed in blood and a separate line is sitting on top of the patient, suction pressure will be halved.

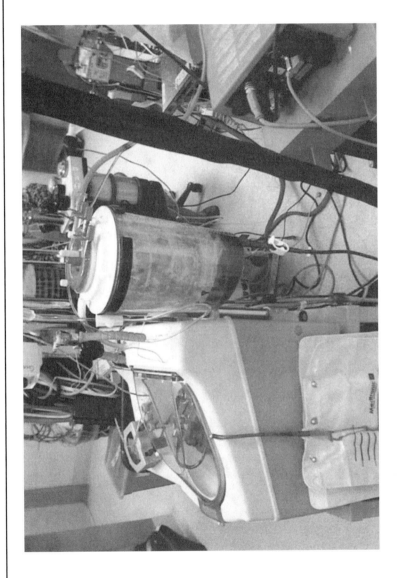

Figure 9-1. Collection component of a blood recovery system.

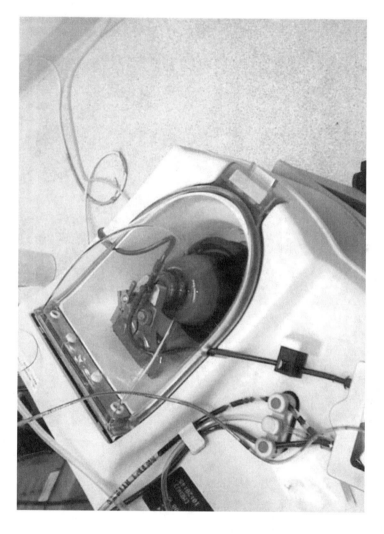

Figure 9-2. Processing component of a blood recovery system.

Suction Tip

Suction-tip style and the method of use can also affect the degree of turbulence and red cell recovery rates. Fine tips create high-shear stress, which can lyse cells during collection. Suction tips should be immersed in the shed blood during collection and should not be dipped in and out. Entrainment of air causes formation and breakage of bubbles, in turn causing cellular destruction. Whenever possible, shed blood should be aspirated immediately and should not be allowed to pool in contact with the wound surface. Prolonging contact time exponentially activates the coagulation system and results in higher loss of otherwise viable cells. Occasional irrigation of the wound with anticoagulant solution will help prevent loss of salvageable blood caused by clot formation.

Gauze pads that have absorbed blood should be soaked in a basin of saline on the sterile field and wrung out before they are discarded. That practice provides a surprisingly rich source of lost blood. It has been estimated that each $18'' \times 18''$ lap sponge can contain up to 100 mL of red cells.

Anticoagulant

The purpose of anticoagulants in blood recovery is to prevent clot formation in the collection reservoir or processing system. Clotting of blood in the collection system will result in loss of otherwise recoverable blood as well as in the need for reservoir and bowl replacement when large clots obstruct blood flow through the system. Either citrate or heparin can be used for anticoagulation during blood recovery. Because of its low cost and ready availability, heparin is most commonly used. Added to a carrier such as normal saline at a dosage of 30,000 units/L of heparin, the solution is then titrated through the aspiration suction system at a rate of 15 mL per 100 mL of collected blood. Overadministration of heparin during shed blood recovery is of no consequence in a cell-washing system. Adequate washout will remove all but a trace of heparin, with less than 10 units remaining in the final blood product.

Citrate has also been used as an anticoagulant. The administration rate for citrate-bearing anticoagulants (eg, acid-citrate-dextrose, citrate-phosphate-dextrose) is 15 mL per 100 mL of collected blood. On reinfusion, rapid liver metabolism makes citrate toxicity difficult to achieve. In patients with compromised liver function, correction with small doses of calcium provides immediate and nontoxic reversal. At some facilities, 7500 units/L of heparin are mixed in a liter of the citrate solution. That solution has been noted to eliminate the commonly observed protein deposits on the interior surface of the processing bowl.

If a leukocyte reduction filter is to be used during blood recovery processing, some thought might be given to the use of heparin rather than citrate. The degree of deformability of leukocytes is reduced in the presence of calcium.[4] If a leukocyte reduction filter is being used to remove bacteria, cancer cells, or amniotic fluid contaminants, the decreased deformability might also affect the contaminants. A decrease in the deformability of these leukocytes may enhance the filter's ability to remove them. Further research is needed in this area.

The low-grade coagulopathy commonly encountered after processing several blood recovery bowls is often attributed, albeit erroneously, to reinfusion of heparin with the packed cells. This coagulopathy rarely occurs with skilled and conscientious operators, however. Loss of platelets and coagulation proteins into the wound and their replacement by crystalloid and colloid solutions lead to a dilutional coagulopathy, requiring treatment with Fresh Frozen Plasma and platelets. Another common source of coagulopathy is the "cell salvage syndrome," which is discussed later in the section titled "Complications of Blood Recovery."

Collection Reservoir

The reservoir is the collection site for blood as it awaits processing. In general, the minimum amount of blood that is needed in the reservoir to fill the processing bowl is equal to three times the size of the bowl. The final product is concentrated into hemoglobin levels that range from 15 to 25 g/dL, depending on the type of machine used. Because blood is lost at hemoglobin levels much lower than those in the desired range, there needs to be enough red cell mass to result in a final hemoglobin level of 15 to 25 g/dL. In addition, some blood is destroyed during processing. Thus, a volume of blood approximately three times the bowl size is needed to process a complete bowl.

The collection reservoirs are generally available with filter sizes ranging from 40 to 120 microns. It is wise to avoid the smaller filters because smaller amounts of residual clot will prevent blood flow through the filter. When inadequate anticoagulation occurs and a clot forms in the collection reservoir, red cells can be trapped in the clot. These red cells can be retrieved by mechanically agitating the reservoir while simultaneously infusing normal saline into the collection reservoir. That procedure can be performed by using one of the suction lines or by infusing saline directly through ports on the top of the reservoir. Ports are available on some manufacturers' reservoirs, but not on all. Surprisingly, large quantities of red cells can be retrieved through this mechanical agitation.

Processing System

The working component of cell washing devices is the separation chamber, which, in essence, is a centrifuge chamber. That component has evolved over the years. Current separation chambers are the Latham-style bowl (Haemonetics Corp, Braintree, MA; Medtronic, Minneapolis, MN; Sorin/Dideco, a member of Sorin Group, Mirandola, Italy), the Baylor bowl (COBE Cardiovascular, member of Sorin Group, Arvada, CO), the "grenade" bowl (Haemonetics Corp, Braintree, MA; Medtronic, Minneapolis, MN), and the continuous disk (Fresenius Medical Care, Bad Homburg, Germany). Regardless of bowl design, all washing systems process blood components according to basic laws of physics.

Processing starts as blood is pumped from the collection reservoir. It enters the bowl through a central straw and exits from the bottom of the bowl while the centrifuge is spinning. The speed at which blood can be moved into and out of the bowl depends partially on the physical characteristics of the straw. For a given pressure generated by the roller pump, the resistance to flow will depend on the length and radius of the straw. Resistance (R) to flow in a straight, unbranched tube is defined as follows:

$$R = (8 \times \text{length} \times \text{viscosity})/[\pi \times (\text{radius})^4].$$

The radius of the straw in the Baylor bowl is greater than that in the typical Latham bowl. Because of the increased radius, there is decreased resistance to flow, making the Baylor bowl ideal for rapid processing.

As the blood enters the processing bowl, the bowl is spinning rapidly to generate centrifugal force. Centrifugation is the process used to separate or concentrate materials suspended in a liquid medium. Separation of recovered blood components depends on the balance between densities of the various constituents of blood (see Table 9-1), the fluid flow rate, and the centrifugal forces applied in the processing bowl. Centrifugal force is described by

$$F = m \, (v^2/r),$$

where m = mass, v = rotation velocity, r = radius of rotation.

Table 9-1. Densities for the Constituents of Blood

Blood Constituent	Density Range
Plasma	1.025 to 1.029 g/dL
Thrombocytes	1.060 to 1.067 g/dL
Leukocytes	1.065 to 1.090 g/dL
Erythrocytes	1.085 to 1.097 g/dL

As the cell separation bowl spins around a central vertical axis, increasingly higher centrifugal forces (g-forces) are generated radially around the central axis of rotation. The centrifugal force generated by the processor is proportional to the rotation rate of the rotor (in revolutions per minute, or rpm) and the distance between the rotor center and the walls of the bowl. That relationship is graphically depicted in Fig 9-3. From the equation, one also recognizes that the force applied to a particle changes depending on its mass. Because red cells are heavier than other blood elements, they will sediment against the walls of the bowl, with the smaller, lighter particles (plasma) sedimenting closer to the core of the bowl.

As blood is pumped into the bowl, hydrostatic force from the pumping will be exerted on the contents of the bowl. Thus, two forces (hydrostatic and centrifugal) will be applied to the bowl contents. Because the plasma, red cell stroma, and other debris have less mass than the red cells, the centrifugal force applied to them is less. Thus, these lighter particles will preferentially exit the bowl. If blood is pumped at too fast a rate or with too great

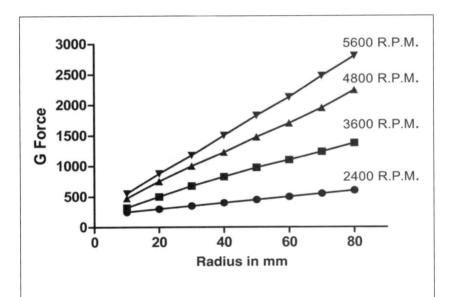

Figure 9-3. G-forces and rpm in a blood recovery processing bowl.

215

a force, the hydrostatic force will overcome the centrifugal force on the red cells and push the cells out of the bowl's top and into the waste bag. Because the hydrostatic force can overcome the centrifugal force when rapid pump speeds are chosen, the bowl pack needs to be observed carefully in order to guarantee that red cells are not being lost during massive blood loss where pumping is rapid.

Concentrating red cells while expressing irrigants and plasma will remove 70% to 90% of the soluble contaminants in recovered blood. However, the most damaging and hazardous contaminants are retained and concentrated in the bowl with the red cells. If reinfused, these contaminants would pose considerable danger to the patient by triggering disseminated intravascular coagulopathy, or what some have labeled the "cell salvage syndrome." These contaminants can be removed with certainty only by cell washing.

Wash solution is introduced into the red cell pack by being pumped through the central straw of the processing bowl. The wash solution is generally normal saline, but one investigator suggests that a more balanced isotonic solution, such as lactated Ringer's solution, may offer slight advantages when compared with normal saline.[5,6] That advantage relates to minimizing the chloride load that would be administered to the patient.

The wash solution percolates through the red cell pack and carries away lighter debris and irregular agglomerates into the wash bag. Washing is considered complete when the effluent line appears clear to the eye and a wash volume of at least three times the bowl volume has been used.

To empty the washed blood, one must reverse the roller pump and aspirate clean, packed red cells from the bowl through the straw and into a holding, or primary reinfusion, bag. Simultaneously, sterile air is drawn from the waste bag back into the bowl. Once the bowl is emptied of blood, another cycle may begin. It is important to move the blood in the holding bag into a transfer bag before readministration. Air will accumulate in the holding bag over time. If blood is administered directly from the holding bag, the patient is placed at risk of air embolism. When a transfer bag is used, blood is moved out of the holding bag, then air is "burped" out of the transfer bag back into the holding bag. Under no circumstances should a pressure cuff be used on the holding bag when blood is being directly reinfused into the patient.

Processing Control

The operator determines collection efficiency and yield of red cells, as well as their cleanliness, through selection of appropriate operational parameters.[7] Not all systems will produce an equivalent product under the same processing conditions, and any given system may perform differently with varying operational parameters.[8,9] The operator's first decision is usually choice of bowl size and is based on anticipated blood loss. Bowls with volumes of 225 to 250 mL are typically used for most cases and require 500 to 750 mL of shed blood, or more, to properly fill. Bowls with volumes of 125 to 135 mL are commonly used for cases of smaller or slower blood loss and require only 250 to 400 mL of shed blood to fill. "Trauma" bowls of about 375 mL are also available for use in high-blood-loss situations, such as trauma or liver surgery. Such bowls require 750 to 1000 mL of shed blood to fill and, therefore, are not applicable to all surgical settings. Selection of fill, wash, and empty flow rates will determine the product's hematocrit, washout efficacy, and residual contaminant level.

Fill Speed

Pump flow rates in modern autotransfusion machines range from 25 to 1500 mL/minute. Operator decisions about the appropriate flow rate for each function and clinical setting should be made to ensure optimal performance. Fill speed directly affects the product's achieved hematocrit in the collection bowl, with slower fill speeds producing higher packed cell densities in the bowl (see Fig 9-4). Faster fill rates produce increased disor-

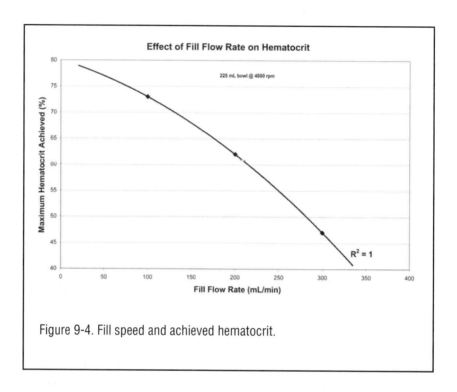

Figure 9-4. Fill speed and achieved hematocrit.

der and lower product hematocrit. The desirable range for bowl hematocrit is 50% to 70%. Hematocrits below or above that range may result in high residual contaminant levels.

Wash Speed and Volume

Wash speed and wash volume also have significant effects on product quality. With the Latham design, wash speeds greater than the fill speed will disrupt the erythrocyte, leading to loss of viable red cells. As seen in Fig 9-5, higher flow rates encourage shunting and incomplete washout, whereas slower flow rates promote a more even distribution of the wash solution through the red cell pack, thereby resulting in a cleaner product for the same total wash volume. In contrast, makers of the BRAT bowl (COBE Cardiovascular), which has more vertical sides, advocate

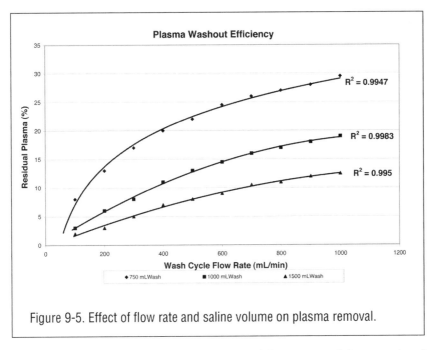

Figure 9-5. Effect of flow rate and saline volume on plasma removal.

using wash flow rates higher than the fill rate to achieve optimal wash efficiency with their system.

Larger wash volumes improve removal of contaminants for all manufacturers' equipment and bowl designs. Under any washing regime, the operator should inspect the effluent line to determine if the volume used has been adequate. The effluent should be clear, without any color or cloudiness, at the end of the wash cycle; if it is not clear, additional washing is indicated.

Speed to Empty

The flow rate to empty the bowl should be set at or below the same rate as the fill cycle. Emptying at a high flow rate risks damaging recovered red cells. In cases where very high hematocrits have been achieved, the empty rate may have to be substantially less than the fill rate to allow for effective recovery from the bowl. An excessive empty rate may cause premature triggering of system air detectors before recovered cells are adequately removed. Although repeat processing does not significantly damage cells, the patient may be denied a timely transfusion of clean red cells.

Partially Filled Bowls

Because the red cell content of recovered blood is seldom known, it is common to process what seems like an adequate amount of collected fluid only to find that not enough recovered blood is present to properly fill the bowl. That situation creates a partial bowl. Partial bowls are difficult or impossible to wash adequately because they allow reinfusion of anticoagulant and other harmful contaminants. Partial bowls produce a very low hematocrit (usually <15%). Transfusion of such clinically insignificant red cell masses with entrained contaminants is rarely indicated.

When partial bowls are encountered, several options are available. If additional blood loss is anticipated, centrifuged cells should be pumped back to the collection reservoir for temporary storage using the "Return" function. With additional shed blood collection, the entire volume can be drawn into the bowl for processing. At the end of a case, washed packed cells in the holding bag can also be returned to fill a partial bowl by using the system's "concentrate" function.

Cell Recovery Efficiency

Mathematical modeling of blood recovery has revealed that small changes in red cell processing efficiency can make large differences in the maximum allowable blood loss that a patient can sustain before allogeneic transfusion therapy becomes necessary.[10] These models suggest that a 70-kg patient with a starting hematocrit of 45% can sustain a blood loss of 9600 mL if a transfusion trigger of 21% is used and if blood recovery captures 60% of lost red cells. The sustainable blood loss rises to 13,750 mL if 70% red cell recovery is achieved. This small change in red cell recovery can have a large effect on the patient's ability to avoid a blood transfusion, which highlights the importance of optimizing the blood recovery system. Figure 9-6 illustrates blood loss calculations.

Patient Factors

Rheologic characteristics of a patient's red cell membrane may make the red cells more or less prone to hemolysis during blood recovery. More hemolysis means fewer red cells to return to the patient. Many factors, including ABO typing, have not been studied, but some work suggests that drug therapy may be used to increase a red cell's ability to sustain hemolytic stress. It is well known that the physical properties of a red cell—such as cell shape, hypotonic lysis resistance, permeability, and cell aggregation—can be altered by the intercalation of amphiphilic molecules into the red cell membrane lipid bilayer.[11] Amphiphilic drugs encompass a variety of therapeutic classes of medications, including antiarrhythmics, antidepressants, neuroleptics, beta-adrenoceptor blocking agents, antihistamines, antimalarial drugs, and anesthetic agents. The rheology of the red cells may also change according to the fluid environment in which they are suspended. The osmotic fragility of erythrocytes can be affected by pH, temperature, and the electrolyte and colloid composition of the suspending medium.[12-15]

In preliminary work performed at the Cleveland Clinic Foundation,[16] an in-vitro model of hemolysis was developed by using a laminar flow chamber. The chamber applies a controlled degree of shear stress onto the red cells. Several different drugs have been tested with this chamber to assess whether they might alter the cells' ability to tolerate shear stress. That work suggests that an anesthetic based on propofol, along with preoperative use of chloroquine, improves red cell recovery. In addition, citrate anticoagulant, compared with heparinized saline, appears to improve red cell recovery. Before widespread application of these findings is undertaken, however, further work needs to be performed in vitro and confirmed in the clinical setting.

$$\text{Blood Loss} = \frac{H_s \times V_b \times N_b}{H_p \times RE}$$

where

H_s = average hematocrit of washed, recovered red cells,
H_p = average patient hematocrit during recycling,
V_b = volume of the processing bowl,
N_b = number of bowls processed, and
RE = estimated recovery efficiency.*

*Recovery efficiencies can vary, depending on vacuum levels, sucker tip size, diligence of recovery efforts, contact time of blood in the wound, and other factors. With good procedural methodology, 80% of lost red cells can be recovered. As the quality of the recovery effort declines, so does efficiency of recovery. Assignment of lower values may be appropriate.

Example 1: During abdominal aortic aneurysm repair, four bowls of 225 mL each were recovered and returned. Low suction levels were used, lap pads (swabs) were washed, and anticoagulation was applied by surgeons to the wound site to prevent clotting. Recovery efficiency was felt to be optimal at about 80%. Measured hematocrit in the washed cells was 61%, 63%, 66%, and 63%, with an average of 63%. Patient hematocrits measured during the respective collection periods were 37%, 33%, 32%, and 30%, averaging 33%. Using these numbers, blood loss was calculated as follows:

$$\text{Blood Loss} = (63\%) \times (225 \text{ mL/bowl}) \times (4 \text{ bowls}) / (33\%) \times (80\%) = 2150 \text{ mL}$$

Example 2: During surgery for a hip revision, blood was fractionated and sequestered, with red cells readministered as needed. Five bowls of 125-mL each were processed. Small suction tips were used with elevated vacuum pressure, and considerable blood was lost to drapes and gauze pads. Recovery efficiency was estimated at 40%. Hematocrit in the bowls was 66%, 70%, 68%, 65%, and 71%, averaging 68%. Concurrent patient values were 32%, 30%, 34%, 30%, and 28%, averaging 30.8%.

$$\text{Blood Loss} = (68\%) \times (125 \text{ mL/bowl}) \times (5 \text{ bowls}) / (30.8\%) \times (40\%) = 3450 \text{ mL}$$

Figure 9-6. Calculation of blood loss derived from recovered blood.

Swab/Sponge Rinsing

Fully soaked gauze pads, lap sponges, or swabs may contain up to 100 mL of blood.[17] Approximately 75% of that blood is retrievable by rinsing the swabs in a basin of isotonic solution (normal saline, Ringer's lactate, Hartmann's solution) and wringing them out before discarding them. The rinse solution is then periodically sucked into the cardiotomy reservoir when the solution appears to be grossly bloody. That practice has been reported to increase red cell retrieval rates by 28%.[18]

Many practitioners are concerned because of the possibility of cotton fibers being entrained into the blood from the sponge or because of the possibility of bacterial contamination being introduced into the system through the sponge. In reviewing unpublished data from the Cleveland Clinic, the authors found that no cotton fibers were retrievable from rinse solutions. The manufacturer, in discussions with the authors, claims that the sponges exhibit no fiber shedding because of the tight weave of the cotton fibers and a double washing process. In addition, macroaggregate filtering at the collection reservoir should remove large particles such as cotton fibers.

Any bacterial contamination that might result from sponge rinsing would come from the surgical wound. Thus, the patient would have already been exposed to the bacteria. It is well documented that blood during recovery is routinely contaminated with bacteria.[19,20] Such contamination has not been correlated with clinical sequelae. If sponges are suspected to be grossly contaminated with bacteria, they should simply be discarded rather than rinsed.

Maximizing Washout Quality

Optimizing the quality of the product readministered to the patient requires as much attention as optimizing the number of red cells returned. The AABB has issued perioperative standards to guide the manufacture of blood recovery products and guidance on how to comply with the standards.[21] Implementation of the standards is necessary if blood recovery is to be performed safely. The primary requirement of the guidelines is that dedicated personnel operate the equipment. Without such dedication, inadequate washing and concentration of the blood being recovered can lead to complications such as disseminated intravascular coagulation or acute renal failure.

Many institutions do not follow the guidelines. Under those circumstances, blood recovery is frequently instituted by the operating room circulating nurse, who has other operating room responsibilities and who frequently has little training in safe blood recovery application. As the surgical procedure proceeds, large quantities of blood will collect in the collection reservoir for blood recovery at the time when the circulating nurse's responsibilities are greatest. Nurses in that situation will process the blood at their convenience, periodically pressing the start button on the blood recovery machine as they pass by while conducting other tasks in the operating room. Thus, no observation takes place regarding the adequacy of processing.

Processing "by convenience" is highlighted by an article on blood recovery from the Cleveland Clinic in an era before dedicated blood recovery personnel existed. O'Hara and colleagues[22] described a lack of red cell avoidance with blood recovery in patients undergoing abdominal aortic aneurysm repair. They reported an average blood recovery unit hematocrit of 31%. Hematocrits of blood that is being recovered should range between 40% and 75%, depending on the method of processing. Lower hematocrits in the recovered unit will hemodilute patients, negating any positive benefit. Furthermore, a lower hematocrit suggests that a partial bowl pack has been washed, thus leaving residual cellular contaminants in the blood that could potentially be harmful to a patient. In the study, the circulating nurse was not observing the equipment, and frequent partial bowls were being washed. That early wash was being triggered by excessive hemolysis in the recovered blood.

The AABB standards, in addition to mandating dedicated personnel for blood recovery equipment, require measurement of the quality and of the concentration of the product produced. Quality indicators are of a controversial nature. Some practitioners advocate periodic albumin washout while others advocate potassium washout. Free hemoglobin has also been advocated. At the Cleveland Clinic, evaluation of the color of the effluent wash solution is used as a measure of the washout quality. That practice stems from a close correlation between the elimination of free hemoglobin and the color of the effluent solution. Many practitioners also periodically measure bacterial contamination. But as previously discussed, bacterial contamination of recovered blood is routine, and little correlation is found with clinical sequelae.

A measurement of concentration is also recommended. Hematocrit or hemoglobin concentration is simply measured and can be performed on all units of blood. Adequate concentration is important to ensure washout of cellular contaminants. Several manufacturers of blood recovery equipment incorporate devices within their systems to measure hematocrit.

Implementation of the AABB standards has significantly reduced plasma and platelet transfusion in surgical procedures where nondedicated nurses were performing blood recovery and were doing so without having measured the quality of the product that they were producing.

Indications for Blood Recovery

In the past, the AABB has recommended the following general indications for blood recovery: 1) the anticipated blood loss is 20% or more of the patient's estimated blood volume, 2) the blood would ordinarily be crossmatched, 3) more than 10% of patients undergoing the procedure require transfusion, and 4) the mean transfusion for the procedure exceeds 1 unit.[23] These recommendations are derived from the comparison of allogeneic blood costs and perceived blood recovery costs. Since these recommendations were developed, the cost of allogeneic blood has escalated while a better understanding has been gained of the costs associated with blood recovery. Therefore, implementation of blood recovery should be considered when much smaller amounts of blood loss are anticipated.

Accurately predicting the probability of significant blood loss and the need for allogeneic transfusion is difficult. Because of the lack of predictability, implementation of blood recovery should start with a collection system that includes a cardiotomy reservoir, a suction line, and an anticoagulant. Such collection or a standby setup is comparable in costs to the reagent costs for typing and crossing 2 units. Hospitals should consider implementation of a standby setup rather than the type and cross, even though that strategy represents a major paradigm shift. In cases where the blood loss is certain, such as in a thoracoabdominal aneurysm repair, it is reasonable to bypass the standby setup and to set up all the components necessary to process blood. Before adoption of such a strategy, it is important to take into account whether the hospital's policy is to contract out the blood recovery or to provide it through an in-house service. It is beyond the scope of this chapter to address all financial permutations of blood recovery services.

Blood recovery might be indicated for many types of cases. Indications for blood recovery should be determined by the institution as well as by the surgeon performing the procedure. The patient's starting hematocrit, gender, age, and body weight can all influence the risk of receiving allogeneic blood.[24] Table 9-2 lists many of the surgical procedures that should be considered before implementation of intraoperative blood recovery.

Contraindications

Possible contraindications to blood recovery are listed in Table 9-3. However, most proposed contraindications are relative rather than absolute, meaning that few data exist to support the dangers associated with them. When a decision is being made whether or not to use blood recovery, it needs to be considered in light of the known risks associated with the alternative therapy—allogeneic blood.

Table 9-2. General Indications for Intraoperative Blood Recovery

Specialty	Surgical Procedure	Comments
Cardiac	Valve replacement Redo bypass grafting Aortic arch aneurysm Coronary artery bypass Cardiac transplant Thoracic trauma	
Orthopedics	Spinal fusion Bilateral knee replacement Laminectomy Revision hip replacement Pelvic fractures Long bone fractures	
Urology	Radical retropubic prostate- ctomy	Individualized by sur- geon
	Cystectomy	Limited to patients with prior radiation ther- apy
	Nephrectomy	When tumor involves major vessels
Neurosurgery	Giant basilar aneurysm	
Obstetrics/ Gynecology	Ectopic pregnancy Hysterectomy	
Vascular	Thoracoabdominal aortic aneurysm repair Aorto-bifemoral grafts Revascularization for femo- ral injuries Liver transplantation	

(Continued)

Table 9-2. General Indications for Intraoperative Blood Recovery (Continued)

Specialty	Surgical Procedure	Comments
	Abdominal aortic aneurysm repair	Should be individualized by surgeon and patient characteristics
Other	Any procedure for a Jehovah's Witness Unexpected massive blood loss Splenectomy	When accepted by patient

Table 9-3. Possible Contraindications to Intraoperative Blood Recovery[25]

Pharmacologic Agents
Clotting agents (Avitene, Surgicel, Gelfoam, etc)
Irrigating solutions (Betadine, antibiotics meant for topical use)
Methylmethacrylate

Contaminants
Bowel contents
Infection
Amniotic fluid

Hematologic Disorders
Sickle cell disease
Thalassemia

Miscellaneous
Catecholamines (pheochromocytoma)
Oxymetazoline (Afrin)

Relative contraindications to blood recovery encompass a wide range of materials that, if incorporated into the recovered blood product, could injure the patient upon readministration. Definite contraindications include anything that results in red cell lysis. In that category are sterile water, hydrogen peroxide, and alcohol. If blood is washed with such solutions or if a hypotonic solution is aspirated into a collection reservoir, red cell hemolysis will occur. Topical additives, including antibiotics, antiseptics, coagulant agents, and various surgical "glues" and polymers, may expose the patient to significant physiologic reactions if they are inadequately removed during cell washing. Table 9-4 identifies some contaminants. In the presence of these contaminants, lysed cells will be washed out if the blood is adequately washed, but it is best to avoid incorporating them into the blood recovery system. Administering blood without adequately washing it could result in renal insufficiency and failure,

Table 9-4. Contaminants Identified in Wound Blood[26-29]

Type of Contaminant	
Solid	**Soluble**
Cells and cellular stroma	Free hemoglobin
Activated leukocytes and platelets	Anticoagulants
Tissue debris	Fats
Implant debris	Fibrin(ogen) split products and D-dimers
Environmental debris	Activated fibrinolytic products (plasmin)
Bacteria	Activated complement ($C3_a$ and $C5_a$)
	Enzymes from cellular disruption
	Endotoxins from bacteria

decreases in hematocrit, elevations in serum lactate dehydrogenase, increases in total serum bilirubin concentration, disseminated intravascular coagulation, and, potentially, death.[30,31]

Many contraindications to blood recovery are not as definitive as those described earlier. That category includes blood aspirated from contaminated or septic wounds, obstetrical procedures, and malignancies. The use of blood recovery in these circumstances is variable from practice to practice, is advocated as safe and effective by some investigators, and is considered dangerous by others. In many circumstances, the physician in charge may make the medical decision to proceed with autotransfusion.

In all circumstances involving possible contamination, blood recovery may be made safer through the use of a double-suction setup. In such a setup, one suction line is connected to the blood recovery reservoir and is used for suctioning of blood, while the other line is connected to the regular wall suction and is used for aspiration of the contaminant.[32-34] The use of separate suction devices minimizes contamination of the blood being recovered. The lesser degree of overall contamination of the recovered red cells results in a lower concentration in the washed product. In general, blood recovery processing is capable of removing significant amounts of these contaminants, but high enough concentrations will overwhelm the system's capabilities. Thus, every effort should be made to minimize the size of the contaminant load.

Bacterial Contamination

In bowel surgery, penetrating trauma to the abdomen, or surgery where an infected wound is involved, shed blood might be contaminated with bacteria. It is thought that readministration of recovered blood in those scenarios could lead to bacteremia or sepsis. No data supporting that concern can be found in the literature, however. The data that can be found suggest that blood recovery in these environments can be performed safely.

Surprisingly, bacterial contamination of recovered blood appears to be routine. Bland et al[35] found that bacterial contamination of recovered blood in cardiac surgery approaches 30% of the units processed and readministered. Kang et al[36] report that 9% of the blood returned to patients undergoing liver transplantation had bacterial contaminants, usually originating from the skin. In these circumstances of bacterial contamination, no clinical sequelae were noted. Contamination from skin flora has been assumed to be inconsequential, but the contaminants of frank stool have been thought to be different. That area has also been investigated primarily in trauma; several authors have reported on frank stool contamination of reinfused, recovered blood, but no increased sepsis rates were noted.[37-39] These studies suggest that blood recovery in the face of bacterial contamination can be performed safely.

The effect of blood recovery processing on blood that has been bacterially contaminated was first investigated by Boudreaux et al[40] who inoculated expired units of blood with bacteria and found that washing was capable of reducing contamination from 5% to 23% of the starting contamination. In a similar study, Waters et al[41] found a reduction of approximately 99% in bacterial contamination when the combination of cell washing and leukocyte reduction filtration was performed. In the same paper, a dose response curve was generated, which showed that a 99% reduction of a starting load of bacteria of 10^7 still left 10^5 bacteria. That level of contamination occurred in surgical procedures where gross fecal contamination of the blood was observed. Differentiating between gross contamination and possible or unobserved contamination is therefore important.

The importance of any remaining bacteria is yet unknown. But bacterial contamination of allogeneic blood, primarily platelets, is of intense interest to the blood-banking community because of the 500 to 750 severe reactions or deaths that occur each year from bacterial contamination of blood products.[42] In a surveillance study by Yomtovian et al,[43] eight bacterially contaminated pools of platelets were administered to patients; five patients had no symptoms, with bacterial loads ranging from 10^2 to 10^{11} cfu/mL, while the others had symptoms, with bacterial loads ranging from 10^6 to 10^8 cfu/mL. That study and others suggest that the type of bacteria is more important than the quantity.[44-46]

During the course of most operations, a bacteremia is present—but it is related to the surgical trauma. Broad-spectrum antibiotics are routinely used to manage routine bacteremia. Several studies have suggested that broad-spectrum antibiotics provide additional safety when contaminated recycled blood is readministered.[47,48]

Dzik and Sherburne,[49] in a review of the controversies surrounding blood recovery, pointed out that allogeneic transfusion leads to an increase in infection rate and that in the face of bacterial contamination of recovered blood, a clinical decision needs to be made as to which therapy offers the least risk to the patient. Known risk exists with allogeneic blood, yet only theoretical risk is associated with recovered blood. Until data are generated supporting the theoretical risk of blood recovery in these circumstances, it seems reasonable to avoid the known risk of allogeneic blood through the use of recovered blood.

Obstetrics

One of the leading causes of death during childbirth is hemorrhage, thus making blood recovery attractive.[50,51] When blood recovery is applied during the peripartum period, shed blood can be contaminated with bacteria, amniotic fluid, and fetal blood. Amniotic fluid contamination is a concern because of the theoretical potential of creating an iatrogenic amniotic fluid embolus. But because amniotic fluid emboli rarely occur (1:8000 to 1:30,000 deliveries), definitive study is impossible. Thus, surrogate markers are sought that might be associated with the syndrome.

Tissue factor is thought to be involved in the disseminated intravascular coagulopathy that typically follows the acute embolic event.[52] Bernstein et al[53] evaluated the washout of tissue factor and found that routine washing eliminated all tissue factor activity. Unfortunately, tissue factor may be only one of many components that lead to the syndrome of amniotic fluid embolism; thus, washing of the tissue factor would not guarantee that amniotic fluid embolism would not occur.[54,55] Several studies assessing the removal of free hemoglobin, bromcresol green dye, and heparin from recovered blood suggest that if one factor is effectively removed, then the other factors are equally removed.[56,57] Those studies would suggest that, if the tissue factor is effectively removed from blood contaminated with amniotic fluid, the other components of amniotic fluid would also be removed or significantly reduced in concentration.

Some investigators feel that particulate contaminants are responsible for amniotic fluid embolization.[58,59] Durand et al[60] showed that cell washing did not remove fetal squamous cells. Waters et al[61] demonstrated that leukocyte reduction filters along with cell washing will remove fetal squamous cells to an extent comparable to the concentration of the cells in a maternal blood sample following placental separation. From that study, it was concluded that the combination of blood recovery washing and filtration produces a blood product comparable to circulating maternal blood, with the exception of fetal hemoglobin contamination.

Isoimmunization can occur from exposure to fetal hemoglobin, leading to erythroblastosis in subsequent pregnancies. ABO incompatibility tends to be a minor problem when compared with Rh incompatibility. To prevent isoimmunization, calculation of Rh Immune Globulin and administration to the mother should occur after recovered blood has been administered so that the dose is adequate to neutralize these additional cells.

Support for the use of blood recovery in obstetric hemorrhage now encompasses 390 reported cases where blood contaminated with amniotic fluid has been washed and readministered without filtration.[62-64]

Malignancy

The last area of controversy is blood recovery in cancer surgery. As mentioned earlier, immunomodulation occurs with allogeneic transfusion. The issue of whether immunomodulation affects tumor growth is unresolved; however, there is evidence to suggest outcome is worse for patients undergoing cancer surgery when they receive allogeneic blood.[65-67] Thus, avoidance of allogeneic blood is important. Likewise, administration of tumor-laden blood from a recovery process would seem to be contradictory to a good outcome for a patient. However, during tumor surgery, hematogenous dissemination of cancer cells is common.[68-70] In fact, it has been demonstrated that a high percentage of patients presenting for cancer surgery have circulating tumor cells, but this presence appears to have no correlation with patient survival.[71] It has been estimated that only 0.01% to 0.000001% of circulating tumor cells have the potential to form metastatic lesions.[72] So, the importance of administration of tumor cells through recovered blood must be questioned.

With this understanding, the use of leukocyte reduction filters is advocated for removal of tumor cells during cancer surgery. Such filters have been used for filtration of malignancy in the clinical settings (blood recovery during urologic surgery[73,74] and pulmonary surgery,[75] and the research setting in a variety of cell lines that were used to contaminate discarded blood[76,77]). These studies have all concluded that leukocyte reduction filters were highly effective at removing tumor cell contamination.

Blood recovery during tumor surgery has been studied in hepatic resection for malignancy and urologic oncology.[78-80] In these uncontrolled studies, actual outcome was compared with expected outcome. No increases in metastasis or death were seen, thus suggesting that diffuse cancer metastasis does not occur following blood recovery use. In those studies, the use of leukocyte reduction filters was not mentioned.

Two studies have been performed to date that evaluate the use of blood recovery in controlled trials. One study was prospective while the other was retrospective.[81,82] In both of the studies, patients undergoing radical retropubic prostatectomy were compared to patients undergoing preoperative autologous donations. Both studies demonstrated that outcome was equivalent. Again, those findings suggest that massive metastasis does not occur because recovered blood was used.

Blood Recovery and the
Jehovah's Witness Patient

Administration of allogeneic blood to the Jehovah's Witness patient is forbidden because of a specific interpretation of Bible scripture. However, normovolemic hemodilution and blood recovery can be accepted with some modifications of technique. Most Jehovah's Witnesses feel that as long as the blood maintains some form of contact with their bodies, the blood is essentially still part of them. For instance, the external tubing of a heart-lung bypass circuit or dialysis tubing is an extension of the individual's own circulatory system. Thus, these techniques will usually be accepted when a continuous connection with the patient is maintained.

Blood recovery for the Jehovah's Witness has been addressed by the church in several church-sponsored publications.[83] Acceptance of blood recovery or normovolemic hemodilution is left to the conscience of the individual. Most Jehovah's Witness patients will accept those techniques, however, when guided by a Jehovah's Witness liaison who has been enlisted by the physician. Jehovah's Witness lay liaisons are typically available at most medical institutions in the United States. Apheresis techniques, discussed in Chapter 8, can also be used with a continuous patient connection so that significant clotting abnormality can be addressed during surgery. Thus, a Jehovah's Witness patient should rarely be at risk during surgical procedures.

Complications of Blood Recovery

The process of blood recovery is associated with a few complications. Air embolism is a concern if the reinfusion bag of the blood recovery circuit is directly connected to the patient's vascular access.[84] That complication can be prevented by simply transferring the blood into a separate blood bag before administration, with the blood bag being burped of its air before sealing.

Similar-looking labels on the 0.9% saline, glycine, and sterile water infusion bags have also led to errors. When investigating those errors, the authors noticed that, in their central storage area, all types of irrigation fluid (0.9% saline and sterile water, and 1.5% glycine) were kept in close proximity to each other. Also, they found that several bags of glycine were stored with 0.9% saline. In 1981, Wang and Turndorf[86] identified that up to 12% of drugs administered in hospitals were in error. Their findings led to an effort to standardize and enhance the labeling of drugs and prefilled syringes.[87] The same effort should be applied to the labeling of irrigation fluids.

References

1. Sutera SP. Flow-induced trauma to blood cells. Circ Res 1977;41:2-8.
2. Gregoretti S. Suction-induced hemolysis at various vacuum pressures: Implications for intraoperative blood salvage. Transfusion 1996;36:57-60.
3. Clague CT, Blackshear PL Jr. A low-hemolysis blood aspirator conserves blood during surgery. Biomed Instrum Technol 1995;29:419-24.
4. Bruil A, Beugeling T, Feijen J, van Aken WG. The mechanisms of leukocyte removal by filtration. Transfus Med Rev 1995;9:145-66.
5. Halpern NA, Alicea M, Seabrook B, et al. Cell saver autologous transfusion: Metabolic consequences of washing blood with normal saline. Trauma 1996; 41:407-15.
6. Halpern NA, Alicea M, Seabrook B, et al. Isolyte S, a physiologic multielectrolyte solution, is preferable to normal saline to wash cell saver salvaged blood: Conclusions from a prospective, randomized study in a canine model. Crit Care Med 1997;25:2031-8.
7. Hood PA, McKenna TR. Quality assessment of washed packed cells produced by centrifugal cell salvage: An in-vitro study. Annviller, PA: American Academy of Cardiovascular Perfusion, 1996.
8. Reeder GD. Principles of autotransfusion. In: Autotransfusion Symposium Reference Manual. 4th ed. Englewood, CO: University of Colorado Health Science Center/Electromedics, 1992:1-225.
9. Reeder GD. Autotransfusion theory of operation: A review of the physics and hematology. Transfusion 2004;44(Suppl 2):10-15.
10. Waters JH, Lee JS, Karafa MT. A mathematical model of cell salvage efficiency. Anesth Analg 2002;95:1312-17.
11. Isomaa B, Hägerstrand H, Paatero G, Engblom AC. Permeability alterations and antihaemolysis induced by amphiphiles in human erythrocytes. Biochim Biophys Acta 1983;860:510-24.

12. Hanzawa K. Fragility of red cells during exercise is affected by blood pH and temperature. Equine Vet J 1999;30:610-11.

13. Sarkar M. Effects of temperature and pH on the osmotic fragility of erythrocytes of yaks. Aust Vet J 1999;77:188-9.

14. Barbee JH. The effect of temperature on the relative viscosity of human blood. Biorheology 1993;10:1-5.

15. Eckman D, Bowers S, Steckner M, Cheung AT. Hematocrit, volume expander, temperature, and shear rate effects on blood viscosity. Anesth Analg 2000;91: 539-45.

16. Waters JH, Kottke-Marchant K, Link E. Modification of cell salvage red cell recovery through red cell membrane stabilizers. Anesthesiology 2003;99: A219.

17. Ronai AK, Glass JJ, Shapiro AS. Improving autologous blood harvest: Recovery of red cells from sponges and suction. Anaesth Intensive Care 1987;15:421-4.

18. Haynes SL, Bennett JR, Torella F, McCollum CN. Does washing swabs increase the efficiency of red cell recovery by cell salvage in aortic surgery? Vox Sang 2005;88:244-8.

19. Kang Y, Aggarwal S, Pasculle AW, et al. Bacteriologic study of autotransfusion during liver transplantation. Transplant Proc 1989;21:35-8.

20. Bland LA, Villarino ME, Arduino MJ, et al. Bacteriologic and endotoxin analysis of salvaged blood used in autologous transfusions during cardiac operations. J Thorac Cardiovasc Surg 1992;103:582-8.

21. Ilstrup S, ed. Standards for perioperative autologous blood collection and administration. 3rd ed. Bethesda, MD: AABB, 2007.

22. O'Hara PJ, Hertzer NR, Santilli PH, Beven EG. Intraoperative autotransfusion during abdominal aortic reconstruction. Am J Surg 1983;145:215-20.

23. Autologous Transfusion Committee. Guidelines for blood recovery and reinfusion in surgery and trauma. AABB, Bethesda, MD: 1997.

24. Scott BH, Seifert FC, Glass PS, Grimson R. Blood use in patients undergoing coronary artery bypass surgery: Impact of cardiopulmonary bypass pump, hematocrit, gender, age, and body weight. Anesth Analg 2003;97:958-63.

25. Waters JH, Gottschall JL, eds. Perioperative blood management: A physician's handbook. Bethesda, MD: AABB/SABM, 2006:62-3.

26. Dietrich W. Pro: Shed mediastinal blood retransfusion should be used routinely in cardiac surgery. J Cardiothorac Vasc Anesth 1995;91:95-9.

27. Mazer CD. Con: Shed mediastinal blood should not be reinfused after cardiac surgery. J Cardiothorac Vasc Anesth 1995;91:100-2.

28. Simonian PT, Robinson RP. Titanium contamination of recycled Cell Saver blood in revision hip arthroplasty. J Arthroplasty 1995;101:83-6.

29. Orr MD, Riester DE, Hultman J. Complement activation in shed blood: Release of C3a and C5a. Implications for autologous transfusion. J Cardiothorac Anesth 1989;35(Suppl 1):85.

30. Pierce LR, Gaines A, Varricchio F, Epstein J. Hemolysis and renal failure associated with use of sterile water for injection to dilute 25% human albumin solution. Am J Health Syst Pharm 1998;55:1057-70.

31. Centers for Disease Control and Prevention. Hemolysis associated with 25% human albumin diluted with sterile water—United States, 1994-1998. JAMA 1999;281:1076-7.

32. Fong J, Gurewitsch ED, Kump L, Klein R. Clearance of fetal products and subsequent immunoreactivity of blood salvaged at cesarean delivery. Obstet Gynecol 1999;93:968-72.

33. Potter PS, Waters JH, Burger GA, Mraovic B. Application of cell-salvage during cesarean section. Anesthesiology 1999;90:619-21.

34. Rebarber A, Lonser R, Jackson S, et al. The safety of intraoperative autologous blood collection and autotransfusion during cesarean section. Am J Obstet Gynecol 1998;179:715-20.

35. Bland LA, Villarino ME, Arduino MJ, et al. Bacteriologic and endotoxin analysis of salvaged blood used in autologous transfusions during cardiac operations. J Thoracic Cardiovasc Surg 1992;103:582-8.

36. Kang Y, Aggarwal S, Pasculle AW, et al. Bacteriologic study of autotransfusion during liver transplantation. Transplant Proc 1989;21:35-8.

37. Ozman V, McSwain NE, Nichols RL, et al. Autotransfusion of potentially culture-positive blood in abdominal trauma: Preliminary data from a prospective study. J Trauma 1992;32:36-9.

38. Schwieger IM, Gallager CJ, Finlayson DC, et al. Incidence of cell saver contamination during cardiopulmonary bypass. Ann Thorac Surg 1989;48:51-3.

39. Timberlake GA, McSwain NE. Autotransfusion of blood contaminated by enteric contents: A potentially life-saving measure in the massively hemorrhaging trauma patient. J Trauma 1988;28:855-7.

40. Boudreaux JP, Bornside GH, Cohn I Jr. Emergency autotransfusion: Partial cleansing of bacteria-laden blood by cell washing. J Trauma 1983;23:31-5.

41. Waters JH, Tuohy MJ, Hobson DF, Procop G. Bacterial reduction by cell salvage washing and leukocyte depletion filtration. Anesthesiology 2003;99:652-5.

42. Jacobs MR, Palavecino E, Yomtovian R. Don't bug me: The problem of bacterial contamination of blood components—challenges and solutions. Transfusion 2001;41:1331-4.

43. Yomtovian R, Lazarus HM, Goodnough LT, et al. A prospective microbiologic surveillance program to detect and prevent the transfusion of bacterially contaminated platelets. Transfusion 1993;33:902-9.

44. Do A, Jarvid WR. Transfusion-related infection. In: Schlossberg D, ed. Current therapy for infectious disease. St. Louis, MO: Mosby-Yearbook 1996:340-3.

45. Sapatnekar S, Wood EM, Miller JP, et al. Methicillin-resistant Staphylococcus aureus sepsis associated with the transfusion of contaminated platelets: A case report. Transfusion 2001;41:1426-30.

46. Kuehnert MJ, Jarvis WR, Schaffer DA, Chaffin DJ. Platelet transfusion reaction due to *Yersinia enterocolitica.* JAMA 1997;278:550-1.

47. Smith RN, Yaw PB, Glover JL. Autotransfusion of contaminated intraperitoneal blood: An experimental study. J Trauma 1978;18:341-4.

48. Wollinsky KH, Oethinger M, Büchele M, et al. Autotransfusion-bacterial contamination during hip arthroplasty and efficacy of cefuroxime prophylaxis. Acta Orthop Scand 1997;68:225-30.

49. Dzik WH, Sherburne B. Intraoperative blood salvage: Medical controversies. Transfus Med Rev 1990;4:208-35.

50. Berg CJ, Chang J, Callaghan WM, Whitehead SJ. Pregnancy-related mortality in the United States, 1991-1997. Obstet Gynecol 2003;101:289-96.

51. Chang J, Elam-Evans LD, Berg CJ, Herndon J, et al. Pregnancy-related mortality surveillance—United States, 1991-1999. Morb Mortal Wkly Rep Surveill Summ 2003;52:1-8.

52. Lockwood CJ, Bach R, Guha A, et al. Amniotic fluid contains tissue factor, a potent initiator of coagulation. Am J Obstet Gynecol 1991;165:1335-41.

53. Bernstein HH, Rosenblatt MA, Gettes M, Lockwood C. The ability of the Haemonetics 4 cell saver system to remove tissue factor from blood contaminated with amniotic fluid. Anesth Analg 1997;85:831-3.

54. Halmagyi DFJ, Starzecki B, Shearman RP. Experimental amniotic fluid embolism: Mechanism and treatment. Am J Obstet Gynecol 1962;84:251-6.

55. Morgan M. Amniotic fluid embolism. Anaesthesia 1979;34:20-32.

56. Kling D, Börner U, Bormann VB, Hempelmann G. Heparin elimination and free hemoglobin following cell separation and washing of autologous blood with Cell Saver 4. Anasth Intensivther Notfallmed 1988;23:88-90.

57. Umlas J, O'Neill TP. Heparin removal in an autotransfusor device. Transfusion 1981;21:70-3.

58. Maleck WH, Petroianu GA. Autologous blood transfusion. Br J Anaesth 1999; 82:154.

59. Petroianu GA, Altmannsberger SHG, Maleck WH, et al. Meconium and amniotic fluid embolism: Effects on coagulation in pregnant mini-pigs. Crit Care Med 1999;27:348-55.

60. Durand F, Duchesne-Gueguen M, Le Bervet JY, et al. Rheologic and cytologic study of autologous blood collected with Cell Saver 4 during cesarean. Rev Fr Transfus Hemobiol 1989;32:179-91.

61. Waters JH, Biscotti C, Potter P, Phillipson E. Amniotic fluid removal during cell-salvage in the cesarean section patient. Anesthesiology 2000;92:1531-6.

62. Rainaldi MP, Tazzari PL, Scagliarini G, et al. Blood salvage during caesarean section. Br J Anaesthesia 1998;80:195-8.

63. Grimes DA. A simplified device for intraoperative autotransfusion. Obstet Gynecol 1988;72:947-50.

64. Jackson SH, Lonser RE. Safety and effectiveness of intracesarean blood salvage (letter). Transfusion 1993;33:181.

65. Francis DM. Relationship between blood transfusion and tumour behavior. Br J Surg 1991;78:1420-8.

66. Vamvakas EC. Perioperative blood transfusion and cancer recurrence: Meta-analysis for explanation. Transfusion 1995;35:760-8.

67. Blumberg N, Heal JM. Effects of transfusion on immune function: Cancer recurrence and infection. Arch Pathol Lab Med 1994;118:371-9.

68. Oefelein MG, Kaul K, Herz B, et al. Molecular detection of prostate epithelial cells from the surgical field and peripheral circulation during radical prostatectomy. J Urol 1996;155:238-42.

69. Roberts S, Watne A, McGrath R, et al. Technique and results of isolation of cancer cells from the circulating blood. Arch Surg 1958;76:334-6.

70. Fisher ER, Turnbull RB Jr. Cytologic demonstration and significance of tumor cells in the mesenteric venous blood in patients with colorectal carcinoma. Surg Gynecol Obstet 1955;100:102-5.

71. Klimberg IW. Autotransfusion and blood conservation in urologic oncology. Semin Surg Oncol 1989;5:286-92.

72. Weiss L. Metastatic inefficiency: Causes and consequences. Cancer Rev 1986; 3:1-24.

73. Edelman MJ, Potter P, Mahaffey KG, et al. The potential for reintroduction of tumor cells during intraoperative blood salvage: Reduction of risk with use of the RC-400 leukocyte depletion filter. Urology 1996;47:179-81.

74. Wiesel M, Gudemann C, Hoever KH, et al. Separation of urologic tumor cells from red blood cells by the use of a cell-saver and membrane filters. Investig Urol (Berl) 1994;5:244-8.

75. Perseghin P, Vigano M, Rocco G, et al. Effectiveness of leukocyte filters in reducing tumor cell contamination after intraoperative blood salvage in lung cancer patients. Vox Sang 1997;72:221-4.

76. Kongsgaard UE, Wang MY, Kvalheim G. Leucocyte depletion filter removes cancer cells in human blood. Acta Anaesthesiol Scandi 1996;40:118-20.

77. Torre GC, Ferrari M, Favre A, et al. A new technique for intraoperative blood recovery in the cancer patient. Eur J Surg Oncol 1994;20:565-70.

78. Zulim RA, Rocco M, Goodnight JE, et al. Intraoperative autotransfusion in hepatic resection for malignancy. Arch Surg 1993;128:206-11.

79. Klimberg I, Sirois R, Wajsman Z, Baker J. Intraoperative autotransfusion in urologic oncology. Arch Surg 1986;121:1326-9.

80. Hart OJ, Klimberg IW, Wajsman Z, Baker J. Intraoperative autotransfusion in radical cystectomy for carcinoma of the bladder. Surg Gynecol Obstet 1989; 168:302-6.

81. Gray CL, Amling CL, Polston GR, et al. Intraoperative cell salvage in radical retropubic prostatectomy. Urology 2001;58:740-5.

82. Davis M, Sofer M, Gomez-Marin O, et al. The use of cell salvage during radical retropubic prostatectomy: Does it influence cancer recurrence? Br J Urol 2003; 91:474-6.

83. Jehovah's Witnesses and the question of blood. Brooklyn, NY: Watchtower Bible and Tract Society, 1977:1-64.

84. Williamson KR, Taswell HF. Intraoperative blood salvage: A review. Transfusion 1991;31:662-75.

85. Smith DF, Mihm FG, Mefford I. Hypertension after intraoperative autotransfusion in bilateral adrenalectomy for pheochromocytoma. Anesthesiology 1983; 58:182-4.

86. Wang BC, Turndorf H. Prevention of medication error. N Y State J Med 1981; 81:395-402.

87. Rendell-Baker L. Better labels will cut drug errors. Anesthesia Patient Safety Foundation Newsletter 1987;2:29-40.

In: Waters JH, ed.
Blood Management: Options for Better Patient Care
Bethesda, MD: AABB Press, 2008

10

Quality Systems in the Perioperative Setting

JUDITH A. SULLIVAN, MS, MT(ASCP)SBB, CQA(ASQ)

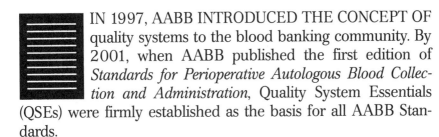 IN 1997, AABB INTRODUCED THE CONCEPT OF quality systems to the blood banking community. By 2001, when AABB published the first edition of *Standards for Perioperative Autologous Blood Collection and Administration*, Quality System Essentials (QSEs) were firmly established as the basis for all AABB Standards.

What is a quality system? In *Standards for Perioperative Autologous Blood Collection and Administration* (or *Perioperative Standards*), AABB defines a quality system as "the organizational structure, responsibilities, policies, processes, procedures, and resources established by executive management to achieve quality."[1(p43)] In essence, it is the support structure put in place by those in authority to ensure that a quality product or service can be provided to a customer on a consistent basis.

Judith A. Sullivan, MS, MT(ASCP)SBB, CQA(ASQ), Manager, Accreditation Programs, AABB, Bethesda, Maryland

One could question the applicability of a quality systems approach in the perioperative arena. After all, a surgical suite is not the same as an automobile manufacturing plant. Surgical personnel do not provide a product that can be reproduced within certain tolerance limits. However, the inherent variability of the products produced in the perioperative setting is what necessitates the implementation of a quality system. Providing the best possible product in any kind of reproducible manner demands a quality framework that should include the following:

- Management knowledgeable in, and committed to, quality concepts.
- Well-developed policies, processes, and procedures.
- Staff who are trained and competent, and who follow processes and procedures as written.
- Equipment that is selected with care, qualified before use, and well maintained.
- Quality supplies from qualified vendors.
- Processes to make changes in a controlled manner and to manage documents and records.
- A means to identify and correct errors so that they do not recur.
- Methods to assess effectiveness and to continuously improve.
- An environment that is safe for personnel and patients.

Accrediting organizations such as AABB, the College of American Pathologists (CAP), and The Joint Commission have established requirements for the implementation of quality functions that support operations. AABB defines 10 QSEs that form the framework for a quality system. (See Table 10-1.) These elements, integrated into the day-to-day activities of a perioperative program, provide the structure that allows the provision of consistent, quality products.

Organization

An effective quality system is not merely a vague notion that is discussed at periodic meetings. It must be defined and docu-

Table 10-1. Quality System Essentials	
1	Organization
2	Resources
3	Equipment
4	Supplier and customer issues
5	Process control
6	Documents and records
7	Deviations, nonconformances, and adverse events
8	Assessments: internal and external
9	Process improvement
10	Facilities and safety

mented, then implemented and maintained. The development, implementation, and maintenance of a quality system rest with executive management: the personnel within the organization with the authority to establish or change quality policy. For a quality system to be truly effective, the oversight of and responsibility for it must reside at the highest possible level within the program. "Executive management" may be one individual or a group of individuals. In either case, the perioperative program must clearly define its executive management. However, the quality system cannot reside with executive management alone. All personnel must be trained so that they 1) know what the quality system is, 2) understand its importance, and 3) recognize and act on their role in the system.

Other important elements under the QSE "organization" include those described below.

Defined Structure. The perioperative program must identify the individuals responsible for providing the perioperative products and services, the individuals responsible for key quality functions, and the relationship among personnel. Organizational charts are often used to visually define personnel and relationships.

Medical Director Responsibilities. The medical director has ultimate responsibility for the establishment of policies, processes, and procedures of the perioperative program.

Management Review of the Quality System. A quality system must be evaluated periodically if it is to provide any lasting benefit to the organization. Executive management is responsible for evaluating the effectiveness of the quality system on an ongoing basis and for making changes to the system on the basis of results of the review. Effectiveness of the quality system may be evaluated through reviews such as these:

- Findings from internal and external assessments and subsequent follow-up actions.
- Error reports, root cause analysis, and corrective action.
- Customer surveys and complaints.
- Process improvement activities.

Reviews must be documented, along with any changes to the quality system resulting from the review.

Policies, Processes, and Procedures. Written policies, processes, and procedures form the backbone of any quality system, thereby providing consistent practice within the perioperative program. Personnel perform their functions not on the basis of hearsay, but on the basis of clear written instructions. Processes are well defined so that they can be followed the same way by everyone. When new personnel are trained, they are given accurate information. Consistent execution of policies, processes, and procedures leads to consistent products and services.

AABB *Perioperative Standards* defines *policy* as "a documented general principle that guides present and future decisions." It expresses the commitment and the intent of the organization regarding a quality element. A *process* is "a set of related tasks and activities that accomplish a work goal." It usually involves more than one person or one group within a program. Processes are often depicted by flow charts. A *procedure* is "a series of tasks usually performed by one person according to instructions."[1(p42)] Procedures are to the perioperative program what recipes are to cooks. See Table 10-2 for examples of a policy, a process, and a procedure as they relate to equipment.

Table 10-2. Policy, Process, and Procedure	
Policy: Equipment *(Rule)*	The perioperative service at XYZ hospital identifies equipment that is critical to the provision of services and ensures that calibration, maintenance, and monitoring of equipment conform to specified requirements.
Process: Equipment selection *(What we do)*	1. Establish equipment need. 2. Determine if item is in budget. 3. Identify vendors. 4. Perform site visits to evaluate. 5. (etc)
Procedure: Setting up a blood recovery machine *(How we do things)*	1. Assemble disposables. 2. Record lot numbers on form. 3. Open package and inspect for defects. 4. Place bowl in machine. 5. (etc)

Policies, processes, and procedures must be in writing, and they must be followed. Personnel must be trained not to deviate from written processes and procedures. Processes and procedures must be written in such a way that they are easy to understand and easy to follow.

Exceptions to Policies, Processes, and Procedures. Given a particular clinical situation or patient, the medical director can justify and approve exceptions to policies, processes, and procedures. This approval must occur before the event's occurrence and must be in writing. Exceptions must be monitored; if recurring, they should be evaluated for incorporation into existing policies, processes, and procedures.

Resources

The primary resource in a perioperative program is the personnel hired to perform the functions of the program. All personnel must be qualified, trained, and competent.

Qualifications. The perioperative program must define in writing the qualifications needed for an individual to be hired for a specific position. Usually, these qualifications are included as part of a job description. AABB *Perioperative Standards* does not specify who may or may not work in a perioperative program (perfusionist, autotransfusionist, registered nurse, medical technologist, etc). Rather, each program must define the level of education, training, experience, or a combination of these that are needed to qualify for each position. This way, each institution has the flexibility to hire individuals that best fit the needs of the particular program.

Training. Once qualified personnel are hired, the perioperative program must have a written process for training each individual according to the policies, processes, and procedures of that program. Simply because a new hire has 5 years of experience in performing blood recovery does not mean that he or she is ready to perform that function in any given program using that program's equipment and procedures. Training for program-specific policies, processes, and procedures ensures a common understanding among the staff as well as consistent implementation. When new processes or procedures are introduced, or when existing ones are changed, the program must also have a process for identifying and assessing training needs and for providing additional training as necessary.

Competency. Because an individual has been trained in a specific task does not necessarily guarantee that he or she is competent (that is, capable of independently performing the task according to procedure). Therefore, the program must have a process for assessing competency before releasing an individual to work independently. Methods of competency assessment may include a combination of these[2]:
- Direct observation of task performance.
- Monitoring of the recording and reporting of test results.
- Review of worksheets, quality control records, and preventive maintenance records.
- Direct observation of performance of instrument maintenance and function checks.
- Assessment of problem-solving skills.

If one is to ensure that individuals remain competent in assigned tasks, competency must be assessed at least annually. Written records of the assessment must be maintained. If the assessment indicates that an individual is not competent, documentation of follow-up actions must also be maintained.

Equipment

Personnel can be only as good as the equipment they operate. Equipment that is not carefully selected, qualified, calibrated, and maintained is incapable of providing a consistent and high-quality product, regardless of the skills of the individual operating the equipment.

Selection

The perioperative program must define a process that is used to select equipment. The process should allow for a deliberate consideration of all elements necessary for selection. The following are examples:
- What is my budget?
- How will this equipment be used?
- What specifications must the equipment meet?
- Who will operate it?
- How often will it be used?
- What kind of support will the manufacturer provide in installation and ongoing maintenance?
- What types of disposables will be needed, and how easy is it to acquire them?
- What experiences (positive and negative) have other users had with this equipment?
- How reliable is the manufacturer?

A defined process ensures that the best selection is made. It also takes into account all critical parameters, especially for those times when equipment must be purchased on an emergency basis.

Qualification

Once the equipment is purchased, it must be qualified (that is, it must be evaluated to ensure it will work as expected *before* it is used in a patient procedure). A qualification plan must be developed, approved, implemented, and evaluated before equipment use. Qualification involves three stages:

- Installation Qualification (IQ). This process ensures that the equipment is installed according to requirements (operator's manual, applicable standards and regulations, fire code, etc).
- Operational Qualification (OQ). This process ensures that the equipment does what the manufacturer says it can do. Do all the buttons have the desired effect when pushed? Does the centrifuge spin? Can the blood recovery device wash and concentrate blood? Does a platelet separator indeed separate platelets?
- Performance Qualification (PQ). This process answers the question "Does this equipment perform as expected in this environment, using these procedures and these personnel?" It may involve testing various scenarios to determine if the equipment will function as expected under different circumstances.

Once qualification is complete, the plan is reviewed to ensure that it was followed as written, that expected results were achieved, that any discrepancies were identified and addressed, and that documentation is complete.

Calibration

If a piece of equipment requires calibration, a process must be defined to ensure that calibration occurs 1) before use, 2) after activities that may affect calibration, and 3) at specified intervals. Safeguards must be in place to ensure that calibration settings cannot be inadvertently changed. If it is discovered that a piece of equipment is out of calibration, the equipment must be removed from service, and a process must be followed to assess the effect of the calibration change on any products that may have been produced.

Preventive Maintenance

To ensure that equipment continues to yield good products, the perioperative program must define a process and schedule for preventive maintenance. At a minimum, the manufacturer's recommendations for the type and frequency of maintenance must be followed. Records of preventive maintenance must be maintained.

Supplier and Customer Issues

As with equipment, the final perioperative product will be only as good as the critical materials used in its manufacture. When the perioperative program 1) qualifies its suppliers of equipment, materials, and services; 2) defines agreed-upon expectations; and 3) verifies the acceptability of the supplies before use, it has taken steps to ensure a consistent supply of quality critical materials and services.

Supplier Qualification

Critical materials are defined as those that can affect the quality of the perioperative program's products or services. The program is responsible for identifying those materials it considers to be critical and for qualifying the suppliers of the materials. "Qualify" in this situation means to determine—before entering into a contract—that a supplier can consistently provide materials that meet the program's requirements.

The AABB *Guidance for Standards for Perioperative Autologous Blood Collection and Administration*[3] identifies some factors to consider in supplier qualification:

- Licensure, certification, or accreditation by a reputable organization.
- Product requirements.
- Review of a supplier's relevant quality documents.
- Review of the program's experience with the supplier.
- Cost of products or services.
- Delivery arrangements.
- Financial security, market position, and customer satisfaction.
- Postsales support.

The perioperative program must 1) define a process for qualifying new suppliers, 2) maintain a current list of qualified suppliers, and 3) ensure through policy that only qualified suppliers are used. Ongoing monitoring of a supplier's performance must be documented and feedback must be provided, including complaints and quality issues. In situations where the perioperative program does not have direct authority for purchasing decisions, it is essential that the program provide input regarding program requirements and feedback regarding the ability of suppliers to meet requirements to those individuals with contracting authority.

Agreements

After a supplier of equipment, materials, or services has been qualified, agreements are established between the perioperative program and the supplier to define expectations and to reflect that both parties have accepted the terms. Agreements can be as formal as legal contracts or as informal as oral commitments. In any case, the agreement must be reviewed periodically and any changes must be incorporated as needed.

If the program contracts with third-party providers for perioperative services, it is important that the agreement defines the responsibilities of each entity to ensure that all requirements are accounted for. For example, if the third-party provider is responsible for making platelet gel, but hospital personnel are responsible for application, the agreement should define the "hand-off" point and the responsibilities of both the third-party provider and hospital personnel.

Receipt, Inspection, and Testing of Materials and Products

The time to discover that the disposables for the blood recovery machine are defective should not be when the patient is on the operating table. Upon delivery and before use, materials and products must be inspected to ensure that they are acceptable and will function as expected. Depending on the product, inspection may involve visual examination, testing, or receipt of documentation from the supplier that the product has been tested and meets requirements (eg, certificate of analysis). The method of inspection must be defined, and documentation of inspection must be maintained.

Process Control

As mentioned previously, written policies, processes, and procedures form the backbone of the quality system. Process control is the management of these processes and procedures to ensure that they are performed uniformly and as intended, thus resulting in the provision of a consistent, predictable product or service. Elements of process control are described next.

Validation

Once a process or procedure has been written and before it is put into use, the following questions must be asked and answered:
- Is it understandable to those who will use it?
- Is it complete?
- Is it easy to use?
- Does it provide the expected outcome on a consistent basis?

To answer these questions is the purpose of validation. Before a new process or procedure is implemented, a validation plan is developed and carried out. Elements of a validation plan may include the following:

- Purpose of the validation.
- Scope of the plan.
- Definition of responsibilities of the individuals involved.
- Type and extent of activities.
- How the validation will occur.
- Needed resources.
- Expected outcomes.
- Review and approval.

Once the validation has been conducted and documented, results must be reviewed. If expected outcomes were not achieved, changes are made to the process or procedure and then revalidated. Upon successful validation, the process or procedure can be approved, staff can be trained and evaluated for competency, and then the process or procedure can be implemented.

Change Control

When a new process or procedure is implemented, what effect might it have on other parts of the perioperative program, or even on other departments? When changes are made to existing processes or procedures, how does the perioperative program know whether these changes will affect the quality of the product or service related to this process or procedure? How might changes to a process or procedure affect the perioperative program or other departments? How can the perioperative program prevent unauthorized changes to processes and procedures? To answer these questions is the purpose of change control.

Change does not occur in a vacuum; often, change has unexpected consequences. If one is to anticipate and minimize these consequences, change must be planned and controlled, and a change control process must be defined and consistently used. As with new processes and procedures, changes to existing processes and procedures must be validated; the scope of the validation plan should correspond to the significance of the proposed change. For both new and changed processes and procedures, the anticipated effect on other processes, procedures, equipment, and personnel within the perioperative program and other departments must be defined, evaluated, and communicated to all affected parties *before* the process or procedure is implemented. A change control plan must also include how the effectiveness of any changes will be evaluated and over what time period. Unanticipated consequences of the change must be documented and addressed.

Quality Control

The purpose of quality control is to ensure 1) that reagents, equipment, and processes function as expected and 2) that a perioperative product of consistent quality is produced. Each perioperative program must define a quality control program that is based on the products and services it provides. Both the frequency and type of quality control should be defined.

The frequency of measurement for a particular parameter may depend on the confidence the program has in its ability to produce a consistent product. For example, if a program has just instituted blood recovery with processing, it may wish to perform a hematocrit on every product to determine an acceptable range of values. Once it can be demonstrated that this range can be consistently achieved, the program may decide that the hematocrit of only a certain percentage of products will be tested each month. As long as the test values remain within the defined range, sampling continues. However, if products are tested and found to be outside of acceptable limits, the program—upon investigation and resolution of any problems—may wish to increase the number of units tested until confidence in its ability to produce a consistent product is reestablished.

The type of quality control is defined by the products made. Indicators should be selected according to the type of blood or component produced and the manufacturer's recommendations, if available. A definition of acceptable results and documentation of assessment must be maintained. In addition to measurements such as weight or volume, hemoglobin content, free hemoglobin content, fibrinogen level, or platelet count (as appropriate), quality control also includes 1) a visual examination of the product for abnormalities before administration, and 2) a determination that the product has not exceeded the established expiration time.

Use of Materials

When the perioperative program qualifies its suppliers, it specifies its requirements for equipment, supplies, and services. It is then the responsibility of the program to use materials in accordance with the manufacturer's written instructions so that materials will perform as expected. If pharmaceuticals, solutions, testing reagents, or a combination of these are produced in house, the program must define the criteria for these materials and must document that these materials have indeed met the defined criteria.

Sterility

To provide assurance of a sterile product, the perioperative program must define and use appropriate aseptic methods throughout its processes. This approach includes the use of sterile and pyrogen-free equipment and single-use materials.

Identification and Traceability

To allow for the investigation of errors, discrepancies, adverse outcomes, and other problems, the perioperative program must define and use a process to identify and trace perioperative products and the critical materials used in their processing, as well as laboratory samples and patient records. This process must include a means to identify the source, location, and disposition of perioperative products and critical materials. It must also include a means to identify the individual or individuals who performed each critical step in the collection, processing, and administration of each perioperative product, and to note when that step was performed. Identification of individuals can be accomplished through means such as electronic recording, signature file, or identification numbers. The perioperative program must define and use a process for labeling perioperative products. Particularly important if the product and patient are to be separated, all perioperative products must be labeled with the information required to positively identify both the product and the intended recipient.

Inspection

To ensure that a nonconforming perioperative product is detected as early in the process as possible and before administration to the recipient, the perioperative program must define stages in the process at which inspection and testing of the product will occur. The program must have a process to ensure that the final product is acceptable before being handed off for administration. In addition, the program must have a means to ensure that, if a nonconforming product is identified, it is removed in a controlled manner from the process so that it is not inadvertently administered.

Handling, Storage, and Administration

The elements of process control described thus far involve the use of validated procedures performed by trained and competent individuals with qualified, calibrated equipment and acceptable supplies to produce a product of high quality. The perioperative program must also have a process in place to ensure that this product is handled, stored, and administered in a manner that will prevent damage and will limit deterioration, thus providing maximum benefit for the intended recipient. AABB standards defining appropriate storage and expiration for both red cell and non-red-cell products have been established.[1(pp21-25)] In addition, the perioperative program must define and use a process for collecting, handling, labeling, and storing of those perioperative products known to contain infectious agents.

Documents and Records

As mentioned previously, quality system documents include policies, processes, and procedures. To capture the outcome of a process or procedure, the perioperative program designs forms. A form, once completed, becomes a record. (See Figure 10-1.) All documents, including policies, processes, procedures, forms, and labels must be identified and must be approved before their use and again after modification. They must also be controlled; that is, the perioperative program must have a process to ensure 1) that only current documents are available and 2) that obsolete versions cannot be used. Elements of document control are described next.

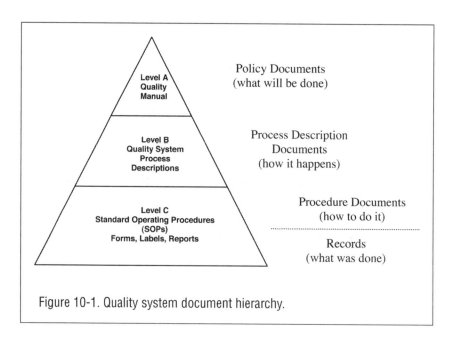

Figure 10-1. Quality system document hierarchy.

Master List of Documents

The master list is "document control at-a-glance." It contains a listing of all policies, processes, procedures, forms, and labels. The following information may be incorporated into the master list:

- Title of the document.
- Current version number.
- Date of implementation.
- Locations of all copies.
- Date the document was retired.

The master list should be a living document: as a new process is written and implemented, it should be added to the list, and the former version should be noted as having been archived.

Standardized Formats for Documents

For ease of development and for ease of use, policies, processes and procedures should be written in standard formats. The perioperative program must define and use its standard format [often called the "SOP (standard operating procedure) for SOPs"]. The standard format should include a means to uniquely identify each document (for example, document control number or version number) and a means to capture the dates the document was created, approved, implemented, and reviewed, as well as review signatures.

Review and Approval of New and Revised Documents Before Use

Before a document is placed in use, it must be reviewed and approved. Validation, change control, and training must also occur as appropriate.

Annual Review

An authorized individual (usually the medical director) must review all policies, processes, and procedures at least annually to ensure that these documents remain relevant to the perioperative program. Documentation of review must be maintained.

Use of Only Current and Valid Documents

Policies, processes, and procedures are of little use if they are not current and if the individuals using them do not have easy access to them. The perioperative program should have a process for the distribution of new or changed documents. In addition, staff should be trained not to add more information to the copies of the documents they use, because this information has not been authorized and is not controlled.

Identification and Archiving of Obsolete Documents

When a new version of a document is to be implemented, the perioperative program must have a process to locate and retrieve all copies of the former version. Documents must be archived in accordance with all applicable standards and federal, state, or local laws.

The documentation showing that an activity has been performed is a record. Records prove that a product or service conforms to specified requirements and that each step of the process was performed. The perioperative program must have policies, processes, and procedures in place for the management of records, including how records will be
- Identified (ie, what records will be maintained).
- Collected.
- Indexed for easy retrieval.
- Accessed in a timely manner only by authorized personnel.
- Filed.

- Stored to ensure confidentiality and protection from damage.
- Retained according to record retention policies.
- Disposed of when appropriate to do so.

In addition, the program's record system must make it possible to trace a perioperative product from source to final disposition, to review the records related to that product, and to investigate any adverse events a patient receiving the product may have experienced.

Deviations, Nonconformances, and Adverse Events

In spite of a perioperative program's best efforts, events will occur that deviate from requirements. The program must define a process to capture adverse events. Staff should be encouraged to report events and should be assured that nobody will be punished. In this way, problems can be identified and used as opportunities for improvement. Once an event is identified, the program must have processes to

- Assess any products or critical materials involved, to establish if they are in conformance with defined acceptance criteria.
- Determine the disposition of the product or critical material.
- Prevent any nonconforming product or critical material from unintentional distribution or use.
- Quarantine, retrieve, and recall nonconforming products or critical materials.
- Report to the customer, supplier, patient's physician, or a combination of these, as applicable, any nonconforming product or critical material that was released.
- Investigate the cause of the adverse event.
- Institute corrective action as appropriate.
- Monitor adverse events to identify trends.

The perioperative program must have a process to evaluate any complications arising from perioperative product administration. The fact that such complications occur rarely only emphasizes the need for an established process so that when the administration is interrupted, the evaluation can be performed effectively and proper clinical management of the patient is not delayed. Of particular concern is the occurrence of a suspected hemolytic reaction. The perioperative program's process for managing such an event must include the following:

- Discontinuation of administration.
- Comparison of the blood container label and other records to the patient's identification.
- Discontinuation of any processing devices involved and evaluation for the cause of the reaction.
- Request for laboratory analysis as needed.
- Documentation and reporting of the event and the investigation.

Assessments

To ensure that both operations and the quality system are functioning effectively, the perioperative program must have processes to assess both of these elements on a routine basis. Although a perioperative program may choose to be assessed by an outside agency, this external audit does not substitute for developing processes to perform the program's own internal operational and quality assessments. Those responsible for performing internal assessments should be knowledgeable about quality principles and trained in auditing principles and communication, and they should not assess areas for which they have direct responsibility. A schedule for assessments must be defined, and appropriate tools and forms must be developed.

When an internal assessment is complete, the results should be communicated to those responsible for the area under assessment. If problems are identified, investigation and corrective action must be instituted. For assessments to be of use to the program, the results of assessments and any related actions must be reviewed by executive management.

A utilization review program must be developed to monitor perioperative collection and administration practices. Policies and their expected use should be defined and overseen by a committee that is responsible for reviewing blood utilization for the organization. Areas to review may include the following:

- Ordering practices and appropriateness of use.
- Significant adverse events, deviations, and near-miss events.
- Ability of the program to provide services when needed.

Process Improvement

The perioperative program must have processes in place to implement corrective and preventive actions that will prevent non-conformances from recurring and that will collect and analyze quality indicator data. Opportunities for process improvement may arise as a result of deviations (both planned and un-planned), nonconformances, adverse events, internal and external assessments, and customer complaints.

Corrective action is taken in response to problems that have been identified. Processes and procedures for corrective action include the following:

- Documentation of the problem.
- Investigation of the cause of the problem.
- Determination of the action to be taken to correct the problem.
- Identification of the individual(s) responsible for implementation.
- Establishment of a time frame for implementation.
- Evaluation of the effectiveness of the action.
- Reevaluation if the action was not effective.

It is important that the extent of investigation and corrective action be in proportion to the importance of the problem so that resources are used effectively. It is equally important that efforts are made to identify the root cause of the problem and that the investigation does not stop at the first obvious answer, which may simply be a symptom of an underlying cause. Although it is easy to lay the cause at the feet of the individuals involved in a problem, most problems are a result of process and system issues. Unless these issues are investigated and addressed, the problem will tend to resurface.

Preventive action is active anticipation of potential problems. It involves monitoring data and identifying trends that may signal that a problem is about to occur. For example, quality control data may be monitored over time. Although data are within acceptable limits, it may be noted that a downward trend has developed, which, if left unaddressed, will eventually lead to a nonconforming product. Viewing the data for trends allows for investigation and resolution even before a problem has occurred. Once a potential problem has been identified, follow-up uses the same processes and procedures described above for corrective action.

The documentation of corrective and preventive actions should be reviewed by executive management in a timely manner. In addition, executive management should actively participate in process improvement by defining quality objectives on an ongoing basis. Quality indicator data must be defined, collected, and evaluated on a scheduled basis, and the results must be communicated to all affected parties.

Safety

It is the responsibility of the perioperative program to provide a safe environment and to develop policies, processes, and procedures that minimize risks to the health and safety of employees, donors, volunteers, patients, and third-party providers. Suitable quarters, environment, and equipment must be available to maintain safe operations. The program must meet all applicable local, state, and federal regulations. In addition, it must monitor adherence to biological, chemical, and radiation safety standards and regulations where applicable. Processes for handling and discarding perioperative products must be defined and implemented to prevent human exposure to infectious agents. Documentation of disposal must be maintained.

Conclusion

The provision of a high-quality product on a consistent basis to the intended recipient is the ultimate goal of a perioperative program. The proper design and implementation of a quality system in the perioperative setting provides the support and framework needed by perioperative personnel to perform their functions effectively on a day-to-day basis. Trained and competent staff who follow validated, current procedures with qualified equipment and supplies and who know how to recognize and resolve problems and how to improve processes are able to provide quality products to patients who need them. A quality system is not only in the best interest of the patient but also in the best interest of the perioperative program.

References

1. Ilstrup S, ed. Standards for perioperative autologous blood collection and administration. 3rd ed. Bethesda, MD: AABB, 2007.
2. Code of federal regulations. Standard: Technical supervisor responsibilities. Title 42 CFR Part 493.1451(b)(8). Washington, DC: US Government Printing Office, 2007 (revised annually).
3. Ilstrup S, ed. Guidance for standards for perioperative autologous blood collection and administration. 3rd ed. Bethesda, MD: AABB, 2007.

In: Waters JH, ed.
Blood Management: Options for Better Patient Care
Bethesda, MD: AABB Press, 2008

11

Topical Hemostatics and Fibrin Sealants

ANTONIO PEPE, MD; FELICIA A. IVASCU, MD;
TIMOTHY J. HANNON, MD; AND
CARL I. SCHULMAN, MD, MSPH

CONTROL OF BLOOD LOSS DURING TRAUMA or surgery is paramount to the success of patient survival and recovery. Methods to control bleeding have existed for many centuries. Efforts to achieve hemostasis have ranged from the use of raw meat by the ancient Egyptians to the use of dried plasma in World War I. In the early part of the 20th century, Bergel[1] reported the hemostatic effects of fibrin. In 1916, Harvey[2] discussed the use of fibrin patches to stop bleeding from solid organs during general

Antonio Pepe, MD, Assistant Professor, Surgery, University of Miami, Miami, Florida; Felicia A. Ivascu, MD, Attending Surgeon/Surgical Intensivist, Division of Trauma Services, William Beaumont Hospital, Royal Oak, Michigan; Timothy J. Hannon, MD, Medical Director, Blood Management Program, Department of Anesthesiology, St. Vincent Hospital and Healthcare Center, Indianapolis, Indiana; and Carl I. Schulman, MD, MSPH, Assistant Professor, Surgery, University of Miami, Miami, Florida surgery. In 1940, Young and Medawar[3] reported an experimental nerve anastomosis by fibrin sealing.

In the early attempts, providers tried to find the ideal biomaterial for hemostasis and wound closure. The basic properties of the ideal biomaterial include promotion of hemostasis and wound healing, complete absorption, and excellent tissue tolerance. Over the past 20 years, a number of hemostatic agents and tissue sealants have been developed and are currently used in the many surgical disciplines. These hemostatic agents provide hemostasis by mechanical properties, by augmenting the coagulation cascade, or—in the case of tissue sealants, which often provide all the components necessary for clot formation—by binding to and closing defects in tissue. Hemostatic agents and tissue sealants are used routinely in preventing excess blood loss and in reconstruction during surgical repair.

Basic Coagulation and Hemostasis

Hemostasis involves the complex interaction between plasma proteins, blood cells, and the coagulation and fibrinolytic cascades. Platelets are activated at the site of injury and provide the initial hemostatic response. The clotting cascade involves the sequential activation of proenzymes in a stepwise response. The final stages of the cascade involve the conversion of fibrinogen to fibrin by thrombin in the presence of calcium ions. The fibrin monomers undergo polymerization to form long fibrin strands that are stabilized by activated Factor XIII. The resulting fibrin clot acts as a primary hemostatic plug and provides a matrix to enhance wound healing.

Research into the mechanism of blood coagulation has led to the development of various topical hemostatics and sealants. Older, first-generation materials include oxidized, regenerated cellulose products such as Surgicel (Johnson & Johnson Gateway, New Brunswick, NJ) and bovine collagen products such as Gelfoam (Pfizer, New York, NY). Newer, second-generation agents, such as the gelatin matrix sealant FloSeal (Baxter, Deerfield, IL) contain a viscous collagen matrix combined with concentrated human thrombin. Another second-generation product, the sealant CoSeal (Baxter), contains two polyethylene glycol polymers. Fibrin sealants such as Tisseel (Baxter) and Evicel (Johnson & Johnson) contain human (Evicel) or bovine (Tisseel) thrombin and fibrinogen in separate syringes that are simultaneously injected at the desired site of action. The compound forms a stable adherent clot that seals small leaks and promotes hemostasis. Figure 11-1 provides an overview as to where in the clotting cascade the various agents exert their effect. The following discussion details the more commonly used agents and their individual properties. Research continues on novel hemostatic agents that are independent of the coagulation cascade.

First-Generation Topical Hemostatics

Gelfoam (gelatin sponge) was introduced in the 1940s for use in neurosurgical procedures. Made of purified porcine skin beaten into a gelatin, Gelfoam stimulates hemostasis by contact activation of the intrinsic pathway and platelets. Because it functions proximally in the coagulation cascade, functioning clotting factors and cofactors are still required to create a clot. Gelfoam absorbs approximately 45 times its weight in blood and can expand to approximately 200% of its original volume. Those properties become problematic when the product is applied to confined spaces such as the spinal foramina or the intracranial space, where it can cause spinal cord nerve compression or brain compression, respectively.[4] The body absorbs it in approximately 4 to 6 weeks. Dry Gelfoam can be applied directly to the bleeding surface or can be moistened with normal saline before application. The addition of topical thrombin also makes an effective combination. A powderlike Gelfoam preparation is available commercially as Surgiflo (Johnson & Johnson). It comes preloaded into a syringe and can be mixed with saline or topical thrombin to achieve the desired consistency. The product can then be applied in a pastelike consistency on surfaces or in hard-to-reach spaces or holes.

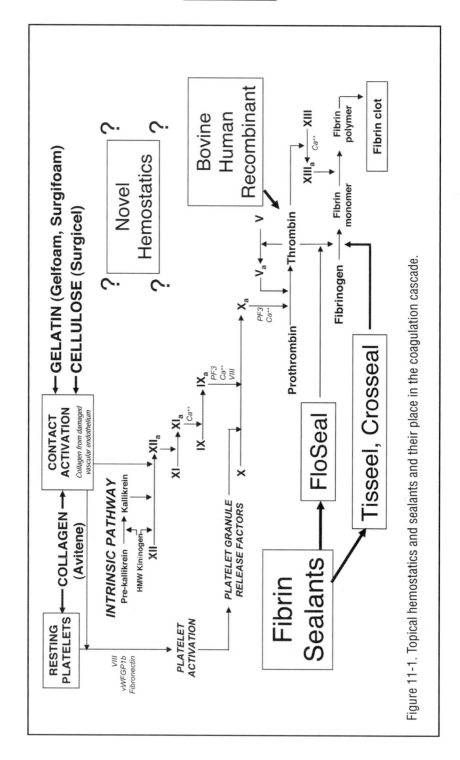

Figure 11-1. Topical hemostatics and sealants and their place in the coagulation cascade.

Surgicel (or Oxycel) is made from oxidized regenerated cellulose. It is derived from alpha cellulose and is plant based. Surgicel has a "knit" form to its structure. Like Gelfoam, Surgicel activates the intrinsic system proximally by contact activation, thus requiring functional clotting factors to form a clot. Surgicel is also thought to have bacteriostatic properties because of its relatively low pH, causing denaturing of bacterial proteins. The product is applied dry and is absorbed by the body within 4 to 8 weeks. Postoperative imaging of recently placed Surgicel may appear as ring-enhancing lesions that can be mistaken for an abscess cavity or tumor recurrence.[5] Although Surgicel has an antimicrobial effect relative to the other hemostatic agents, it can still be a nidus for infection. Therefore, it should always be removed if possible, before the incision is closed. Also, as with any foreign substance, the product causes a certain amount of foreign body reaction and granulation formation.[6]

Avitene (Davol, Murray Hill, NJ), a microfibrillar collagen, is derived from bovine skin. It is most commonly used in a light flour form. It adheres tightly to body surfaces and can be very difficult to manipulate. It is best applied in as dry a field as possible because it must achieve contact with the tissue surface before being washed away. As a collagen, Avitene activates the intrinsic coagulation system proximally by contact activation, and it directly activates platelets. The body absorbs it within 3 months. Avitene has the most significant surrounding edema and foreign body reaction when compared with other agents. It is recommended that pressure be applied until clot formation, thus allowing as much of the product as possible to be removed to minimize foreign body reaction. Arterial embolization and allergic reactions are also reported complications.[4]

Second-Generation Topical Hemostatics

FloSeal, introduced in 1999, is a hemostatic sealant composed of bovine thrombin and cross-linked gelatin granules that are mixed together. FloSeal directly activates fibrinogen and converts it into fibrin monomers, requiring functional fibrinogen for clot formation. FloSeal does not swell to the same extent as Gelfoam does because of the structural cross-linking of the gelatin granules. It can thus be used in more enclosed spaces. It is absorbed in approximately 6 to 8 weeks and is often used in acute anterior epistaxis.[7]

CoSeal is another product in which the mechanism of action depends on host coagulation factors. The product contains two polyethylene glycol polymers that combine to form a covalently bonded gel. It is indicated for use in vascular reconstructions to achieve adjunctive hemostasis by mechanically sealing areas of leakage. CoSeal is stored at room temperature, is easily prepared, and has no animal or human proteins, thus no risk of disease transmission or allergic reaction.

BioGlue (Cryolife, Kennesaw, GA) is a two-component surgical adhesive and sealant composed of bovine serum albumin and glutaraldehyde. Clinical studies have demonstrated that BioGlue is safe and effective at reducing anastomotic bleeding during cardiac procedures.[8] It is stored at room temperature and is easily prepared, with no premixing required. The product has also been shown to be effective in iatrogenic splenic injuries and to help prevent bile leakage after major liver resection.[9,10]

Hydrogen Peroxide

As a topical hemostatic agent, 3% hydrogen peroxide has been applied to tangential excisions of burn patients. It provides an adjunct to topical epinephrine for hemostasis and has been most useful clinically with known platelet dysfunction.[11] Hydrogen peroxide soaks have not resulted in complications related to corrosive damage, oxygen gas formation, or lipid peroxidation, which are associated with high concentrations of hydrogen peroxide. In addition, there are no reports of interference with skin graft take at the wound bed after use of hydrogen peroxide.

Topical Thrombin

Thrombin is a naturally derived enzyme that plays a role in hemostasis, inflammation, and cell signaling. The potent hemostatic properties of thrombin derive from its ability to activate platelets directly, causing them to aggregate and adhere to damaged vessels and to catalyze the formation of a fibrin matrix. Application of exogenous thrombin bypasses the physiologic process of generating a thrombin burst by directly initiating the terminal reactions of clot formation. Thrombin has been purified from numerous sources and used as a clinical aid for topical hemostasis for more than 60 years.

Because of ease of use and apparent effectiveness, thrombin is routinely used as an aid for topical hemostasis in nearly all types of surgical procedures, including, but not limited to, cardiovascular, orthopedic, neurologic, general, gynecologic, and dental procedures. It is estimated that, because of widespread acceptance of thrombin in the surgical setting, at least 1 million patients in the United States are treated with topical applications of thrombin every year.[12] The only thrombin currently approved by the Food and Drug Administration (FDA) as a stand-alone hemostatic product in the United States is derived from bovine sources. Bovine thrombin has potent biologic activity in its ability to convert fibrinogen to fibrin, to activate platelets, and to induce vascular contraction. However, bovine-derived thrombin is a potent stimulator of the immune system and has been associated with clinical syndromes that range from severe postoperative bleeding to high rates of vascular bypass thrombosis and the induction of lupus-like autoimmune syndrome in mice.[12]

The current thrombin used to control surgical bleeding is primarily derived from bovine plasma, with a small percentage from human plasma. Human thrombin isolated from pooled plasma carries the risk of transmission of plasma-borne pathogens or prion disease. The bovine preparations have been associated with protein and preparative contaminants that pose the potential risk of developing cross-reacting antibodies. Recombinant human thrombin has been efficiently produced and is free of process-derived contaminants. It has been described extensively in terms of composition, structure, and enzymatic activity.[13] In-vivo studies have shown that it is effective in achieving hemostasis in a rabbit liver excisional wound model, but clinical studies are ongoing to evaluate its safety and efficacy as an adjunct to hemostasis in patients undergoing surgery.[13]

Fibrin Sealants

Fibrin sealant products contain both thrombin and fibrinogen, thereby effectively bypassing the clotting cascade. They differ in the origin of the fibrinogen and the thrombin used. The earliest form was prepared using the patient's own plasma. The patient's blood was drawn in the operating room and centrifuged to collect the plasma, which was combined with bovine thrombin in double-lumen delivery syringes. The benefit of such autologous donation is that no risk exists for transmission of blood-borne diseases. Products that use heterologous donation (Evicel and Tisseel) are produced from bovine plasma or pooled human plasma from donors who undergo screening and viral testing.

The ideal fibrin sealant should be clinically effective, safe, usable, and cost-effective. Clinical effectiveness is associated with high-molecular bonding and surface-adherence strength. These qualities translate into appropriate clot formation, hemostasis, and tissue healing by fibroblastic growth and adhesiveness. Fibrin sealants should carry no risk of transmission of blood-borne pathogens, such as disease-causing viral uses. The sealants should not have serious side effects and should be biodegradable in a reasonable amount of time. The ideal fibrin sealant is prepared rapidly and simply in the operating room. It should solidify quickly but application time must allow for manipulation. Cost-effectiveness of the product depends not only on the actual cost of the sealant but also on the potential benefits of reduced morbidity and hospital stay.

Commercial Products

Two fibrin sealants are available in the United States for commercial use: Tisseel (bovine-derived) and Evicel (human-derived).

Tisseel is licensed for use as an adjunct to hemostasis in operations involving cardiopulmonary bypass and for treatment of splenic injuries from blunt or penetrating trauma to the abdomen when control of bleeding by conventional techniques is ineffective or impractical. It is also licensed as an adjunct in the closure of colostomies. Tisseel contains bovine-derived components and can cause allergic or anaphylactic reactions in cases of hypersensitivity to bovine proteins or after repeated use.

Evicel, a second-generation fibrin sealant, is licensed as an adjunct to hemostasis in patients undergoing liver surgery when control of bleeding by conventional surgical techniques is ineffective or impractical. Evicel is composed of pooled human fibrinogen and thrombin, as well as synthetic tranexamic acid. Because of the tranexamic acid, the product must not be used in contact with cerebrospinal fluid or dura mater.

Clinical Uses of Fibrin Sealants

The commercial agents that are available for use in the United States are approved for hemostasis during operations such as coronary artery bypass, repair of splenic trauma, liver resection, and sealing of colonic anastomoses at the time of colostomy closure. In cardiac surgery, coagulopathy ensues as a result of fibrinolysis and platelet dysfunction from the cardiopulmonary bypass pump and the use of heparin to prevent clotting in the bypass circuit. Despite the use of protamine to reverse the effect of heparin, a randomized, prospective clinical trial using fibrin sealant reduced the volume of bleeding and the need for reoperation. Although the use of fibrin sealants in a variety of surgical procedures is documented in the literature, sealants are not a substitute for surgical sutures and excellent surgical technique. Sealants will not stop active arterial bleeding when a suture is required.

Reinforcing anastomoses with fibrin sealant before recirculation of blood—by allowing the sealant to polymerize for a period of 1 to 2 minutes—has demonstrated excellent results in achieving hemostasis and has been shown to be superior to the use of manual pressure, bovine thrombin, and oxidized-regenerated cellulose in hand-sewn polytetrafluoroethylene, or PTFE, grafts.[14] With venous microvascular anastomoses, however, the use of fibrin sealant with concentrations of thrombin in excess of 500 IU/mL may contribute to an increased rate of thrombosis.[15] Fibrin sealant has also been reported to be a satisfactory means of providing external support to vein grafts that will be subjected to arterial pressures, and it appears to reduce endothelial cell injury.[16]

Three major applications of fibrin sealant in plastic surgery and burn treatment have been described. First, it can be used as a hemostatic agent following burn debridement, with or without skin grafting.[17,18] Second, it can be used to immediately attach new grafts and to improve graft survival in a variety of clinical situations.[19] In burn wound management, the fibrin sealant helps achieve hemostasis and contributes to the successful placement, attachment, and survival of a skin graft. For instance, fibrin sealants reduce the need for drains in muscle flap procedures and in extensive soft tissue dissections.[20,21] Third, with facelift procedures, the necessity for drains can be eliminated, thereby reducing hematoma formation, edema, and ecchymosis.[22]

In orthopedic surgery, the applications of fibrin sealant are most evident in joint replacement. Patients undergoing such surgeries can have significant blood loss and an increased risk of developing deep venous thrombosis and pulmonary embolism. Fibrin sealants allow for hemostasis and permit the early use of prophylaxis for deep venous thrombosis. Literature has supported significant reductions in blood loss in both knee replacement and hip replacement when fibrin sealants were used.[23,24] Other orthopedic applications and benefits include increased ingrowth during repair of tendons and articular defects, enhanced bone induction, improved bone graft filling, strengthened fracture fixation, improved spinal fusion, and improved implant fixation.[21]

In trauma surgery, fibrin sealant has been a valuable adjunct to both liver and spleen procedures. Evicel and Tisseel have been approved in the United States for use in liver and splenic injuries, respectively. Fibrin sealant is particularly useful in liver injuries, which can be associated with significant blood loss, whereas use in splenic injuries is largely reserved for splenic salvage techniques. Fibrin sealants for use in mass casualty situations are under investigation but have not yet obtained FDA approval for use in the United States.

The currently available fibrin sealants have also been approved for use as adjuncts to colonic anastomosis at the time of colostomy closure. Their use is controversial in many colonic anastomoses, however, especially in challenging situations such as fecal peritonitis and high-risk or hand-sewn anastomoses.[25,26] Their use in laparoscopic treatment of perforated peptic ulcers, bleeding ulcers, and endoscopic control of bleeding peptic ulcers is still investigational. The use of fibrin sealants in the management of anal and colonic fistula has been gaining support in a large body of literature.[27] That support stems from ease of application, absence of pain, and decreased likelihood of causing incontinence, although the long-term success rate has yet to be determined.

The Cochrane Database Review performed a meta-analysis of seven quality trials of fibrin sealants.[28] The reviewing body chose only trials in which fibrin sealant was used as a method to minimize perioperative blood transfusion. It found a reduced rate of exposure to allogeneic blood transfusions by 54% (relative risk = 0.46; 95% confidence interval = 0.32-0.68), coinciding with reduced blood loss (average = 134 mL/patient).[28] The finding suggests that, on the whole, fibrin sealants are effective and can be used to minimize operative blood loss.

Novel Hemostatics

Poly-N-acetyl glucosamine (P-NAG) is a naturally occurring, biodegradable, complex polysaccharide. Found in a variety of marine life, it is commercially obtained by a fermentation process and is isolated from microalgal cultures. P-NAG is called *chitin* when it is acetylated, and *chitosan* when most of the compound is deacetylated. Mechanisms of action are not completely clear but may involve adhesiveness to tissues, attraction of circulating blood cells, nitric oxide scavenging, and vasoconstriction mediated by endothelin-1.[29] Different forms of P-NAG have been used in the control of injury bleeding, including splenic lacerations, esophageal varices, and capillary oozing in neurosurgery. In addition, the Syvek patch (Marine Polymer Technologies, Danvers, MA), which has been available for some time, is used to stop bleeding from blood vessel access sites. The efficacy of chitosan has been demonstrated in one large animal study of uncontrolled, brisk liver bleeding. The study showed a significant decrease in the volume of blood loss and resuscitation volume as well as increased survival in the chitosan group.[30]

QuikClot (Z-Medica, Wallingford, CT), a granular mineral zeolite, has been shown to have excellent hemostatic properties. It is an inert product composed of oxides of silicone, aluminum, sodium, and magnesium as well as small amounts of quartz. The synthetic zeolite acts as a molecular sieve and absorbs water. That process generates heat (exothermic process), which is physical rather than chemical in nature. Maximal temperatures reached are 42 to 44 C for a duration of 30 to 60 seconds. The process concentrates the platelets and clotting factors, thereby promoting rapid clot formation. In animal models of complex, lethal vascular and soft tissue injuries of the groin, application of 3.5 ounces of QuikClot 5 minutes after injury significantly decreased mortality and reduced blood loss compared with application of a standard dressing.[31]

Autologous platelet gel (APG) is a fibrin and platelet tissue adhesive produced from autologous platelet-rich plasma. APG was developed in the early 1990s as a byproduct of platelet-rich plasma sequestration in cardiac surgery.[32,33] The process of sequestration involves removing whole blood from the patient, followed by fractionation into platelet-poor plasma, platelet-rich plasma (PRP), and red cells. The combination of PRP with thrombin and calcium results in the rapid formation of a viscous coagulum (gel). The thrombin can be either autologous or bovine. Soon, there will be a recombinant thrombin available for use.

Devices for application are similar to the devices used for fibrin sealants. APG can be sprayed or squirted onto a tissue surface. PRP can be generated during surgery with a variety of blood recovery machines. Additionally, a number of companies manufacture tabletop devices that can be used to manufacture small amounts of PRP. The Smart PReP (Harvest Technologies, Plymouth, MA), the Biomet GPS II system (Biomet Biologics, Warsaw, IN), and the Dideco Angel (Sorin Group, Mirandola Modena, Italy) are several examples of these tabletop devices. The indications, contraindications, and properties of platelet gel are summarized in Appendix 11-1. Similar to fibrin tissue adhesives, APG is thought to have hemostatic and tissue-sealing properties. APG is also thought to speed wound healing and enhance osteogenesis through concentrated platelet-derived growth factors. At this time, these clinical benefits are purely theoretical and not convincingly demonstrated by clinical trials.

Conclusion

The ideal topical hemostatic should be inexpensive, easily stored and prepared, highly efficacious (even in the absence of clotting factors), bacteriocidal, biodegradable, and free of adverse effects or consequences. While not one of the available topical hemostatics or fibrin sealants meets all of these requirements, each has properties that can be useful in various situations. The choice of a hemostatic agent will be dictated by local availability, expediency (ability to wait for preparation time), and the patient's coagulation status. Familiarity with all of the options—then using the right agent at the right time—is the best approach to optimize hemostasis. Future developments are sure to bring even more complexity to the growing line of hemostatic agents.

References

1. Bergel S. Uber die wirkung des fibrins. Dtsch Med Wochenschr 1909;35:663-5.
2. Harvey S. The use of fibrin paper and forms in surgery. Boston Med Surg J 1916;174:658.
3. Young J, Medawar P. Fibrin suture of peripheral nerves. Lancet 1940;ii:126-32.
4. Schonauer C, Tessitore E, Barbagallo G, et al. The use of local agents: Bone wax, gelatin, collagen, oxidized cellulose. Eur Spine J 2004;13(Suppl 1):S89-96.
5. Sabel M, Stummer W. The use of local agents: Surgicel and Surgifoam. Eur Spine J 2004;13(Suppl 1):S97-101.
6. Tomizawa Y. Clinical benefits and risk analysis of topical hemostats: A review. J Artif Organs 2005;8:137-42.
7. Mathiasen RA, Cruz RM. Prospective, randomized, controlled clinical trial of a novel matrix hemostatic sealant in patients with acute anterior epistaxis. Laryngoscope 2005;115:899-902.
8. Coselli JS, Bavaria JE, Fehrenbacher J, et al. Prospective randomized study of a protein-based tissue adhesive used as a hemostatic and structural adjunct in cardiac and vascular anastomotic repair procedures. J Am Coll Surg 2003; 197:243-52; discussion 252-3.
9. Biggs G, Hafron J, Feliciano J, Hoenig DM. Treatment of splenic injury during laparoscopic nephrectomy with BioGlue, a surgical adhesive. Urology 2005; 66:882.
10. Abouljoud M, Yoshida A, Kim D, Jerius J. Safety and efficacy of BioGlue in preventing bile leakage after major liver resections. Presented at the sixth World Congress of the International Hepato-Pancreato-Biliary Association, Washington, DC, June 2, 2004.
11. Potyondy L, Lottenberg L, Anderson J, Mozingo DW. The use of hydrogen peroxide for achieving dermal hemostasis after burn excision in a patient with platelet dysfunction. J Burn Care Res 2006;27:99-101.
12. Lawson JH. The clinical use and immunologic impact of thrombin in surgery. Semin Thromb Hemost 2006;32(Suppl 1):98-110.
13. Bishop PD, Lewis KB, Schultz J, Walker KM. Comparison of recombinant human thrombin and plasma-derived human alpha-thrombin. Semin Thromb Hemost 2006;32(Suppl 1):86-97.
14. Unlu Y, Vural U, Kocak H, et al. Comparison of the topical haemostatic agents for the prevention of suture hole bleeding: An experimental study. Eur J Vasc Endovasc Surg 2002;23:441-4.
15. Frost-Arner L, Spotnitz WD, Rodeheaver GT, Drake DB. Comparison of the thrombogenicity of internationally available fibrin sealants in an established microsurgical model. Plast Reconstr Surg 2001;108:1655-60.
16. Stooker W, Niessen HW, Wildevuur WR, et al. Perivenous application of fibrin glue reduces early injury to the human saphenous vein graft wall in an ex vivo model. Eur J Cardiothorac Surg 2002;21:212-17.
17. Nervi C, Gamelli RL, Greenhalgh DG, et al. A multicenter clinical trial to evaluate the topical hemostatic efficacy of fibrin sealant in burn patients. J Burn Care Rehabil 2001;22:99-103.

18. McGill V, Kowal-Vern A, Lee M, et al. Use of fibrin sealant in thermal injury. J Burn Care Rehabil 1997;18:429-34.

19. Mittermayr R, Wassermann E, Thurnher M, et al. Skin graft fixation by slow clotting fibrin sealant applied as a thin layer. Burns 2006;32:305-11.

20. Kulber DA, Bacilious N, Peters ED, et al. The use of fibrin sealant in the prevention of seromas. Plast Reconstr Surg 1997;99:842-9; discussion 850-1.

21. Spotnitz WD, Prabhu R. Fibrin sealant tissue adhesive—review and update. J Long Term Eff Med Implants 2005;15:245-70.

22. Oliver DW, Hamilton SA, Figle AA, et al. A prospective, randomized, double-blind trial of the use of fibrin sealant for face lifts. Plast Reconstr Surg 2001;108:2101-5; discussion 2106-7.

23. Curtin WA, Wang GJ, Goodman NC, et al. Reduction of hemorrhage after knee arthroplasty using cryo-based fibrin sealant. J Arthroplasty 1999;14:481-7.

24. Wang GJ, Goldthwaite CA Jr, Burks S, et al. Fibrin sealant reduces perioperative blood loss in total hip replacement. J Long Term Eff Med Implants 2003;13:399-411.

25. Byrne DJ, Hardy J, Wood RA, et al. Adverse influence of fibrin sealant on the healing of high-risk sutured colonic anastomoses. J R Coll Surg Edinb 1992; 37:394-8.

26. van der Ham AC, Kort WJ, Weijma IM, et al. Effect of fibrin sealant on the integrity of colonic anastomoses in rats with faecal peritonitis. Eur J Surg 1993; 159:425-32.

27. Lamont JP, Hooker G, Espenschied JR, et al. Closure of proximal colorectal fistulas using fibrin sealant. Am Surg 2002;68:615-18.

28. Carless PA, Henry DA, Anthony DM. Fibrin sealant use for minimizing peri-operative allogeneic blood transfusion. Cochrane Database Syst Rev 2003;(2): CD004171.

29. Favuzza J, Hechtman HB. Hemostasis in the absence of clotting factors. J Trauma 2004;57(Suppl 1):S42-4.

30. Jewelewicz DD, Cohn SM, Crookes BA, Proctor KG. Modified rapid deployment hemostat bandage reduces blood loss and mortality in coagulopathic pigs with severe liver injury. J Trauma 2003;55:275-80; discussion 280-1.

31. Alam HB, Uy GB, Miller D, et al. Comparative analysis of hemostatic agents in a swine model of lethal groin injury. J Trauma 2003;54:1077-82.

32. Oz MC, Jeevanandam V, Smith CR, et al. Autologous fibrin glue from intraoperatively collected platelet-rich plasma. Ann Thorac Surg 1992;53:530-1.

33. Tawes RL Jr, Sydorak GR, DuVall TB. Autologous fibrin glue: The last step in operative hemostasis. Am J Surg 1994;168:120-2.

Appendix 11-1. Indications, Contraindications, and Properties of Platelet Gel

	Properties
Indications	
Hemostasis	Binding of tissues
	Activates coagulation cascade locally
	Adheres platelets to wound surfaces
	Has high concentration of fibrinogen and platelets
Wound healing	Use for liver, spleen, pancreas, kidney, lung, dura
	Has high concentration of PDGF for impaired wound healing (caused by DM, PVD, radiation, chemotherapy, malnutrition, steroids, smoking)
Bone graft/osteogenesis	Augments osteogenesis in cancellous bone grafts (with platelet gel)
	Augments osteogenesis in large osseous defects, multilevel spinal fusions, nonunions (with osteogenic bone gel)
Nonhealing Wounds	Improves nonhealing wounds with PDGF and platelets
	Warrants further study
Contraindications	
Coagulation defects	Thrombocytopenia
	Hypofibrinogenemia
	Anticoagulation use
Hypersensitivity	Hypersensitivity to bovine thrombin
Technical factors (insufficient plasma sample)	Poor venous access
	Patient size

PDGF = platelet-derived growth factor; DM = dermatomyositis; PVD = peripheral vascular disease.

In: Waters JH, ed.
Blood Management: Options for Better Patient Care
Bethesda, MD: AABB Press, 2008

12

Ancillary Techniques

GREGORY A. NUTTALL, MD, AND WILLIAM C. OLIVER, MD

A HIGH PERCENTAGE OF ALLOGENEIC BLOOD is given to patients in the operating room, especially to patients undergoing cardiac surgery and liver transplantation.[1,2] Multiple surgical and nonsurgical factors can affect blood loss and blood transfusion in surgery. This chapter addresses several common factors and ancillary techniques that are used during surgery to reduce bleeding and transfusion requirements.

Gregory A. Nuttall, MD, and William C. Oliver, MD, Associate Professors of Anesthesiology, The Department of Anesthesiology, Mayo College of Medicine, Rochester, Minnesota

Volume Expanders and Choice of Infusion Fluids

Management of fluid therapy is a key component of the care of surgical patients. Fluid therapy is used to maintain effective intravascular volume. Patients who undergo surgery with significant bleeding and tissue injury usually receive large amounts of fluid. Maintaining normovolemia minimizes the occurrence of hypoperfusion and ischemia as well as subsequent reperfusion injury. Hypovolemia can lead to organ dysfunction, which increases morbidity and mortality, whereas adequate circulating blood volume improves outcome.[3]

Intravenous fluid is used in the operating room to restore and maintain intravascular volume and hemodynamic stability. In situations of excessive blood loss, the ideal fluid to maintain an effective circulating volume is whole blood because it is being lost. Unfortunately, however, allogeneic transfusions are complicated by infectious risks, allergic reactions, and expense.[4] Furthermore, many blood banks do not provide whole blood for transfusion purposes. Other fluids such as crystalloids, colloids, or a combination of the two have consequently been adopted to meet volume replacement demands associated with surgical procedures. The most commonly administered fluids for perioperative volume replacement in the United States are 1) the colloids, 5% albumin and hydroxyethyl starch (HES), and 2) crystalloids such as lactated Ringer's (LR) solution and normal saline.

Crystalloids

Crystalloid solutions of various electrolyte compositions, particularly LR, have been advocated for fluid resuscitation and maintenance of intravascular volume with surgical hemorrhage for years.[5] Crystalloid solutions are thought to equilibrate between the extravascular and intravascular spaces according to a defined ratio. Early work indicated that as little as 9% of crystalloid remained intravascularly, while 90% leaked into the interstitium. Other studies have reported that 25% of crystalloid volume remains intravascularly, thereby accounting for the widely held recommendation of replacing 1 mL of blood loss with 4 mL of crystalloid.[6] The body's ability to retain certain fluids appears to be altered by hemorrhage, whereby nearly 50% of LR may effectively remain in the plasma volume during hemorrhage. But over time, the plasma volume expands only by 20%. More recently, the 4:1 ratio of LR to blood loss replacement has been challenged on the basis of data that indicate LR may expand the intravascular volume by 50%.[7] Therefore, these studies suggest that LR replacement of blood loss should occur in a ratio of 2:1 or even 1:1, instead of 4:1. Furthermore, the blood-expanding effect of crystalloid was very short lived. The uncertainty regarding the amount of crystalloid necessary to replace ongoing blood loss and maintain effective circulating volume is a drawback for crystalloid resuscitation.

Because of the distribution problems described above, large volumes of crystalloid may be required to maintain intravascular volume in situations of blood loss and tissue damage. Large volumes of crystalloid may lead to the accumulation of extravascular lung water, resulting in interstitial edema and possibly pulmonary edema. Pulmonary edema may compromise oxygenation and oxygen delivery in the operating room and the intensive care unit (ICU). It also can prolong the duration of ventilation and ICU stay, as well as morbidity and mortality.[8] The expansion of blood volume with colloid is more than twice the expansion possible with crystalloid rapid infusion. McIlroy et al[9] found 6% HES to be significantly more effective as a blood volume expander than crystalloid in healthy volunteers made moderately hypovolemic by phlebotomy of 1000 mL of blood.

Colloids

Colloids have been advocated for volume expansion and resuscitation for many years.[10] The primary colloids in routine clinical use worldwide are albumin, HES, dextran, and gelatin. Colloid fluids have been added or substituted for crystalloid fluids in an effort to control the distribution of water between the interstitial and intravascular spaces. The basis for colloid administration is the importance of colloid oncotic pressure (COP) in modulating fluid flux between the vascular and interstitial spaces. The greater COP observed with colloid fluids allows expansion of plasma volume to a greater degree than their administered volume without expanding interstitial space to the same extent as crystalloid fluids. An increased intravascular volume may partially account for recent evidence demonstrating that colloids or whole blood maintained hemodynamics more effectively than crystalloids, thus resulting in less end-organ damage during excessive bleeding and trauma.

The two most commonly used colloid fluids in the United States are albumin and HES. Albumin has historically been considered the most beneficial colloid because it is a naturally occurring protein. It binds cations and anions and may act as a scavenger of free radicals, potentially benefiting patients who develop inflammatory reactions.[11] Albumin may pass through damaged capillary membranes to remain in the interstitium, attracting additional fluid, so the advisability of giving albumin to patients with inflammatory reactions is uncertain. Other concerns of albumin usage include shortages, Creutzfeldt-Jakob disease transmission, anaphylactic reactions, and greater expense.

HES is a synthetic colloid substituted for albumin. It is available in many different forms, reflecting both average molecular weight and extent of molar substitution. In the United States, only the 6% HES of high molecular weight (450 kDa) and 0.7 molar substitution ratio has been used in routine fluid management.[12] It is inexpensive, widely available, devoid of infectious risks, and long acting.[13] In the United States, dextran is less extensively used for fluid management than is HES, and gelatin is unavailable for clinical use.

Numerous studies have indicated that HES administration can lead to reduction in circulating Factor VIII and von Willebrand factor levels; to impairment of platelet function, resulting in prolongation of partial thromboplastin time and activated partial thromboplastin time; and to an increase in bleeding complications.[14] Problems with coagulopathy and excessive bleeding associated with the use of HES occur predominantly in cardiac surgery with cardiopulmonary bypass (CPB).[12,15-17] CPB induces transient-acquired platelet dysfunction and dilution of both platelet count and coagulation factor concentrations, which may be aggravated by the use of HES. The effects of HES on clinical bleeding in cardiac surgery depend on the volume of HES administered; however, excessive postoperative bleeding has been reported with less than the recommended maximum HES doses.[18]

Comparison of Infusion Fluids

Because of those concerns, a debate has continued for more than 30 years as to which fluid is superior for volume resuscitation: crystalloids or colloids. Until recently, the majority of studies have had small samples that were underpowered for detecting clinically significant differences in patient outcome. This has resulted in the use of meta-analysis in an effort to resolve the issue.[19-22] The results of the meta-analysis studies have varied over a wide range. The Cochrane Injuries Group Albumin Reviewers published a meta-analysis that included 24 studies involving a total of 1419 patients. The reviewers found that—compared with normal saline—albumin administration was associated with a 6% increased risk of death (relative risk = 1.68; 95% confidence interval, 1.26-2.23). Similar findings were noted for patients with hypovolemia, hypoproteinemia, and burns.[19] As a result of that study, the Food and Drug Administration (FDA) sent a "Letter to Healthcare Providers" on August 19, 1998, in which the agency expressed serious concern over the safety of albumin administration in the critically ill population and urged treating physicians to exercise discretion in its use.[23] A subsequent meta-analysis of 55 trials that involved a total of 3504 patients examined the effect of resuscitation with albumin-containing fluid on the risk of death in a general population of patients and did not find a significant increase in the risk of death.[22] The conflicting results of these meta-analyses have left many clinicians unsure about the effect of albumin-containing fluids on survival in critically ill patients.

The largest study to date to compare the use of crystalloid vs colloid for resuscitation,[24] was performed by the Saline vs Albumin Fluid Evaluation (SAFE) Study in 16 ICUs in Australia and New Zealand. It randomly assigned 6997 ICU patients to either 4% albumin or normal saline for vascular fluid resuscitation over a period of 28 days. The primary outcome measure was death from any cause during the 28-day period following randomization. The study was not blinded. The two groups had similar baseline characteristics. There were 726 deaths in the albumin group, and 729 deaths in the saline group (relative risk of death = 0.99; 95% confidence interval, 0.91-1.09; p = 0.87). There was no difference in the proportion of patients with new single-organ and multiple-organ failure in the two groups (p = 0.85). There also were no significant differences between the groups in the mean (± standard deviation, or SD) number of days spent in the ICU (6.5 ±6.6 in the albumin group and 6.2 ±6.2 in the saline group; p = 0.44), hospital days (15.3 ±9.6 and 15.6 ±9.6, respectively; p = 0.30), days of mechanical ventilation (4.5 ±6.1 and 4.3 ±5.7, respectively; p = 0.74), or days of renal dialysis (0.5 ±2.3 and 0.4 ±2.0, respectively; p = 0.41).

A secondary analysis of prespecified subgroups of patients with adult respiratory distress syndrome, severe sepsis, and trauma were consistent overall with those findings. In addition, an exploratory analysis of trauma patients with concomitant traumatic brain injury showed increased mortality in the albumin treatment arm (relative risk of mortality = 1.36; 95% confidence interval, 0.99-1.86). A higher survival rate was observed in the albumin-treated patients with severe sepsis, but because that finding was not statistically significant (p = 0.09), its clinical significance remains uncertain. SAFE Study Investigators concluded that—for ICU patients—use of either 4% albumin or normal saline for fluid resuscitation results in similar outcomes at 28 days.

On May 16, 2005, the FDA issued a notice to revise the agency's previous advice regarding the safety of albumin administration in critically ill patients.[25] That action was taken following the FDA's review of recent studies on the safety of albumin. The FDA's revised position is consistent with recommendations made on March 17, 2005, by members of the Blood Products Advisory Committee (BPAC), who voted unanimously that the SAFE study had resolved the prior safety concerns raised by the Cochrane Injuries Group in 1998. BPAC noted that the relative safety of albumin for use in patients with burns cannot be determined at this time because that group was excluded from the SAFE study. BPAC also noted that further evaluation of albumin in patients with traumatic brain injury and septic shock will have to be performed to ascertain the safety of albumin administration in these patient populations.

Another concern with the use of intravenous fluids is dilutional coagulopathy. Administration of non-blood intravenous fluids is known to result in dilution of humeral and cellular blood elements.[26,27] Administration of Red Blood Cells (RBCs) with fluids will result in dilution of coagulation factors and platelet count because RBCs have very little plasma or platelets. Therefore, when large volumes of intravenous fluids with or without RBCs are administered, a dilutional coagulopathy can result.

Dilutional coagulopathy is especially a problem with massive trauma. There are multiple causes of coagulopathy in trauma patients, and dilution is certainly a contributor. Usually, the injured patient initially bleeds without any replacement. The patient then receives crystalloids en route to the hospital and blood only when he or she is in the operating room. In the era of whole blood transfusion, thrombocytopenia was the initial event of dilutional coagulopathy.[28] With the use of RBC transfusions today, dilution of clotting factors is the initial event.[29] The problem must be anticipated and corrected in patients who require large volumes of fluid for volume resuscitation.

Deliberate Hypotension

One method of reducing intraoperative blood loss and transfusion requirements during anesthesia for major surgery is the use of controlled, deliberate hypotension.[30] This strategy can also produce a drier field, thereby increasing the ease of surgery and the likelihood of a good surgical result. The technique has been used with many surgical procedures, especially major spinal surgery.[31] One study involving blood loss in spinal surgery found that reducing mean arterial blood pressure by 20 mm Hg resulted in a 50% reduction in blood loss and a 36% reduction in the need for blood transfusions.[32] Another study involving posterior spinal fusion patients found that reducing mean arterial pressure to less than 80 mm Hg resulted in a 33% reduction in blood loss.[33] Hypotension may be achieved with increased doses of volatile anesthetic agents or by continuous infusion of vasodilating drugs such as nitroprusside. Safe application of deliberate hypotension requires knowledge of the physiology of hemorrhagic shock and close, usually invasive intraoperative monitoring to avoid vasoconstriction and end-organ ischemia.

The benefits of deliberate hypotension must be weighed against the risks of inadequate cerebral, myocardial, or renal perfusion, especially as they relate to ischemic optic neuropathy. In normotensive young patients who are healthy, those risks are minimal, but patients with long histories of hypertension show signs of cerebral ischemia at higher pressures because of up-regulation of organ autoregulation. Such patients are probably at higher risk of complications from deliberate hypotension. Ischemic optic neuropathy is a rare but devastating complication that has resulted in blindness in patients undergoing spinal surgery.[34-36] Possible contributing causes of ischemic optic neuropathy include both lower mean arterial blood pressure associated with deliberate hypotension and increases in intraocular pressure from prone positioning that result in reduced perfusion of the optic nerve, especially when combined with anemia and atherosclerotic disease.[37,38]

Positioning

Positioning of the patient before surgery is an important step in the overall surgical procedure, especially for spine surgery. The ideal patient position should facilitate surgical exposure, minimize both bleeding and damage to vital structures, and allow adequate perfusion of the organs and ventilation of the lungs.[39] Many patient positions can be used for various surgical procedures. Each position has advantages from the standpoint of surgical exposure. Each also has disadvantages that may result in patient injuries such as nerve damage and compression of vessels resulting in ischemia. The focus of this section is the effect of positioning on blood loss and specifically the use of the prone position for spine surgery.

Elevation of the operative site relative to the heart will reduce bleeding by reducing hydrostatic pressure, although there is a risk of venous air embolism (VAE). VAE can be a lethal complication of surgical procedures.[40] It results when the venous pressure at the site of surgery is subatmospheric or when gas is forced under pressure into a body cavity. VAE is classically associated with neurosurgery, especially when the patient is in the sitting position, but it is also a potential complication of laparoscopic, pelvic, and orthopedic procedures.[41]

Neither the supine nor the lateral positions affect intraoperative bleeding because neither directly alters cardiopulmonary physiology. The prone position is frequently used for posterior spine surgery, and it can result in increased bleeding secondary to engorgement of vertebral veins. Near the vertebrae is a plexus of thin-walled, valveless veins known as Batson's plexus, which normally has low pressure. The vertebral veins connect to the veins in the chest, abdomen, and pelvis through intercostals. It has been shown that, in cases of inferior vena cava (IVC) obstruction, the venous return from the lower parts of the body can divert into the vertebral venous system and can return blood to the heart.[39] Pressure on the anterior abdominal is transmitted to the IVC to the point where moderate external pressure results in a big rise in IVC pressure.[40] Abdominal compression in the prone position, especially in obese patients, will also decrease respiratory compliance through displacement of the diaphragm into the chest. The reduced respiratory compliance results in high airway pressures, which in turn compromise adequate ventilation of the lungs, impairing venous return to the heart. The net effect is reduced cardiac output and increased venous pressure.[42] Through both of those mechanisms, blood flow and pressure through the venous plexus in the area vertebrae are increased—as is the possibility of intraoperative blood loss during posterior spine surgery.

Because of the mechanisms described above, intra-abdominal pressure (IAP) may influence blood loss during posterior spinal surgery.[43] In an effort to reduce intraoperative blood loss and subsequent engorgement of the vertebral veins with such surgery, multiple positions and frames have been developed. The ideal positioning should provide good surgical exposure and normal sagittal spinal alignment and should reduce IAP. The positioning in posterior spine surgery can be further complicated by the need to use a C-arm for fluoroscopy.

McNulty et al[44] performed a prospective, randomized study of the hemodynamic effects of the prone position in 18 patients randomized to one of three different prone support systems (Andrews spinal surgery frame, Cloward surgical saddle, and longitudinal bolsters). The researchers measured IVC and superior vena cava (SVC) pressures and mean arterial pressures in the supine and prone positions, as well as after repositioning. They examined the validity of measuring central venous pressure (CVP) for determining the ideal positioning of the patient, and they studied the relationships among frame type, blood loss, and hemodynamic measurements. Patients positioned on the Andrews frame had decreased mean SVC and IVC pressures when changing from the supine position to the prone position and had the lowest prone-position CVP. Blood loss was higher in the Cloward group than in the Andrews and bolsters groups.

Lee et al[45] performed a prospective, observational study of IVC pressure of 20 patients undergoing lumbar spine surgery under controlled isoflurane-induced hypotension in different positions and with different levels of blood pressure. In each patient, the IVC pressure was measured when the patient was supine, prone on a conventional pad, and prone on a Relton-Hall frame. The IVC pressure achieved a mean of 15.3 mm Hg when patients were positioned prone on a conventional pad.

When they were subsequently positioned prone on a Relton-Hall frame, the IVC pressure decreased to a mean of 8.2 mm Hg.

Park[43] performed a prospective randomized trial in 40 patients having posterior lumbar fusion. IAP was measured with a rectal balloon pressure catheter. For an examination of the relationship of IAP changes to blood loss, patients were randomly assigned to narrow (group 1) or wide (group 2) pad support widths of the Wilson frame. IAP was measured when the patient was supine after the induction of anesthesia, then prone on a gurney, prone on the Wilson frame before and after incision, and finally again supine after tracheal extubation. IAP for patients in the prone position on the Wilson frame in group 2 was significantly less than for patients in group 1. Intraoperative blood loss per vertebra in group 2 was significantly less than in group 1. There was a significant correlation between blood loss and IAP for patients in the prone position on the Wilson frame in group 1. It was concluded that IAP and intraoperative blood loss were significantly less in the wide than in the narrow pad support of the Wilson frame. Blood loss increased with an increase in IAP in the narrow pad support of the Wilson frame.

Choice of Anesthesia

The choice of anesthesia for surgery can influence surgical blood loss. Most of the studies related to choice of anesthesia have focused on the difference in blood loss between general and regional anesthesia, especially spinal and epidural anesthesia. Spinal anesthesia and epidural anesthesia are thought to reduce intraoperative surgical blood loss through reduction of afterload and, subsequently, blood pressure; to improve perioperative hemodynamic stability; and to reduce pain in the immediate postoperative period.[46]

Salonia et al[47] performed a prospective randomized study to evaluate the effect of general anesthesia vs spinal anesthesia on intraoperative and postoperative outcome in 72 patients undergoing radical retropubic prostatectomy. The overall blood loss was significantly less in the spinal group. The authors concluded that spinal anesthesia rather than general anesthesia allowed good muscle relaxation and resulted in less intraoperative blood loss, less postoperative pain, and a faster postoperative recovery.

Dunet et al[48] performed a retrospective study of 62 consecutive patients who underwent radical retropubic prostatectomy over a 2-year period. Nineteen patients who received epidural anesthesia in association with general anesthesia were compared with 43 patients who received only general anesthesia. Operative time was longer in the "general anesthesia only" group. Significantly less blood loss and lower blood transfusion rates were found in the "epidural with general anesthesia" group compared with the "general anesthesia only" group. The study authors concluded that epidural anesthesia associated with general anesthesia generated better intra- and postoperative management and resulted in significantly lower morbidity in patients undergoing radical retropubic prostatectomy, compared with those who underwent general anesthesia only.

Lertakyamanee et al[49] performed a prospective, randomized trial to compare the effectiveness of general and regional anesthesia for cesarean section; 341 patients were randomized into groups receiving general anesthesia, epidural anesthesia, or spinal anesthesia. General anesthesia resulted in significantly more blood loss, lower postoperative hematocrit, and a higher proportion of patients who had postoperative hematocrit $<30\%$ than either epidural or spinal anesthesia.

In contrast, Slappendel et al[50] used a relational database containing information about 28,861 orthopedic surgery patients to determine when and how to improve guidelines for transfusions. Their survey showed the circumstances surrounding a high incidence of allogeneic red cell infusions: failure to follow the established guidelines, preoperative use of nonselective nonsteroidal anti-inflammatory drugs, low preoperative hemoglobin levels, failure to retrieve blood, and high cutoff values for allogeneic red cell transfusion. The type of anesthesia had no blood-sparing effect.

Maintenance of Normothermia

Hypothermia is common during extensive and prolonged surgical procedures.[51] General anesthesia impairs central thermoregulation, which redistributes body heat to maintain temperature irrespective of the ambient temperature. The operating room has cool ambient temperatures, and the administration of high-volume cold fluid may also contribute to accelerated heat loss. Other factors that contribute to hypothermia, beyond a long and extensive surgical procedure, include the prolonged time required for induction of anesthesia, patient positioning, shaving, skin disinfection, and exposure of large areas of the body surface to the ambient temperature.

Different systems have been developed to prevent and control intraoperative hypothermia. Patients can be warmed 1) with a convective forced-air warming system[52,53] (Warm-Touch system, Mallinckrodt, St. Louis, MO; Bair Hugger, Arizant, Eden Prairie, MN), 2) with resistive-heating, electric carbon-fiber blankets[54] (Thermamed SmartCare OP system, Medeqco, Bad Oeynhausen, Germany), or 3) with a disposable, circulating-water warming garment[55] (Allon 2001 system, MTRE Advanced Technologies, Or-Akiva Industrial Park, Israel). Actively warming the patient causes a significant danger of skin burns, which must be avoided.[51]

Even mild hypothermia is thought to significantly increase blood loss and to augment allogeneic transfusion requirements and myocardial dysfunction.[56,57] The molecular pathophysiology of the coagulopathic effect remains to be elucidated, but hypothermia is thought to impair coagulation factor and platelet function.[56,58-60] Schmied et al[61] demonstrated that even mild hypothermia increases blood loss. In that study, patients were randomly assigned to normothermia or mild hypothermia during elective primary hip arthroplasty. A decrease of just 1.6 C core hypothermia increased blood loss by 500 mL (30%) and significantly increased allogeneic transfusion requirements. These results were confirmed by the same group in a retrospective analysis that demonstrated the hemostatic benefits of maintaining intraoperative normothermia.[62] Hofer et al[63] randomly assigned 90 patients who presented for elective, multiple, off-pump, coronary artery bypass grafting to one of the three warming systems. They found that normothermia could be sufficiently maintained during the operation only by the Allon 2001 system. They also found that the final body core temperatures were 34.7 C ±0.9 C (Warm-Touch), 35.6 C ±0.8 C (Thermamed SmartCare OP), and 36.5 C ±0.4 C (Allon 2001) (p <0.001). Perioperative blood loss and transfusion requirements were less with the Allon 2001 system.

In contrast, Johansson et al[64] studied patients who were undergoing primary prosthetic hip surgery under spinal anesthesia and who were randomized to receive forced-air warming (n = 25) or not to receive it (n = 25) during the procedure. Core temperature, as measured by the tympanic membrane, among controls decreased by 1.3 C ±0.6 C (mean ±SD). The core temperature decreased by 0.5 C ±0.4 in the warmed patients (p <0.0001). There was no difference between the groups in blood loss or in the number of allogeneic units transfused.

Perioperative hypothermia also has other adverse effects. As noted by Doufas,[65] it triples the incidence of adverse cardiac events in high-risk patients. Hypothermia adversely affects antibody- and cell-mediated immune defenses. It adversely affects the oxygen availability in the peripheral wound tissues as well and has been associated with an increased rate of surgical wound infection.[66] Kurz et al found that decreasing core hypothermia by only 1.9 C triples the incidence of surgical wound infection following colon resection and increases the duration of hospitalization by 20%. Mild perioperative hypothermia also changes the action and pharmacokinetics of various anesthetic and paralyzing agents, increases thermal discomfort, and delays recovery following anesthesia. Finally, mild hypothermia influences pulse oximetry monitoring and various electrophysiological indices of the nervous system, which can obscure interpretation of these tests and thereby can result in a delay or complete lack of therapy.

Conclusion

Blood loss and transfusion requirements in the operating room can be affected by multiple ancillary techniques. Infusion of either crystalloid or colloid fluid is necessary during surgery to maintain adequate intravascular volume. Use of some fluids for volume expansion has been associated with increased blood loss and transfusion requirements. Induction of deliberate hypotension has been successfully used to reduce blood loss, especially in spine surgery, but the benefits of that technique must be balanced against the potential risk of organ ischemia and injury. Patient positioning influences blood loss, especially if abdominal compression is present in spine surgery. Use of spinal or epidural anesthesia rather than general anesthesia has been thought to reduce intraoperative bleeding in certain operations. Although hypothermia is common during extensive and prolonged surgical procedures, efforts can be taken to minimize it. Even mild hypothermia may significantly increase blood loss, allogeneic transfusion requirements, and myocardial dysfunction.

References

1. Goodnough LT, Johnston MF, Toy PT. The variability of transfusion practice in coronary artery bypass surgery. JAMA 1991;265:86-90.
2. Stover EP, Siegel LC, Parks R, et al. Variability in transfusion practice for coronary artery bypass surgery persists despite national consensus guidelines: A 24-institution study. Institutions of the Multicenter Study of Perioperative Ischemia Research Group. Anesthesiology 1998;88:327-33.
3. Gan TJ, Soppitt A, Maroof M, et al. Goal-directed intraoperative fluid administration reduces length of hospital stay after major surgery. Anesthesiology 2002;97:820-6.
4. Nicholls MD. Transfusion: Morbidity and mortality. Anaesth Intensive Care 1993;21:15-19.
5. Choi PT, Yip G, Quinonez LG, Cook DJ. Crystalloids vs. colloids in fluid resuscitation: A systematic review. Crit Care Med 1999;27:200-10.
6. Hahn RG. Volume effect of Ringer's solution in the blood during general anaesthesia. Eur J Anaesthesiol 1998;15:427-32.
7. Riddez L, Hahn RG, Brismar B, et al. Central and regional hemodynamics during acute hypovolemia and volume substitution in volunteers. Crit Care Med 1997;25:635-9.

8. Boyd O, Grounds RM, Bennett ED. A randomized clinical trial of the effect of deliberate perioperative increase of oxygen delivery on mortality in high-risk surgical patients. JAMA 1993;270:2699-707.

9. McIlroy DR, Kaharasch ED. Acute intravascular volume expansion with rapidly administered crystalloid or colloid in the setting of moderate hypovolemia. Anesth Analg 2003;96:1572-7.

10. Velanovich V. Crystalloid versus colloid fluid resuscitation: A meta-analysis of mortality. Surgery 1989;105:65-71.

11. Boldt J, Muller M, Mentges D, et al. Volume therapy in the critically ill: Is there a difference? Intensive Care Med 1998;24:28-36.

12. Barron ME, Wilkes MM, Navickis R. A systematic review of the comparative safety of colloids. Arch Surg 2004;139:552-63.

13. Tigchelaar I, Gallandat Huet RCG, Korsten J, et al. Hemostatic effects of three colloid plasma substitutes for priming solution in cardiopulmonary bypass. Eur J Cardiothorac Surg 1997:11:626-32.

14. Jonville-Béra A, Autret-Leca E, Gruel Y. Acquired type I von Willebrand's disease associated with highly substituted hydroxyethyl starch. N Engl J Med 2001;345:622-3.

15. Cope J, Banks D, Mauney M, et al. Intraoperative hetastarch infusion impairs hemostasis after cardiac operations. Ann Thorac Surg 1997;63:78-83.

16. Knutson JE, Deering JA, Hall FW, et al. Does intraoperative hetastarch administration increase blood loss and transfusion requirements after cardiac surgery? Anesth Analg 2000;90:801-7.

17. Wilkes MM, Navickis RJ, Sibbald WJ. Albumin versus hydroxyethyl starch in cardiopulmonary bypass surgery: A meta-analysis of postoperative bleeding. Ann Thorac Surg 2001;72:527-33; discussion 534.

18. Herwaldt L, Swartzendruber S, Edmond M, et al. The epidemiology of hemorrhage related to cardiothoracic operations. Infect Control Hosp Epidemiol 1998;19:9-16.

19. Reviewers. Human albumin administration in critically ill patients: Systematic review of randomised controlled trials. BMJ 1998;317:235-40.

20. Bunn F, Alderson P, Hawkins V. Colloid solutions for fluid resuscitation. Cochrane Database Syst Rev 2003;1:CD001319-CD001319.

21. Perel P, Roberts I. Colloids versus crystalloids for fluid resuscitation in critically ill patients (review). Cochrane Database Syst Rev 2007;Oct 17:CD000567.

22. Wilkes M, Navickis R. Patient survival after human albumin administration: A meta-analysis of randomized, controlled trials. Ann Intern Med 2001;135: 149-64.

23. Feigal D. Medical Deputy Director, Center for Biologics Evaluation and Research, Food and Drug Administration. Letter to healthcare providers. (August 19, 1998; updated May 16, 2005) Rockville, MD: CBER, 1998 [Available at http://www.fda.gov/cber/ltr/albumin.htm.]

24. Finfer S, Bellomo R, Boyce N, et al. A comparison of albumin and saline for fluid resuscitation in the intensive care unit. N Engl J Med 2004;350:2247-56.

25. Food and Drug Administration. Safety of albumin administration in critically ill patients. Rockville, MD: CBER, 2005. [Available at http://www.fda.gov/cber/infosheets/albsaf051605.htm.]

26. Svensen C, Hahn R. Volume kinetics of Ringer solution, dextran 70, and hypertonic saline in male volunteers. Anesthesiology 1997;87:204-12.

27. Counts R, Haisch C, Simon T, et al. Hemostasis in massively transfused trauma patients. Ann Surg 1979;190:91-99.

28. Miller R, Robbins T, Tong M, Barton S. Coagulation defects associated with massive blood transfusion. Ann Surg 1971;174:794-801.

29. Murray D, Pennel B, Weinstein S, Olson J. Packed red cells in acute blood loss: dilutional coagulopathy as a cause of surgical bleeding. Anesth Analg 1995; 80:336-342.

30. Dutton R. Controlled hypotension for spinal surgery. Eur Spine J 2004;13 (Suppl 1):S66-71.

31. Rosenblatt M. Strategies for minimizing the use of allogeneic blood during orthopedic surgery. Mt Sinai J Med 2002;69:83-7.

32. Mandel R, Brown M, McCollough NR, Pallares V, Varlotta R. Hypotensive anesthesia and autotransfusion in spinal surgery. Clin Orthop Relat Res 1981; 154:27-33.

33. Lawhon S, Kahn AR, Crawford A, Brinker M. Controlled hypotensive anesthesia during spinal surgery: A retrospective study. Spine 1984;9:450-3.

34. Stevens W, Glazer P, Kelley S, et al. Ophthalmic complications after spinal surgery. Spine 1997;22:1319-24.

35. Dilger J, Tetzlaff J, Bell G, et al. Ischaemic optic neuropathy after spinal fusion. Can J Anaesth 1998;45:63-6.

36. Lee A. Ischemic optic neuropathy following lumbar spine surgery: Case report. J Neurosurg Anesth 1995;83:348-9.

37. Potarazu S. Ischemic optic neuropathy: Models for mechanism of disease. Clin Neurosci 1997;4:264-9.

38. Nuttall G, Garrity J, Dearani J, et al. Risk factors for ischemic optic neuropathy after cardiopulmonary bypass: A matched case/control study. Anesth Analg 2001;93:1410-16.

39. Schonauer C, Bocchetti A, Barbagallo G, et al. Positioning on surgical table. Eur Spine J 2004;13:S50-5.

40. Pearce D. The role of posture in laminectomy. Proc R Soc Med 1957;50:109-12.

41. Black S, Ockert D, Oliver WJ, Cucchiara R. Outcome following posterior fossa craniectomy in patients in the sitting or horizontal positions. Anesthesiology 1988;69:49-56.

42. Palmon S, Kirsch J, Depper J, Toung T. The effect of the prone position on pulmonary mechanics is frame-dependent. Anesth Analg 1998;87:1175-80.

43. Park C. The effect of patient positioning on intraabdominal pressure and blood loss in spinal surgery. Anesth Analg 2000;91:552-7.

44. McNulty S, Weiss J, Azad S, et al. The effect of the prone position on venous pressure and blood loss during lumbar laminectomy. J Clin Anesth 1992;4:220-5.

45. Lee T, Yang L, Chen H. Effect of patient position and hypotensive anesthesia on inferior vena caval pressure. Spine 1998;15:941-7.

46. Jellish W, Shea J. Spinal anaesthesia for spinal surgery. Best Pract Res Clin Anaesthesiol 2003;17:323-34.

47. Salonia A, Crescenti A, Suardi N, et al. General versus spinal anesthesia in patients undergoing radical retropubic prostatectomy: Results of a prospective, randomized study. Urology 2004;64:95-100.

48. Dunet F, Pfister C, Deghmani M, et al. Clinical results of combined epidural and general anesthesia procedure in radical prostatectomy management. Can J Urol 2004;11:2200-4.

49. Lertakyamanee J, Chinachoti T, Tritrakarn T, et al. Comparison of general and regional anesthesia for cesarean section: Success rate, blood loss, and satisfaction from a randomized trial. J Med Assoc Thai 1999;82:672-80.

50. Slappendel R, Dirksen R, Weber E, Van der Shaaf DB. An algorithm to reduce allogeneic red blood cell transfusions for major orthopedic surgery. Acta Orthop Scand 2003;74:569-75.

51. Gali B, Findlay J, Plevak D. Skin injury with the use of a water warming device. Anesthesiology 2003;98:1509-10.

52. Matsuzaki Y, Matsukawa T, Ohki K, et al. Warming by resistive heating maintains perioperative normothermia as well as forced air heating. Br J Anaesth 2003;90:689-91.

53. Taguchi A, Ratnaraj J, Kabon B, et al. Effects of a circulating-water garment and forced-air warming on body heat content and core temperature. Anesthesiology 2004:1058-64.

54. Camus Y, Delva E, Bossard A, et al. Prevention of hypothermia by cutaneous warming with new electric blankets during abdominal surgery. Br J Anaesth 1997;79:796-7.

55. Nesher N, Insler S, Sheinberg N, et al. A new thermoregulation system for maintaining perioperative normothermia and attenuating myocardial injury in off-pump coronary artery bypass surgery. Heart Surg Forum 2002;5:373-80.

56. Rohrer M, Natale A. Effect of hypothermia on the coagulation cascade. Crit Care Med 1992;20:1402-5.

57. Greene P, Cameron D, Mohlala M, et al. Systolic and diastolic left ventricular dysfunction due to mild hypothermia. Circulation 1989;80(5,Pt 2):III44-8.

58. Frelinger A III, Furman M, Barnard M, et al. Combined effects of mild hypothermia and glycoprotein IIb/IIIa antagonists on platelet-platelet and leukocyte-platelet aggregation. Am J Cardiol 2003;92:1099-101.

59. Yenari M, Palmer J, Bracci P, Steinberg GK. Thrombolysis with tissue plasminogen activator (tPA) is temperature dependent. Thromb Res 1995;77:475-81.

60. Valeri R, Cassidy G, Khuri S, et al. Hypothermia-induced reversible platelet dysfunction. Ann Surg 1987;205:175-81.

61. Schmied H, Kurz A, Sessler D, et al. Mild intraoperative hypothermia increases blood loss and allogeneic transfusion requirements during total hip arthroplasty. Lancet 1996;347:289-92.

62. Schmied H, Schiferer A, Sessler D, Maznik C. The effects of red-cell scavenging, hemodilution, and active warming on allogeneic blood requirement in patients undergoing hip or knee arthroplasty. Anesth Analg 1998;86:387-91.

63. Hofer C, Worn M, Tavakoli R, et al. Influence of body core temperature on blood loss and transfusion requirements during off-pump coronary artery bypass grafting: A comparison of 3 warming systems. J Thorac Cardiovasc Surg 2005;129:838-43.

64. Johansson T, Lisander B, Ivarsson I. Mild hypothermia does not increase blood loss during total hip arthroplasty. Acta Anaesthesiol Scand 1999;43:1005-10.

65. Doufas A. Consequences of inadvertent perioperative hypothermia. Best Pract Res Clin Anaesthesiol 2003;17:535-49.

66. Kurz A, Sessler D, Lenhardt R. Study of wound infections and temperature group: Perioperative normothermia to reduce the incidence of surgical-wound infection and shorten hospitalization. N Engl J Med 1996;334:1209-15.

In: Waters JH, ed.
Blood Management: Options for Better Patient Care
Bethesda, MD: AABB Press, 2008

13

Point-of-Care Testing

GREGORY A. NUTTALL, MD, AND
PAULA SANTRACH, MD

A LARGE PERCENTAGE OF ALLOGENEIC BLOOD is transfused to patients in the operating room, especially to patients undergoing cardiac surgery and liver transplantation.[1,2] It has been estimated that 20% of blood transfused in that population is thought to be inappropriate.[3] By the year 2010, it is projected that there will be large deficiencies in the blood supply in the United States as a result of the aging of the country's population.[4,5] Throughout the United States, there have already been delays in elective surgical procedures at many institutions because of shortages of blood components.[6]

Gregory A. Nuttall, MD, Associate Professor of Anesthesiology, and Paula Santrach, MD, Associate Professor of Laboratory Medicine, the Departments of Anesthesiology and Laboratory Medicine and Pathology, The Mayo Clinic, Rochester, Minnesota

Many consensus conferences and task forces of specialty societies have published recommendations for the transfusion of different blood components. They all have advocated the use of hemoglobin and coagulation tests to guide red cell and non-red-cell transfusions. But a recent survey of anesthesiologists indicates that such testing still may not be commonly performed.[7] According to the survey, the major reasons for lack of testing are as follows: 1) the time it takes for the test results to become available, 2) the unavailability of tests in the operating room, and 3) the long time required for blood components to become available. Point-of-care testing (POCT) of hemoglobin or hematocrit and coagulation allows rapid test results to be available for clinical decision making in the operating room.

POCT has matured recently from a novelty to an accepted and commonly used patient care tool. POCT is a means of providing laboratory testing at or near the site of patient care. POCT has the potential to improve patient outcome from earlier treatment by providing rapid results.[8,9] Coagulation assessment is one of the most common categories of POCT performed in the United States. POCT for hemoglobin and coagulation is most useful in certain patient populations, especially surgical patients. The combination of having an open surgical wound and the multifactorial nature of the bleeding (lack of surgical hemostasis, hypothermia, dilutional and consumptive coagulopathy, fibrinolysis, platelet dysfunction, and thrombocytopenia) make the need for information on coagulation status imperative. The time-sensitive nature of the operating room requires decisions be made in minutes. A compounding factor is the time it takes to get allogeneic blood ready for transfusion, especially for platelets, which must be pooled, and for Fresh Frozen Plasma (FFP), which must be thawed. Knowing test results quickly is a major advantage of POCT in that it can reduce the time the patient experiences blood loss without proper transfusion therapy.

The surgical patients who most benefit from POCT for hemoglobin and coagulation are generally those patients at high risk for transfusion. In that category are trauma victims and patients undergoing cardiac surgery, liver transplantation, and vascular surgery.[10-12] The majority of studies involve patients who have had cardiac surgery and liver transplantation. Goodnough et al,[3] in a multicenter study of coronary artery bypass grafting surgery, found inappropriate transfusions for 47% of platelet transfusions, 32% of FFP transfusions, and 15% of red cell transfusions. Also, there are large differences among institutions in the percentage of patients who are transfused for cardiac surgery and for liver transplant surgery.[1,13,14] Given the rising cost of blood transfusions, the challenges with the blood supply, and the significant variations in clinical transfusion practice, the need for objective decision making is compelling.[15,16]

Preanalytical Issues in Point-of-Care Coagulation Testing

Even before the actual analysis, a number of factors can affect the results of coagulation testing. Such issues are critical for both test operators and clinicians to understand for accurate testing and interpretation. With POCT, the effect may be greater because of small sample sizes, alternative collection techniques, and a lack of familiarity with potential problems. The possible causes of variability in coagulation test results are 1) biologic variation, 2) sample variation, 3) reagent and instrument variation, and 4) nontraditional test operators.

Biologic Variation

Patient-related factors can significantly influence test results. Ongoing illness can alter the patient's baseline hemostatic function: patients with liver disease may appear hypocoaguable and cancer can induce a hypercoaguable state. Acute illness can also have an effect. Both diet and medications can influence hemostasis; that knowledge is particularly important for patients on anticoagulation therapy with warfarin.

Sample Variation

In the laboratory, citrated plasma is the specimen of choice for most coagulation-based testing. However, in POCT, fresh whole blood is much more commonly used. Fresh blood requires rapid initiation of testing for accuracy. With citrated samples, the volume of specimen in relation to the amount of citrate present in the collection tube is very important; significant alterations in the ratio of blood to anticoagulant can markedly affect results. Results from whole blood specimens are often different than results from plasma samples. Collection techniques also play an important role. Capillary specimens are subject to technique variability, specimens collected from indwelling catheters may be contaminated by flush solution, and difficulty with venous or arterial collection may result in premature activation of the coagulation system. Sample size is also important in relation to the amount of reagent in the test cartridge. Specimens that are too large or too small can produce inaccurate results.

Reagent and Instrument Variation

Different reagents may be used to perform the same test, and these reagents may have varying sensitivities to factor deficiency and anticoagulant effect. Furthermore, each reagent and instrument combination can produce somewhat different results—and standardization is typically not possible. Consequently, tests from POCT and from the laboratory do not match. Therefore, a test method must be chosen, and clinical decision points must be validated for that method. Providers must be aware of the appropriate decision points and must maintain consistency in testing (POCT or laboratory) in order to avoid confusion.

Nontraditional Test Operators

With POCT, test operators are typically physicians, nurses, perfusionists, and other allied health-care personnel who are not familiar with the effect of preanalytical variables. There may also be significant variations in technique with multiple operators, particularly if testing is infrequent. Therefore, training and on-going competency assessment of test operators are crucial.

Regulatory and Accreditation Issues

POCT is subject to the regulatory requirements outlined by the Clinical Laboratory Improvement Amendments (CLIA). Many of the tests are categorized as "waived," which means that the requirements are limited. The basic mandate is that manufacturers' directions must be followed. Other tests fall into the "nonwaived" category, which tends to indicate that they are more complex. Most point-of-care coagulation tests fall into that category. For nonwaived tests, CLIA has specific requirements related to test orders, operator training and competency assessment, test validation, quality control, and test reporting. The POCT program must be aware of the CLIA classification of each test that is performed and must have a CLIA certificate appropriate for the level of testing being performed.

The Joint Commission has accreditation requirements for hospital- and clinic-based POCT, including both waived and nonwaived tests. Many facilities limit their POCT to the waived category and use The Joint Commission as their accrediting organization. The College of American Pathologists (CAP) also offers accreditation with a checklist specific for POCT. These organizations have standards that may be similar to or even exceed the minimum CLIA requirements.

For nonwaived testing, certification requires periodic inspection to assess the program's compliance with regulatory requirements. Certification may be performed directly by the Centers for Medicare and Medicaid Services (CMS) or through "deemed" agencies such as state departments of health, The Joint Commission, and CAP. Facilities with only waived testing do not require periodic inspection by CMS; however, CMS does perform validation inspections of waived as well as nonwaived testing programs.

Most institutions have an established oversight program for POCT that is managed by one or more point-of-care coordinators. These individuals are laboratory personnel or nurses who have POCT experience and manage the daily program operations while working to ensure compliance in practice and with documentation. Laboratory directors and multidisciplinary institutional committees typically provide the governance and policy setting for such programs. Participation in the oversight system brings numerous advantages, including established methods for ordering, reporting, training, competency assessment, validation, quality control, and billing. Good collaboration and communication between the POCT program and the testing sites and operators are important keys to success.

Hemoglobin

There are multiple POCT devices or tests for determining blood hemoglobin and hematocrit (H/H) levels that provide rapid patient assessment, including assessment of the need for transfusion of red cells. These tests are very useful in situations where decisions based on H/H are time sensitive. For that reason, there is a lot of interest in the use of point-of-care H/H testing in the operating room, the intensive care unit, and the emergency room.

Point-of-care hemoglobin monitoring has a useful role during acute isovolemic hemodilution. Acute isovolemic hemodilution involves the use of acute intraoperative withdrawal of blood with simultaneous infusion of crystalloid or colloid to achieve isovolemic filling of the heart. The blood is then stored and reinfused during the part of the operation when there is large loss of blood. The purpose is to reduce transfusion of allogeneic red cells by decreasing the hemoglobin content of the blood shed during the surgical procedure. Acute isovolemic hemodilution is controversial and relatively underused.

Acute isovolemic hemodilution has been used successfully to decrease the number of allogeneic blood transfusions in cardiac, vascular, hepatic, spinal, and prostate surgery. The average blood savings have been between 1.5 and 3.5 units or between 500 and 1200 mL of allogeneic blood transfusions.[17,18] Periodic hemoglobin determinations during the procedure allow volume modification of the whole blood collection to more accurately achieve the patient's target hemoglobin and to prevent excessive blood withdrawal.

Although POCT is being used increasingly as a basis for deciding on perioperative red cell transfusion, the accuracy of H/H measurements by point-of-care devices needs to be established. There are optical- and conductivity-based methods of blood H/H determinations. Conductivity-based methods can be influenced by plasma protein concentration.[19]

Hopfer et al[19] assessed H/H levels at varying protein concentrations using two POCT instruments: iSTAT-1 (conductivity method; Abbott, Inc, Abbott Park, IL) and HemoCue (optical method; HemoCue, Inc, Lake Forest, CA). These H/H results were compared with results obtained by a laboratory hematology analyzer. Comparability between the HemoCue system and the laboratory analyzer was good, with a mean bias of 0.34 g/dL at protein concentrations ranging from 0.7 to 6.2 g/dL. Correlations were excellent when hemodilution was performed with either saline ($r = 0.999$) or lactated Ringer's solution ($r = 1.000$). The iSTAT-1 results showed slightly less correlation with those of the laboratory analyzer ($r = 0.978$-0.980) over the same protein range. However, the iSTAT-1 results were generally 1 g/dL lower than the laboratory results, with discrepancies up to 2 g/dL for hemoglobin values and up to 4% for hematocrits at the lowest protein concentration. Corresponding results were documented by Connelly et al,[20] but the discrepancies seen with low protein levels could be corrected by using algorithms.

Gehring et al[21] determined the accuracy and precision of POCT for blood hemoglobin concentration measurements in 50 blood samples from 50 postoperative patients requiring intensive care. Hemoglobin values from two blood gas analyzers—the HemoCue system and an automated hematology analyzer—were compared with results obtained with the cyanmethemoglobin method, the reference "gold standard" procedure. The hemoglobin concentrations of the reference measurements ranged from 73.9 to 159.4 g/L. Although the results generally compared well, there were some differences in terms of precision and bias among the methods. An earlier study that examined conductivity, adjusted conductivity, and photometric and centrifugation methods as compared with an automated hematology analyzer noted similar differences.[22]

In general, point-of-care H/H testing is reliable and clinically useful for managing both acute isovolemic hemodilution and red cell transfusion therapy. However, users must be aware of the distinctive characteristics of the method they are using and of the patient's potential for hypoproteinemia so that the result can be interpreted appropriately.

Hemostasis

Coagulation Cascade

There are multiple tests to measure the coagulation cascade. The prothrombin time (PT)/international normalized rate and activated thromboplastin time (aPTT) are two laboratory tests commonly used to examine the extrinsic and intrinsic coagulation pathways, respectively. These tests are useful for the management of warfarin and heparin therapies as well as for the guidance of transfusion therapy. Versions of the PT and aPTT tests have been developed for POCT and incorporated into transfusion algorithms in the operating room. Use of POCT based-transfusion algorithms have been associated with reduced allogeneic transfusions, especially in cardiac surgical procedures.[23,24]

Multiple studies have addressed the accuracy of these point-of-care-based PT and aPTT tests relative to tests performed in the hospital laboratory.[25-30] In the latest study, Chavez et al[31] performed a prospective, blinded study of 32 patients scheduled for elective cardiac surgery involving cardiopulmonary bypass. Arterial blood samples were drawn at four points: before surgery, after induction of anesthesia, and at 10 minutes and 60 minutes after reversal of heparin with protamine. PT and aPTT were measured with the CoaguChek Pro DM (Roche Diagnostics, Basel, Switzerland) and the MD180 laboratory analyzers (bioMérieux, Durham, NC). Although the correlations between the two methods were strong for the aPTT and the PT ($r^2 = 0.83$ and 0.92, respectively), the results were not identical. The largest difference was seen in the aPTT at 10 minutes after protamine reversal; at that time, the mean lab aPTT was 48.9 ±12.7 seconds and the mean point-of-care aPTT was 36.1 ±9.4 seconds. The turnaround time was significantly shorter for the point-of-care system (average <10 min) than for the laboratory (average >30 min).

The POCT tests PT and aPTT produced results more quickly than the standard laboratory tests. However, most of the POCT had bias relative to the hospital laboratory because of differences in reagents and instruments. Therefore, method-specific decision points are critical for appropriate clinical use.

Heparin Anticoagulation Testing

Systemic anticoagulation with high-dose intravenous, unfractionated heparin, usually 300 units/kg, is required for cardiopulmonary bypass (CPB) to prevent thrombus formation within the CPB pump. Inhibition of thrombin and clot formation is the foremost function of heparin anticoagulation during CPB. Unfractionated heparin is composed of heterogenous groups of polysaccharides. A unique pentasaccharide sequence of heparin interacts with the serine protease enzyme antithrombin (AT).[32,33] The interaction of heparin with AT enhances the anticoagulant activity of AT. The activated AT binds to thrombin (Factor II), Factor IX, and Factor X and inhibits their activity. Thrombin is the key element in the coagulation amplification process, resulting in fibrin generation as well as activation of platelets and fibrinolysis. Despite heparin therapy during CPB, thrombin is continuously generated.[34] Thrombin formation stimulates consumption of hemostatic components, which increase the risk of coagulopathy, excessive bleeding, and perioperative allogeneic blood transfusion.

Because very large doses of heparin are used for CPB, standard monitoring of heparin with the aPTT test is not possible. In 1975, Bull et al[35,36] introduced a simple and safe point-of-care test for high-dose, unfractionated heparin monitoring called the activated clotting time (ACT) test. A baseline ACT is measured. Following heparin administration, another ACT is obtained to determine if anticoagulation is adequate for commencement of CPB. Additional heparin is given to maintain the ACT at or above a certain value during CPB, usually 450 seconds.

Culliford et al,[37] along with others, have shown that factors other than plasma heparin concentration, including hypothermia and hemodilution, have an influence on the ACT during CPB.[38] Furthermore, the credibility of the "safe" ACT for anticoagulation during CPB was challenged when Young et al[39] demonstrated the presence of fibrin monomer in animals with so-called safe ACT values during CPB. These results have been confirmed by Slaughter et al,[40] and even subclinical, inadequate anticoagulation has been shown to increase the likelihood of coagulopathy after CPB.

Subsequently, the merits of the ACT vs heparin concentration to monitor the adequacy of anticoagulation during CPB in relation to bleeding and transfusion are important considerations. The Hepcon hemostasis management system [HMS (Medtronic Blood Management, Parker, CO)] is a point-of-care monitoring device that generates both ACT and an accurate whole blood heparin concentration measurement through an automated protamine titration method. In 1990, Gravlee et al[41] compared standard heparin dosing and ACT monitoring to heparin dosing with heparin concentration by using the Hepcon in a randomized trial of 21 cardiac surgical patients. Patients managed with heparin concentration received the largest amount of heparin and had the highest postoperative blood loss. In another subsequent study of 63 adults undergoing cardiac surgery, Gravlee et al[42] concluded that heparin dosing and heparin concentration monitoring did not significantly influence postoperative blood loss or transfusion requirements.

In 1995, Jobes et al[43] found that the 24-hour mediastinal chest tube drainage (MCTD) and transfusion requirements were less in the heparin concentration group, thus concluding that heparin concentration monitoring was responsible for improved hemostasis in cardiac surgical patients. However, heparin concentration monitoring identifies only the amount of heparin in the blood and does not reflect the extent of anticoagulation. As noted earlier, the anticoagulant activity of heparin is mediated by AT. Patients can develop an acquired AT deficiency through prior heparin, nitroglycerin, or intra-aortic balloon pump use.

It is possible to determine a patient's in-vivo thrombin activity by performing a heparin dose response (HDR) test to identify a *specific* heparin concentration that will achieve adequate anticoagulation. A study by Despotis et al[44] randomized 254 patients requiring CPB either to a fixed dose of 250 units/kg of heparin or to a treatment group receiving an initial heparin dose based on an automated HDR and heparin concentration. Patients in the heparin concentration group had significantly fewer FFP and platelet transfusions than control patients had, but MCTD in the intensive care unit was similar in the first 8 and 24 hours. Control patients had indirect evidence of increased clotting factor consumption. In a randomized prospective study, Koster et al[45] compared the influence of anticoagulation with a Hepcon HMS heparin concentration-based system to that of ACT-based management on the activation of the hemostatic-inflammatory system. The study involved CPB in 200 elective patients (100 in each group) undergoing standard cardiac surgery in normothermia. After CPB, the Hepcon HMS group had a significant reduction in thrombin generation, D-dimers, and neutrophil elastase. There was no difference in blood loss or transfusion requirements.

Cardiac catheterization also requires systemic anticoagulation to prevent intracoronary thrombosis during the procedure. The standard anticoagulant is unfractionated heparin, and monitoring is done at the point of care using the ACT test. Because the cardiac catheterization procedure tends to be shorter than CPB and usually does not require CPB, less intense anticoagulation is acceptable. The optimal level of heparinization is somewhat controversial. Usually, an initial bolus of heparin (10,000 units or 100 units/kg) is followed by an infusion to keep the ACT >300 seconds.[46,47] The optimal protection against postprocedural ischemia seems to occur with an ACT of 350 to 375 seconds according to a recent study.[48] But other investigators have had success with only a 2500-unit bolus and an average ACT of 185 seconds.[49] Regardless of which protocol is selected, the decision points should be validated for the particular ACT test system in use because the results may vary depending on the nature of the reagent (kaolin vs celite) and the instrument.[48,50,51]

At the conclusion of the procedure, the femoral sheath is left in place until anticoagulation is reduced as indicated by an ACT of <180 seconds. Femoral hematomas may still occur, though, because the standard ACT test is not sensitive to low levels of heparin (<1 unit/mL). Therefore, some investigators have used either a point-of-care-based aPTT test or an ACT test modified to be more heparin sensitive.

Platelet Function

Another important aspect of hemostasis assessment in cardiac catheterization patients is platelet function. Platelets perform an active and complex role in clot formation. When the endothelium becomes damaged and the subendothelial surfaces are exposed, platelets adhere to the von Willebrand factor in the subendothelial surfaces through the glycoprotein Ib receptors. The platelets are activated and release their granules and express their glycoprotein IIb/IIIa (GP IIb/IIIa) receptors. The surface of the platelet acts as the catalyst for the contact, intrinsic, and extrinsic coagulation pathways, resulting in generation of thrombin and, subsequently, fibrin formation. The GP IIb/IIIa receptors bind fibrinogen and mediate platelet aggregation and subsequent clot propagation. The fibrin produced by the coagulation pathways also reinforces the strength of the clot.

The growing realization that the skin bleeding time is often an unreliable measure of platelet function has prompted efforts to identify ways to assess qualitative platelet dysfunction. Qualitative platelet dysfunction can result from multiple disease states and special surgical techniques such as CPB. Furthermore, multiple drugs have recently been developed that impair different aspects of platelet function.

The benefit of aspirin use in the emergent care of acute coronary syndrome (ACS) has been well established.[52] Because of the success of aspirin therapy in ACS, interest in other antiplatelet therapies has been great, and multiple studies have been performed. Aspirin and the thienopyridines are oral antiplatelet agents that interfere with platelet activation in complementary, but separate, pathways. The thienopyridines (ticlopidine, clopidogrel) are thought to induce irreversible alteration of the platelet receptor P2Y12, which mediates the inhibition of stimulated adenylyl cyclase activity by adenosine diphosphate (ADP), thereby resulting in platelet function inhibition.[53] Combination therapy of aspirin with other antiplatelet agents has demonstrated a benefit for the management of ACS.

Another class of drugs that has been very beneficial for the management of ACS is made up of the platelet GP IIb/IIIa inhibitors (abciximab, eptifibatide, and tirofiban), which are now being used routinely to prevent recurrent ischemic events after percutaneous coronary revascularization with or without stent placement.[54] GP IIb/IIIa is the platelet receptor for fibrinogen; the receptor blockade prevents the binding of fibrinogen and, thus, clot formation beyond initial platelet aggregation. Although such agents have been shown to be effective,[55,56] questions remain about the degree of inhibition that is required for a good clinical outcome with minimal risk of hemorrhagic events.[57] Multiple studies with the more powerful GP IIb/IIIa receptor antagonists have shown that these new drugs are superior in preventing ischemic complications after percutaneous coronary interventions, compared with standard antiplatelet therapy using aspirin and ticlopidine or clopidogrel (risk reduction up to 50%).[58]

The benefits of the new GP IIb/IIIa inhibitors and the thienopyridines in interventional cardiology have raised the issue of the possible need to monitor platelet function during therapy. A number of platelet function tests have been studied, but their clinical utility has not been firmly established. It has been shown that platelet receptor density and function can vary significantly between patients.[59] Patrono et al have shown that the metabolism of the thienopyridines varies between patients,[52] and patients ingesting clopidogrel show large variability in platelet inhibition.[60] Indeed, the variability in response to the original antiplatelet therapy, aspirin, has been recognized for nearly 40 years.[61]

Furthermore, bleeding is a complication of current therapies for ACS, and excessive response to antiplatelet drugs could increase the risk of that complication. A study by Rao et al[62] of patients who had ACS found that there were stepwise increases in the adjusted hazards of 30-day mortality [mild bleeding, hazard ratio (HR) 1.6; moderate bleeding, HR 2.7; severe bleeding, HR 10.6] and 6-month mortality (mild bleeding, HR 1.4; moderate bleeding, HR 2.1; severe bleeding, HR 7.5) as bleeding severity increased. The study authors found that the Global Use of Strategies to Open Occluded Coronary Arteries (GUSTO) bleeding classification identified patients who are at risk for short- and long-term adverse events.

Because of the high cost of intravenous GP IIb/IIIa agents and the possible grave consequences of incorrect dosing of those drugs, developing POCT methods to assess the effect of GP IIb/IIIa inhibition has also stimulated interest in developing fast and simple platelet function testing. Such testing might also be useful in the assessment of patients who are on therapy and who need emergent invasive procedures—should they receive prophylactic treatment to reverse the platelet inhibition before the procedure? Finally, development of point-of-care platelet function tests would be useful for patients with other qualitative platelet function defects, such as the defects that result from CPB.

Multiple techniques have been developed to measure platelet adhesion, platelet aggregation, platelet contraction, the ability of platelets to retard or stop flow, and the contribution of platelets to in-vitro clot formation. Only point-of-care tests approved by the Food and Drug Administration are discussed below.

Thromboelastogram

The thromboelastogram [TEG (Haemoscope, Skokie, IL)] was first developed in the 1940s. The test measures the clot's physical properties. A small quantity (0.36 mL) of whole blood is placed in a cylindrical cup, and a pin is suspended in the blood. The cup is rotated through an angle of 4 degrees, 45', and as the blood clots, that motion is imparted to the pin, which results in the characteristic TEG clot signature (see Fig 13-1).[63] The five parameters most frequently discussed in the literature are R, R+K, alpha, MA, and A60. The R value is the time from sample placement until initial pin deflection, and the R+K is the time from initial sample placement until the pin is deflected 20 mm. Alpha is the angle formed by the tangent of the tracing's amplitude at the initial pin deflection. The MA is the maximal amplitude of the deflection, and the A60 is the amplitude of the tracing 60 minutes following the MA. The five TEG parameters are not independent variables. They are interdependent, and a change in one aspect of the coagulation system frequently af-

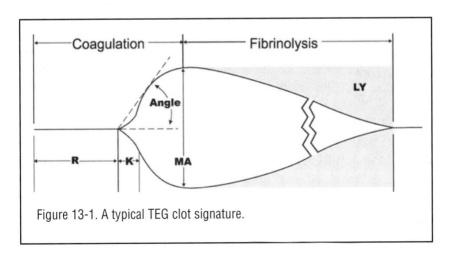

Figure 13-1. A typical TEG clot signature.

fects many of the variables. The most important variables that affect clot strength and the subsequent MA of the TEG tracing are the fibrinogen concentration and the platelet function and count.[64,65]

Several activators, such as tissue factor and celite, are sometimes added to the whole blood to speed the time to get TEG results. The TEG can also be modified by adding other drugs to increase the ability to test other aspects of platelet function and to increase the TEG's correlation with platelet aggregometry.[66-69] The in-vitro addition of abciximab results in significant concentration-dependent reductions in the MA.[70] The ability of the TEG to measure the effects of the different GP IIb/IIIa receptor antagonists has recently been found to depend on the agent used.[71] The TEG has been successfully used to predict excessive bleeding and to guide transfusion therapy in cardiac surgical patients.[23,72-74]

Sonoclot Coagulation Analyzer

The Sonoclot coagulation analyzer (Sienco, Arvada, CO) is another device that measures the clot's physical properties. A small quantity (0.4 mL) of whole blood is placed in a cylindrical cuvette in which a vertically vibrating probe (200 Hz, distance = 1 μm, temperature = 37 C) is suspended. The changes in mechanical impedance over time exerted on the probe by the viscoelastic properties of the forming clot produce a qualitative graph, known as the Sonoclot signature (see Fig 13-2). The analyzer also generates quantitative results on the clot formation time (ACT at onset), the rate of fibrin polymerization (clot rate, or the gradient of the primary slope), time to peak (TP), and peak amplitude (PA).[75] Platelet dysfunction results in a lack of an inflection point between R1 and R2, a prolongation of the time to peak, and a missing downslope after the maximal peak of R3.[76] One of the biggest problems with the Sonoclot test is high variability of results. Improvement of the activator in the Sonocuvette, use of native whole blood, and repeated Sonoclot analyses would lessen variability of results.[77] The Sonoclot vari-

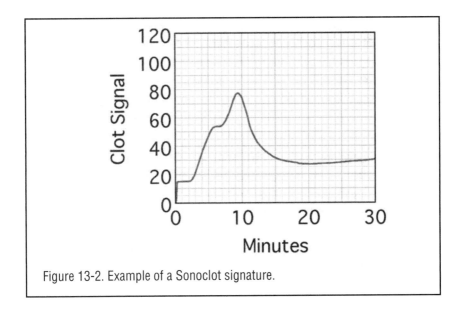

Figure 13-2. Example of a Sonoclot signature.

ables are also affected by hemoglobin levels, age, and gender.[78] The addition of tirofiban has been shown to slow the onset and rate of fibrin formation on Sonoclot analyses.[79]

The Sonoclot has been used to detect hypercoagulability in cancer patients,[80,81] to monitor antiplatelet effects of eptifibatide,[82] and to predict excessive bleeding and guide transfusion therapy in cardiac surgical patients.[83,84] Finally, the Sonoclot has recently been modified to produce a new "aprotinin-insensitive" ACT test for heparin monitoring in cardiac surgery (aiACT).[85]

Plateletworks

The ICHOR/Plateletworks analyzer (Helena Laboratories, Beaumont, TX) is an automated point-of-care platelet function test based on a Coulter counter and the platelet count ratio.[86] The device produces an aggregation result as a percentage that is similar to platelet aggregometry. It uses collagen or ADP as agonists. The device is designed to count only single platelets. Once the agonist is added to the platelets, the platelets aggregate, thus causing the number of single platelets to decrease. The platelet count ratio is calculated as follows:

$$\frac{\text{Baseline Platelet Count} - \text{Agonist Platelet Count}}{\text{Baseline Platelet Count}} \times 100 = \% \text{ Aggregation}$$

The Plateletworks has a good correlation with traditional platelet aggregometry. A study of in-vitro addition of eptifibatide, tirofiban, or abciximab to whole blood demonstrated that platelet inhibition measured by the Plateletworks mirrored the level obtained with traditional light transmission aggregometry.[87] A study of 75 patients who received standard-dose abciximab therapy during percutaneous coronary interventions evaluated platelet inhibition as measured by Plateletworks and by whole blood aggregation.[88] Patients above the lowest quartile of inhibition with Plateletworks demonstrated a relative risk of 0.48 (confidence interval = 0.23-0.99) for experiencing return of angina within 30 days. The study authors concluded that measurements with Plateletworks reflect platelet activation suppression and that higher Plateletworks measurements were associated with a decreased risk of return of angina.

In a study by Ostrowski et al,[89] of 35 patients undergoing cardiac surgery with CPB, the Plateletworks demonstrated a statistically significant change in platelet function with the ADP reagent tube from the preoperative period to the removal of the aortic cross clamp (p = 0.011). A significant correlation was found between Plateletworks collagen reagent tubes before surgery and chest tube drainage (p = 0.048, r = −0.324). There was no statistical correlation between TEG parameters and chest tube drainage at any time interval. The preoperative TEG MA showed a correlation to receipt of blood components (p = 0.016).

Conversely, Lennon et al[90] studied 50 consecutive adult patients undergoing elective cardiac surgery for coronary artery bypass grafting or cardiac valve replacement. Both Plateletworks and turbidimetric platelet aggregometry stimulated with collagen showed poor correlation to chest tube drainage. The correlation coefficient between preoperative Plateletworks and preoperative turbidimetric platelet aggregometry with postoperative mediastinal blood loss was 0.07 (p = 0.58) and −0.31 (p = 0.03), respectively. Following completion of surgery, the correlation coefficients were 0.14 (p = 0.34) and −0.29 (p = 0.08), respectively.

HemoSTATUS Platelet Function Test

The hemoSTATUS (Platelet ACT) (Medtronic, Parker, CO) is an assay of platelet function using a modified Hepcon HMS device. Platelet procoagulant activity is determined by measuring the shortening of the kaolin ACT induced by the platelet activating factor (PAF). PAF is a potent, endogenous platelet activator that stimulates in-vitro thrombosis, thus indicating platelet responsiveness. There are six channels in the device, with increasing doses of PAF in channels three to six. The clot ratio values are thought to reflect platelet function. The clot ratio is calculated by the following formula for each respective PAF concentration: clot ratio = 1 − (ACT/control ACT). In a study by Despotis et al,[91] the clot ratio in channels five and six were found to have a good correlation with blood loss and high sensitivity and specificity for predicting bleeding following cardiac surgery, but multiple other studies showed a poor correlation and poor sensitivity and specificity.[92-96] The hemoSTATUS has been used to guide desmopressin therapy to treat excessive bleeding in cardiac surgical patients.[97] It has also been shown to change with platelet count and in-vitro additions of abciximab.[98,99]

PFA-100

The Platelet Function Analyzer (PFA-100, Dade Behring, Miami, FL) is a semiautomatic device that reproduces in-vivo conditions and is thought of as an in-vitro simulation of bleeding time. It uses high shear rates of citrated whole blood suctioned through a capillary device and an aperture coated with collagen and other agonists to stimulate clotting.[100] The PFA-100 measures the closure time. In this device, blood is drawn through a capillary tube that has platelet agonists embedded within its surface. The "closure time" endpoint occurs when platelet adhesion and aggregation obstruct blood flow through the tube. The device uses two different cartridges, both of which have a membrane that is covered with a layer of fibrillar Type I collagen. The membrane in one of the cartridges is also covered with epinephrine and in the other with ADP. An alteration of platelet function is thought to be indicated when both epinephrine and adenosine closure times are prolonged. Aspirin therapy is thought to prolong only the epinephrine closure time.[101] The maximum closure time provided by PFA-100 is 300 seconds. In practice, any value >250 seconds may be considered maximally prolonged (equivalent to nonocclusion).[101]

This test is significantly prolonged during GP IIb/IIIa inhibition therapy, but it may be too sensitive for routine use as a monitor for GP IIb/IIIa receptor antagonist therapy.[102-105] The value of PFA-100 lies in the detection of aspirin-induced platelet secretion defect,[106-108] von Willebrand disease,[109,110] and other platelet disorders.[111,112] Using both types of PFA-100 cartridges, a study by Kerenyi et al[113] demonstrated that impaired platelet function caused by thrombolytic therapy and the effectiveness of aspirin could be assessed in parallel.

VerifyNow (Ultegra) System

The VerifyNow (Ultegra) System is also called the Ultegra Rapid Platelet Function Assay (Accumetrics, San Diego, CA). It is an assay that directly measures platelet agglutination. It can be configured to measure activation of the GP IIb/IIIa receptors, aspirin therapy, or clopidogrel therapy. A sample of citrated blood, 0.16 mL, is drawn into two sample channels in a disposable cartridge. The blood is mixed with a lyophilized peptide that activates the thrombin receptor, (iso-S)FLLRN, and fibrinogen-coated polystyrene beads for 70 seconds by movement of a microprocessor-driven steel ball.[114] Light transmission through the sample is measured. Agglutination occurs between the activated platelets and the fibrinogen-coated beads. Agglutination causes the beads to fall out of suspension, thereby leading to an increase in light transmission. The rate and extent of agglutination are used to calculate the platelet aggregation unit (PAU), which decreases in the presence of GP IIb/IIIa antagonists, because agglutination occurs in direct proportion to the number of unblocked GP IIb/IIIa receptors on the activated platelets.[115] Clopidogrel therapy is measured by use of a specific activator for the P2Y12 pathway.

The Ultegra, which has been shown to have a dose-dependent decrease in agglutination during inhibitor therapy, has been used to monitor the inhibitory effects of the GP IIb/IIIa antagonists abciximab,[116] tirofiban, and eptifibatide[117,118] in comparison to platelet aggregometry during percutaneous coronary interventions. Steinhubl et al[119] have shown that the level of platelet function inhibition varies both among patients and by agent used. Tirofiban and eptifibatide demonstrate an inhibition profile that is different from abciximab. The study suggests that the degree of platelet inhibition, as measured by the Ultegra at 10 minutes after the start of therapy, is significantly associated with the likelihood of a major cardiac adverse event within 7 days of the catheterization procedure.

Platelet Function Summary

The ideal POCT of platelet function would be specific, reliable, technically simple, and rapid and would interrogate the aspect of platelet function that is dysfunctional. Those ideals are challenged by the complexity of platelet function and the multiplicity of tests, both currently available and in development, that try to reflect such complexity. A growing number of agents also exist that alter platelet function in a multitude of ways. There may be no single test that is universally helpful. It is more likely that specific therapies and tests will need to be matched to best determine the clinical utility under various clinical situations.

Conclusion

POCT has numerous applications in patient care, especially in the cardiovascular arena. In many cases, outcome studies have been able to document clinical utility despite increased test costs. At the same time, these tests are subject to great variability because of methodological differences, preanalytic specimen collection and handling, and nontraditional operators. Therefore, validation of test performance, clinical decision points, and operator competency are crucial to the effective implementation of point-of-care tests.

References

1. Goodnough LT, Johnston MF, Toy PT. The variability of transfusion practice in coronary artery bypass surgery. JAMA 1991;265:86-90.
2. Stover EP, Siegel LC, Parks R, et al. Variability in transfusion practice for coronary artery bypass surgery persists despite national consensus guidelines: A 24-institution study. Institutions of the Multicenter Study of Perioperative Ischemia Research Group. Anesthesiology 1998;88:327-33.
3. Goodnough LT, Soegiarso RW, Birkmeyer JD, Welch HG. Economic impact of inappropriate blood transfusion in coronary artery bypass graft surgery. Am J Med 1993;94:509-14.
4. Simon T. Where have all the donors gone? A personal reflection on the crisis in America's volunteer blood program. Transfusion 2003;43:273-8.
5. Vamvakas EC, Taswell HF. Epidemiology of blood transfusion. Transfusion 1994;34:464-70.
6. Marcus AD. Blood supply at its lowest level in 9 years; surgeries cancelled. The Wall Street Journal. June 26, 2002; Sect. D-1.
7. Nuttall G, Stehling L, Beighley C, Faust R. Current transfusion practices of members of the American Society of Anesthesiologists: A survey. Anesthesiology 2003;99:1433-42.
8. Nichols J. Quality in point-of-care testing. Expert Rev Mol Diagn 2003;3:563-72.
9. Price C. Point-of-care testing: Impact on medical outcomes. Clin Lab Med 2001;21:285-303.
10. Wudel J, Morris JJ, Yates K, et al. Massive transfusion: Outcome in blunt trauma. J Trauma 1991;31:1-7.
11. DeLoughery T. Coagulation defects in trauma patients: Etiology, recognition, and therapy. Crit Care Clin 2004;20:13-24.

12. Donica S, Roberts L, Duke P, et al. Blood transfusion in orthotopic liver transplantation: Six-year experience. Transpl Int 1992;5(Suppl 1):S214.

13. Stover E, Siegel L, Body S, et al. Institutional variability in red blood cell conservation practices for coronary artery bypass graft surgery. J Cardiothorac Vasc Anesth 2000;14:171-6.

14. Ozier Y, Pessione F, Samain E, Courtois F. Transplantation: Institutional variability in transfusion practice for liver transplantation. Anesth Analg 2003; 79:671-9.

15. Amin M, Fergusson D, Aziz A, et al. The cost of allogeneic red blood cells: A systematic review. Transfus Med 2003;13:275-85.

16. Willson K, Hebert P. The challenge of an increasingly expensive blood system. CMAJ 2003;168:1149-50.

17. Waters J, Lee J, Karafa M. A mathematical model of cell salvage efficiency. Anesth Analg 2002;95:1312-7.

18. Weiskopf R. Mathematical analysis of isovolemic hemodilution indicates that it can decrease the need for allogeneic blood transfusion. Transfusion 1995; 35:37-41.

19. Hopfer S, Nadeau F, Sundra M, Makowski G. Effect of protein on hemoglobin and hematocrit assays with a conductivity-based point-of-care testing device: Comparison with optical methods. Ann Clin Lab Sci 2004;34:75-82.

20. Connelly N, Magee M, Kiessling B. The use of the iSTAT portable analyzer in patients undergoing cardiopulmonary bypass. J Clin Monit 1996;12:311-5.

21. Gehring H, Hornberger C, Dibbelt L, et al. Accuracy of point-of-care-testing (POCT) for determining hemoglobin concentrations. Acta Anaesthesiol Scand 2002;46:980-6.

22. McNulty S, Torjman M, Grodecki W, et al. A comparison of four bedside methods of hemoglobin assessment during cardiac surgery. Anesth Analg 1995;81: 1197-202.

23. Nuttall GA, Oliver WC, Santrach PJ, et al. Efficacy of a simple intraoperative transfusion algorithm for nonerythrocyte component utilization after cardiopulmonary bypass. Anesthesiology 2001;94:773-81.

24. Despotis GJ, Santoro SA, Spitznagel E, et al. Prospective evaluation and clinical utility of on-site coagulation monitoring in cardiac surgical patients. J Thorac Cardiovasc Surg 1994;107:271-9.

25. Despotis GJ, Santoro SA, Spitznagel E, et al. On-site prothrombin time, activated partial thromboplastin time, and platelet count: A comparison between whole blood and laboratory assays with coagulation factor analysis in patients presenting for cardiac surgery. Anesthesiology 1994;80:338-51.

26. Nuttall GA, Oliver WC Jr, Beynen FM, et al. Intraoperative measurement of activated partial thromboplastin time and prothrombin time by a portable laser photometer in patients following cardiopulmonary bypass. J Cardiothorac Vasc Anesth 1993;7:402-9.

27. Samama C, Quezada R, Riou B, et al. Intraoperative measurement of activated partial thromboplastin time and prothrombin time with a new compact monitor. Acta Anaesthesiol Scand 1994;38:232-7.

28. Zalunardo M, Zollinger A, Seifert B, et al. Perioperative reliability of an on-site prothrombin assay under different haemostatic conditions. Br J Anaesth 1998; 81:533-6.

29. Johi R, Cross M, Hansbro S. Near-patient testing for coagulopathy after cardiac surgery. Br J Anaesth 2003;90:499-501.

30. Fitch J, Mirto G, Geary K, et al. Point-of-care and standard laboratory coagulation testing during cardiovascular surgery: Balancing reliability and timeliness. J Clin Monit Comput 1999;15:197-204.

31. Chavez J, Weatherall J, Strevels S, et al. Evaluation of a point-of-care coagulation analyzer on patients undergoing cardiopulmonary bypass surgery. J Clin Anesth 2004;16:7-10.

32. Horlocker TT, Heit JA. Low molecular weight heparin: Biochemistry, pharmacology, perioperative prophylaxis regimens, and guidelines for regional anesthetic management. Anesth Analg 1997;85:874-85.

33. Hirsh J. Heparin. N Engl J Med 1991;324:1565-74.

34. Despotis GJ, Gravlee G, Filos K, Levy J. Anticoagulation monitoring during cardiac surgery: A review of current and emerging techniques. Anesthesiology 1999;91:1122-51.

35. Bull BS, Huse WM, Brauer FS, Korpman RA. Heparin therapy during extracorporeal circulation. II: The use of a dose-response curve to individualize heparin and protamine dosage. J Thorac Cardiovasc Surg 1975;69: 685-9.

36. Bull BS, Korpman RA, Huse WM, Briggs BD. Heparin therapy during extracorporeal circulation. I: Problems inherent in existing heparin protocols. J Thorac Cardiovasc Surg 1975;69:674-84.

37. Culliford A, Gitel S, Starr N, et al. Lack of correlation between activated clotting time and plasma heparin during cardiopulmonary bypass. Ann Surg 1981; 193:105-11.

38. Despotis GJ, Summerfield AL, Joist JH, et al. Comparison of activated coagulation time and whole blood heparin measurements with laboratory plasma anti-Xa heparin concentration in patients having cardiac operations. J Thorac Cardiovasc Surg 1994;108:1076-82.

39. Young JA, Kisker CT, Doty DB. Adequate anticoagulation during cardiopulmonary bypass determined by activated clotting time and the appearance of fibrin monomer. Ann Thorac Surg 1978;26:231-40.

40. Slaughter TF, LeBleu TH, Douglas JM Jr, et al. Characterization of prothrombin activation during cardiac surgery by hemostatic molecular markers. Anesthesiology 1994;80:520-6.

41. Gravlee GP, Haddon WS, Rothberger HK, et al. Heparin dosing and monitoring for cardiopulmonary bypass: A comparison of technique with measurement of subclinical plasma coagulation. J Thorac Cardiovasc Surg 1990;99:518-27.

42. Gravlee G, Rogers A, Dudas L, et al. Heparin management protocol for cardiopulmonary bypass influences postoperative heparin rebound but not bleeding. Anesthesiology 1992;76:393-401.

43. Jobes D, Aitken G, Shaffer G. Increased accuracy and precision of heparin and protamine dosing reduces blood loss and transfusion in patients undergoing primary cardiac operations. J Thorac Cardiovasc Surg 1995;110:35-45.

44. Despotis G, Joist J, Hogue C Jr, et al. The impact of heparin concentration and activated clotting time monitoring on blood conservation: A prospective, randomized evaluation in patients undergoing cardiac operation. J Thorac Cardiovasc Surg 1995;110:46-54.

45. Koster A, Fischer T, Praus M, et al. Hemostatic activation and inflammatory response during cardiopulmonary bypass: Impact of heparin management. Anesthesiology 2002;97:837-41.

46. Ferguson JJ, Dohmen P, Wilson JM, et al. Results of a national survey on anticoagulation for PTCA. J Invas Cardiol 1995;7:136-41.

47. Klein LW, Agarwal JB. When we "act" on ACT levels: Activated clotting time measurements to guide heparin administration during and after interventional procedures. Cathet Cardiovasc Diagn 1996;37:154-7.

48. Chew DP, Bhatt DL, Lincoff M, et al. Defining the optimal activated clotting time during percutaneous coronary intervention. Circulation 2001;103:961-6.

49. Kaluski E, Krakover R, Cotter G, et al. Minimal heparinization in coronary angioplasty: How much heparin is really warranted? Am J Cardiol 2000;85:953-6.

50. Bowers J, Ferguson JJ. The use of activated clotting times to monitor heparin therapy during and after interventional procedures. Clin Cardiol 1994;17:357-61.

51. Popma JJ, Prpic R, Lansky AJ, Piana R. Heparin dosing in patients undergoing coronary intervention. Am J Cardiol 1998;82:19P-24P.

52. Patrono C, Coller B, FitzGerald GA, et al. Platelet-active drugs: The relationships among dose, effectiveness, and side effects. The Seventh ACCP Conference on Antithrombotic and Thrombolytic Therapy. Chest 2004;126:234S-64S.

53. Antithrombotic Trialists' Collaboration. Collaborative meta-analysis of randomised trials of antiplatelet therapy for prevention of death, myocardial infarction, and stroke in high risk patients. BMJ 2002;324:71-86.

54. Singh S, Gopal A, Bahl V. Glycoprotein IIb/IIIa receptor antagonists: Are we ignoring the evidence. Indian Heart J 2005;57:201-9.

55. Ellis S, Lincoff A, Miller D, et al. Reduction in complications of angioplasty with abciximab occurs largely independently of baseline lesion morphology: EPIC and EPILOG Investigators. Evaluation of 7E3 for the prevention of ischemic complications and evaluation of PTCA to improve long-term outcome with abciximab gpiib/iiia receptor blockade. J Am Coll Cardiol 1998;32:1619-23.

56. Manoharan G, Maynard S, Adgey A. The therapeutic use of glycoprotein IIb/IIIa inhibitors in acute coronary syndromes. Expert Opin Investig Drugs 1999;8:555-66.

57. Harrington RA, Kleiman NS, Granger CB, et al. Relation between inhibition of platelet aggregation and clinical outcomes. Am Heart J 1998;136:S43-S50.

58. Claeys M, Van der Planken M, Bosmans J, et al. Does pre-treatment with aspirin and loading dose clopidogrel obviate the need for glycoprotein IIb/IIIa antagonists during elective coronary stenting? A focus on peri-procedural myonecrosis. Eur Heart J 2005;26:567-75.

59. Di Castelnuovo A, de Gaetano G, Benedetta Donati M, Iacoviello L. Platelet glycoprotein IIb/IIIa polymorphism and coronary artery disease: Implications for clinical practice. Am J Pharmacogenomics 2005;5:93-9.

60. Jaremo P, Lindahl T, Fransson S, Richter A. Individual variations of platelet inhibition after loading doses of clopidogrel. J Intern Med 2002;252:233-8.

61. Quick A. Salicylates and bleeding: The aspirin tolerance test. Am J Med Sci 1966;252:265-9.

62. Rao S, O'Grady K, Pieper K, et al. Impact of bleeding severity on clinical outcomes among patients with acute coronary syndromes. Am J Cardiol 2005;96:1200-6.

63. Shore-Lesserson L. Evidence based coagulation monitors: Heparin monitoring, thromboelastography, and platelet function. Semin Cardiothorac Vasc Anesth 2005;9:41-52.

64. Katori N, Tanaka K, Szlam F, Levy J. The effects of platelet count on clot retraction and tissue plasminogen activator-induced fibrinolysis on thrombelastography. Anesth Analg 2005;100:1781-5.

65. Bowbrick V, Mikhailidis D, Stansby G. Influence of platelet count and activity on thromboelastography parameters. Platelets 2003;14:219-24.

66. Craft R, Chavez J, Bresee S, et al. A novel modification of the Thrombelastograph assay, isolating platelet function, correlates with optical platelet aggregation. J Lab Clin Med 2004;143:301-9.

67. Greilich P, Alving B, O'Neill K, et al. A modified thromboelastographic method for monitoring c7E3 Fab in heparinizated patients. Anesth Analg 1997; 84:31-8.

68. Carroll R, Craft R, Chavez J, et al. A Thrombelastograph whole blood assay for clinical monitoring of NSAID-insensitive transcellular platelet activation by arachidonic acid. J Lab Clin Med 2005;146:30-5.

69. Tanaka K, Szlam F, Kelly A, et al. Clopidogrel (Plavix) and cardiac surgical patients: Implications for platelet function monitoring and postoperative bleeding. Platelets 2004;15:325-32.

70. Greilich P, Alving B, Longnecker D, et al. Near-site monitoring of the antiplatelet drug abciximab using the Hemodyne analyzer and modified Thromboelastograph. J Cardiothorac Vasc Anesth 1999;13:58-64.

71. Bailey L, Sistino J, Uber W. Is platelet function as measured by Thrombelastograph monitoring in whole blood affected by platelet inhibitors? J Extra Corpor Technol 2005;37:43-7.

72. Hertfelder H, Bos M, Weber D, et al. Perioperative monitoring of primary and secondary hemostasis in coronary artery bypass grafting. Semin Thromb Hemost 2005;31:426-40.

73. Cammerer U, Dietrich W, Rampf T, et al. The predictive value of modified computerized thromboelastography and platelet function analysis for postoperative blood loss in routine cardiac surgery. Anesth Analg 2003;96:51-7.

74. Shore-Lesserson L, Manspeizer H, DePerio M, et al. Thromboelastography-guided transfusion algorithm reduces transfusions in complex cardiac surgery. Anesth Analg 1999;88:312-19.

75. Furuhashi M, Ura N, Hasegawa K, et al. Sonoclot coagulation analysis: New bedside monitoring for determination of the appropriate heparin dose during haemodialysis. Nephrol Dial Transplant 2002;17:1457-62.

76. Hett D, Walker D, Pilkington S, Smith D. Sonoclot analysis. Br J Anaesth 1995;75:771-6.

77. Ekback G, Carlsson O, Schott U. Sonoclot coagulation analysis: A study of test variability. J Cardiothorac Vasc Anesth 1999;13:393-7.

78. Horlocker TT, Schroeder DR. Effect of age, gender, and platelet count on Sonoclot coagulation analysis in patients undergoing orthopedic operations. Mayo Clin Proc 1997;72:214-19.

79. Tanaka K, Katori N, Szlam F, et al. Effects of tirofiban on haemostatic activation in vitro. Br J Anaesth 2004;93:263-9.

80. Francis J, Francis D, Gunathilagan G. Assessment of hypercoagulability in patients with cancer using the Sonoclot Analyzer and thromboelastography. Thromb Res 1994;15:335-46.

81. Pivalizza E, Abramson D, Harvey A. Perioperative hypercoagulability in uremic patients: A viscoelastic study. J Clin Anesth 1997;9:442-5.

82. Waters J, Anthony D, Gottlieb A, Sprung J. Bleeding in a patient receiving platelet aggregation inhibitors. Anesth Analg 2001;93:878-82.

83. Tuman K, Spiess B, McCarthy R, Ivankovich A. Comparison of viscoelastic measures of coagulation after cardiopulmonary bypass. Anesth Analg 1989; 69:69-75.

84. Saleem A, Blifield C, Saleh SA, et al. Viscoelastic measurement of clot formation: A new test of platelet function. Ann Clin Lab Sci 1983;13:115-24.

85. Ganter M, Dalbert S, Graves K, et al. Monitoring activated clotting time for combined heparin and aprotinin application: An in vitro evaluation of a new aprotinin-insensitive test using Sonoclot. Anesth Analg 2005;101:308-14.

86. Carville D, Schleckser P, Guyer K, et al. Whole blood platelet function assay on the ICHOR point-of-care hematology analyzer. J Extra Corpor Technol 1998; 30:171-7.

87. White M, Krishnan R, Kueter T, et al. The use of the point of care Helena ICHOR/Plateletworks and the Accumetrics Ultegra RPFA for assessment of platelet function with GPIIB-IIIa antagonists. J Thromb Thrombolysis 2004; 18:163-9.

88. Ray M, Walters D, Bett N, et al. Point-of-care testing shows clinically relevant variation in the degree of inhibition of platelets by standard-dose abciximab therapy during percutaneous coronary intervention. Catheter Cardiovasc Interv 2004;62:150-4.

89. Ostrowsky J, Foes J, Warchol M, et al. Plateletworks platelet function test compared to the thromboelastograph for prediction of postoperative outcomes. J Extra Corpor Technol 2004;36:149-52.

90. Lennon M, Gibbs N, Weightman W, et al. A comparison of Plateletworks and platelet aggregometry for the assessment of aspirin-related platelet dysfunction in cardiac surgical patients. J Cardiothorac Vasc Anesth 2004;18:136-40.

91. Despotis GJ, Levine V, Filos KS, et al. Evaluation of a new point-of-care test that measures PAF-mediated acceleration of coagulation in cardiac surgical patients. Anesthesiology 1996;85:1311-23.

92. Ereth MH, Nuttall GA, Klindworth JT, et al. Does the platelet activated clotting test (HemoSTATUS) predict blood loss and platelet dysfunction associated with cardiopulmonary bypass? Anesth Analg 1997;85:259-64.

93. Ereth MH, Nuttall GA, Santrach PJ, et al. The relation between the platelet activated clotting test (HemoSTATUS) and blood loss after cardiopulmonary bypass. Anesthesiology 1998;88:962-9.

94. Shore-Lesserson L, Ammar T, DePerio M, et al. Platelet-activated clotting time does not measure platelet reactivity during cardiac surgery. Anesthesiology 1999;91:362-8.

95. Forestier F, Coiffic A, Mouton C, et al. Platelet function point-of-care tests in post-bypass cardiac surgery: Are they relevant? Br J Anaesth 2002;89:715-21.

96. Isgro F, Rehn E, Kiessling A, et al. Platelet function test HemoSTATUS 2: Tool or toy for an optimized management of hemostasis? Perfusion 2002;17:27-31.

97. Despotis G, Levine V, Saleem R, et al. Use of point-of-care test in identification of patients who can benefit from desmopressin during cardiac surgery: A randomised controlled trial. Lancet 1999;354:106-10.

98. Despotis G, Ikonomakou S, Levine V, et al. Effects of platelets and white blood cells and antiplatelet agent c7E3 (Reopro) on a new test of PAF procoagulant activity of whole blood. Thromb Res 1997;86:205-19.

99. Coiffic A, Cazes E, Janvier G, et al. Inhibition of platelet aggregation by abciximab but not by aspirin can be detected by a new point-of-care test, the hemoSTATUS. Thromb Res 1999;95:83-91.

100. Kundu S, Sio R, Mitu A, Ostgaard R. Evaluation of platelet function by PFA-100. Clin Chem 1994;40:1827-8.

101. Favaloro E. Clinical application of the PFA-100. Curr Opin Hematol 2002; 9:407-15.

102. Madan M, Berkowitz S, Christie D, et al. Determination of platelet aggregation inhibition during percutaneous coronary intervention with the platelet function analyzer PFA-100. Am Heart J 2002;144:151-8.

103. Madan M, Berkowitz SD, Christie DJ, et al. Rapid assessment of glycoprotein IIb/IIIa blockade with the platelet function analyzer (PFA-100) during percutaneous coronary intervention. Am Heart J 2001;141:226-31.

104. Hezard N, Metz D, Nazeyrollas P, et al. Use of the PFA-100 apparatus to assess platelet function in patients undergoing PTCA during and after infusion of cE3 fab in the presence of other antiplatelet agents. Thromb Haemost 2000;83:540-4.

105. Hezard N, Metz D, Nazeyrollas P, et al. PFA-100 and flow cytometry: Can they challenge aggregometry to assess antiplatelet agents, other than GPIIbIIIa blockers, in coronary angioplasty? Thromb Res 2002;108:43-7.

106. Bohner J, von Pape K, Wiebersinsky W, et al. Serial assessment of platelet function with the PFA-100 test system following a single 300 mg dose of acetylsalicylic acid. Clin Lab 1997;43:673-5.

107. Coma-Canella I, Velasco A, Castano S. Prevalence of aspirin resistance measured by PFA-100. Int J Cardiol 2005;11:71-6.

108. Coakley M, Self R, Marchant W, et al. Use of the platelet function analyser (PFA-100) to quantify the effect of low dose aspirin in patients with ischaemic heart disease. Anaesthesia 2005;60:1173-8.

109. Fressinaud E, Veyradier A, Truchaud F, et al. Screening for von Willebrand disease with a new analyser using high shear stress: A study of 60 cases. Blood 1998;91:1325-31.

110. Franchini M. The platelet function analyzer (PFA-100): An update on its clinical use. Clin Lab 2005;51:367-72.

111. Mammen E, Comp P, Gosselin R, et al. PFA-100 system: A new method for assessment of platelet dysfunction. Semin Thromb Hemost 1998;24:195-202.

112. Kerényi A, Schlammadinger Á, Ajzner É, et al. Comparison of PFA-100 closure time and template bleeding time of patients with inherited platelet function disorders. Thromb Res 1999;96:487-92.

113. Kerenyi A, Soltesz P, Veres K, et al. Monitoring platelet function by PFA-100 closure time measurements during thrombolytic therapy of patients with myocardial infarction. Thromb Res 2005;116:139-44.

114. Rand M, Leung R, Packham M. Platelet function assays. Transfus Apher Sci 2003;28:307-17.

115. Steinhubl S, Kereiakes D. Ultegra rapid platelet function analyzer. San Diego, CA: Academic Press, 2002.

116. Kereiakes D, Mueller M, Howard W, et al. Efficacy of abciximab induced platelet blockade using a rapid point of care assay. J Thromb Thrombolys 1999; 7:265-75.

117. Kereiakes DJ, Broderick TM, Roth EM, et al. Time course, magnitude, and consistency of platelet inhibition by abciximab, tirofiban, or eptifibatide in patients with unstable angina pectoris undergoing percutaneous coronary intervention. Am J Cardiol 1999;84:391-5.

118. Simon D, Liu C, Ganz P, et al. A comparative study of light transmission aggregometry and automated bedside platelet function assays in patients undergoing percutaneous coronary intervention and receiving abciximab, eptifibatide, or tirofiban. Cathet Cardiovasc Intervent 2001;52:425-32.

119. Steinhubl S, Talley J, Braden G, et al. Point-of-care measured platelet inhibition correlates with a reduced risk of an adverse cardiac event after percutaneous coronary intervention: Results of the GOLD (AU-Assessing Ultegra) multicenter study. Circulation 2001;103:2572-8.

In: Waters JH, ed.
Blood Management: Options for Better Patient Care
Bethesda, MD: AABB Press, 2008

14

Postoperative Blood Management Strategies

ARYEH SHANDER, MD, FCCM, FCCP;
TANUJA RIJHWANI, MBBS, MPH;
ROBERT DYGA, RN, CCP; AND
JONATHAN H. WATERS, MD

THE END OF THE SURGICAL PROCEDURE does not signify the end of blood loss. Postoperative blood loss can take place through wound drains, third spacing into traumatized tissue, or aggressive phlebotomy during the postoperative period. This chapter discusses several strategies that can be used to minimize the need for allogeneic transfusion in the postoperative period.

Aryeh Shander, MD, FCCM, FCCP, Chief, Department of Anesthesiology, Englewood Hospital and Medical Center, Englewood, New Jersey; Tanuja Rijhwani, MBBS, MPH, Director, Clinical Research, Department of Anesthesiology, Englewood Hospital and Medical Center, Englewood, New Jersey; Robert Dyga, RN, CCP, Director, Biologic Therapy, University of Pittsburgh Medical Center/BioTronics, Pittsburgh, Pennsylvania; and Jonathan H. Waters, MD, Chief and Visiting Associate Professor, Department of Anesthesiology, Magee-Womens Hospital, University of Pittsburgh Medical Center, Pittsburgh, Pennsylvania

Postoperative Blood Recovery

Postoperative blood recovery is a well-recognized and common practice. In this technique, blood from a postoperative drain or chest tube is collected and either is reinfused with microaggregate filtering alone or is reinfused after the blood is washed and concentrated. This technique has been applied after total joint replacement, spinal surgery, abdominal aortic aneurysm repair, aorto-femoral bypass, and cardiac, trauma, cancer, and abdominal surgery.[1] Today it is predominantly used following cardiac[2] and orthopedic procedures[3] because the volume of shed blood is significant. (For cardiac surgery, see Thurer et al—523 mL,[4] Eng et al—371 mL,[5] and Roberts et al—553 mL,[6] and for orthopedic surgery, see Ritter et al—166 mL,[7] Faris et al—750 mL,[8] and Clements et al—475 mL.[9]) Although it is controversial, the most common practice is to reinfuse this collected blood with simple microaggregate filtering and no washing.

Criteria for Use

As with most blood management techniques, postoperative blood recovery should meet certain criteria for use. The primary criteria is that there should be adequate amounts of blood that can be collected. Orthopedic and cardiac uses are the most common. One might question the utility of postoperative recovery in orthopedic surgery. For total knee arthroplasty, the blood loss has been reported to average 378 mL; for total hip arthroplasty, the blood loss averaged 203 mL.[10] Authors studying postoperative blood recovery in orthopedics have reported the hematocrit of this shed blood to range from 20% to 30%.[11,12] Thus, the volume of red cells returned is generally small. Despite this small volume of recovered cells, meta-analysis incorporating data from 16 studies concluded that postoperative recovery is efficacious for these procedures.[13] For cardiac surgery, postoperative mediastinal drainage can be much more significant with respect to the volume of blood lost. Consensus guidelines developed by the Society of Thoracic Surgeons have concluded that postoperative blood recovery is an effective technique for transfusion avoidance; however, the guidelines supported only the use of a washed recovered product.[14]

Postoperative Blood Recovery Devices

On the basis of function, two types of devices exist: those that reinfuse the shed blood without washing and those that concentrate and wash the blood. Further classification identifies four distinct systems that are currently in use (described below).

Type I: Unprocessed Blood

Type I includes products such as the Boehringer AutoVac (Boehringer Laboratories Inc, Norristown, PA), Gish Orthofuser (Gish Biomedical Inc, Rancho Santa Margarita, CA), Snyder Hemovac (Zimmer Corporate, Warsaw, IN), Davol Suretrans (Davol Inc, a subsidiary of C.R. Bard Inc, Murray Hill, NJ), Astra Bellovac ABT (Astra Tech AB, Möindal, Sweden), Stryker ConstaVac (Stryker Corp, Kalamazoo, MI), and the DONOR Autologous Blood Reinfusion System (Van Straten Medical, Nieuwegein, The Netherlands/Pall Medical, Portsmouth, UK/Medinorm AG, Quierschied, Germany). This class dominates the market primarily because of simplicity, cost, and ease of use. In 2005, approximately 320,000 of these postoperative unwashed blood recovery devices were sold.[15] Thus, the prevalence of use of these "flip-n-drip" systems is extensive.

The type I device is generally composed of 1) an inlet that connects to the wound drain, 2) a gross contamination filter that usually removes contaminants larger than 100 to 200 microns, 3) a collection reservoir, and 4) an access port for connection of an intravenous (IV) administration set. (See Fig 14-1.) More sophisticated devices add desirable safety features that include vacuum regulation, fat-specific filtration, a label, an anti-air embolism valve, a check valve, and access to add an anticoagulant.

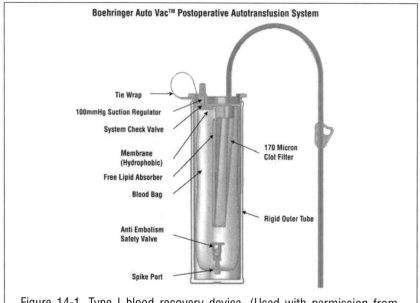

Figure 14-1. Type I blood recovery device. (Used with permission from Boehringer Laboratories, Inc.)

Citrate is the most commonly used anticoagulant but is not generally used here because most wound blood is already defibrinated, eliminating clot formation. Typical costs associated with this device total around $110 to $130.

Type II: Processed Blood at Point of Care

In the type II device, the blood is collected in a fashion similar to a type I device except that the blood is subsequently washed and concentrated before readministration. Only two devices are available that would fall into this category; both are manufactured by Haemonetics Inc (Braintree, MA): the OrthoPat and the CardioPat. These devices incorporate a "dynamic disk" (see Fig 14-2) for washing the shed blood. Because of the small size of this device, it can be mounted on an IV pole and easily moved along with the patient through the perioperative period. All shed blood is processed using a dynamic disk yielding a concentrated, washed red cell volume. Analysis performed by the

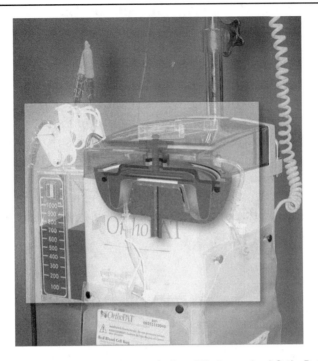

Figure 14-2. Type II blood recovery device. (Photograph of OrthoPat used with permission from Haemonetics Corp.)

Mayo Clinic in 1996 showed the following parameters in the final product: 77% hematocrit, red cell recovery 83%, albumin removal 99.1%, heparin removal 99.8%, and free hemoglobin removal 97.3% (P Santrach, personal communication). Typical cost for the disposable used in this device ranges from $400 to $600.

Type III: Processed Blood with Bench Instrument

Type III devices are typically used intraoperatively. They include the Sorin/COBE BRAT II (Bridgepoint Gambro Inc, Lakewood, CO), Medtronic Autolog (Medtronic, Minneapolis, MN), Fresenius CATS Continuous Auto Transfusion System (Fresenius HemoCare, Redmond, WA) and the Haemonetics CS5+ (Haemonetics Inc, Braintree, MA). (See Fig 14-3.) These instruments use different centrifugation methods based on the Latham bowl, the BRAT bowl, the Autolog bowl, or continuous autotransfusion system (CAT). Each design offers unique methods that provide effective concentration and washing. Because the devices are designed for intraoperative use, two issues must be addressed. First, a sterile and secure connection to the wound drain must be created. Second, each device has a large footprint so use in the postanesthesia care unit (PACU)/intensive care unit (ICU) environment can be cumbersome. Typical cost for the disposable used with one of these devices is $200.

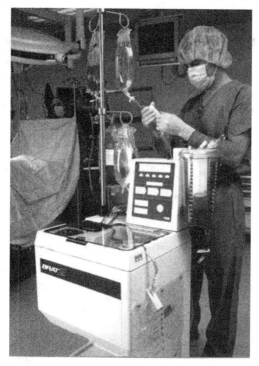

Figure 14-3. Type III blood recovery device. (Used with permission from the Sorin Group.)

Type IV: Processed Blood Combining Types I and III Devices

This approach incorporates the best features of the types I and III devices. A type I device is initially implemented. If adequate blood is lost, then processing takes place by moving the blood from the type I device to the type III device for washing. If small amounts of blood are collected, the device is simply discarded. In this way, the cost of the processing can be staged across the least-expensive devices. An alternative process would be to take the type I device to the blood bank for washing, using standard blood bank washing devices.

Device Selection

The three most common reasons for selecting a particular device are ease of use, cost, and product quality. Type I devices require the least amount of preparation, management, and cost. Types II, III, and IV require additional training and are more costly, but they yield a processed end product with reduced undesirable wound contaminants.

Safety of Unwashed Blood

Controversy surrounds the safety of administering an unwashed, shed blood product. Safety concerns are related to the use of type I devices yielding unprocessed blood with various inflammatory mediators,[16,17] fibrin split products,[18-20] complement fractions,[21-23] interleukins,[24-26] tumor necrosis factor alpha,[16] and fat particles[2] in multiple degrees higher than circulating levels.

In 2004, Hansen and Pawlik[27] reported an extensive list of reasons against the transfusion of unwashed wound blood. This list included the following problems associated with an unwashed blood recovery product:
- Cannot meet modern transfusion standards.

- Quality variable, mostly bad.
- Individual burden of contamination is unknown.
- Serious complications reported but incidence is unknown.
- No safe retransfusion volume is recognized.
- Quality is not controllable.
- Blood saving effect is small to absent.

The most commonly reported complication following unwashed, postoperative shed blood reinfusion is a febrile reaction. The reported rates of febrile reactions following postoperative recovery readministration vary from 4% to 12%.[9,28-30] In one study, Clements et al[9] observed severe hypotension in 2 patients (in a small series of 16 patients), which resolved upon stopping the shed blood readministration. The hypotension reoccurred when the blood was started again. A different patient was reported to have delayed hypotension 5 hours after readministration, which progressed to death from myocardial infarction. This death may have been unrelated to the unwashed product, but no study has been performed to date that was powered enough to evaluate the effect of unwashed blood on thromboembolic events.

In contrast to the hypotensive events reported by Clements, Krohn et al[31] reported a transient increase in pulmonary vascular and systemic vascular resistance during transfusion of unwashed, shed blood. This study was performed in cardiac patients where mediastinal wound blood was reinfused. For many patients, these changes in vascular resistance would be inconsequential; however, in patients with limited cardiac reserve, these afterload changes could be disastrous.

In a Cochrane systematic review, Carless et al[32] reviewed complications from all available studies on perioperative recovery. They assessed total complications, wound infections, stroke and deep venous thrombosis, and thromboembolic events, which included nonfatal myocardial infarction. They found no difference in any of these events between patients who had recovered blood readministered vs those who had not. A flaw in this work was that the researchers mixed washed with unwashed recovered blood, so it is difficult to ascertain the risk specific to an unwashed product.

In orthopedic surgery, venous thromboembolism (VTE) is of particular concern when administering an unwashed, shed blood product. In general, the rates of deep venous thrombosis are reported to be 2.27% in hip arthroplasty and 1.79% in knee arthroplasty, with a fatal pulmonary embolism rate of 0.22%.[33] One could easily postulate that the infusion of an unwashed product loaded with tissue factor would increase the rates of VTE. Only two reports have evaluated this issue. In one study,[34] 20 patients who underwent total knee replacement and who had unwashed recovered blood readministered were compared to 20 control patients. In this study, both groups had two deep vein thromboses. Another study[35] included 35 patients in each group, but no deep vein thromboses were found. If one is to detect changes in incidence of this complication, samples of a much larger size are needed than the samples present in the two currently published reports.

Another area of concern is that of renal dysfunction, which might result from significant amounts of free hemoglobin being readministered through these devices. The effect of poorly washed shed cells on renal function is reported to be dose related.[36,37] This effect can be enhanced by the combination of endotoxin and free hemoglobin.[38] Endotoxin concentrations in unwashed, postoperative shed blood have not been measured. Most likely, significant concentrations may exist in an unwashed shed product. Despite what would appear to be a significant concern regarding the effect of unwashed, shed blood on renal function, the data are of limited numbers.[39,40] In unpublished work from the University of Pittsburgh, a comparison between washed and unwashed blood in total knee replacement found no difference in renal function following readministration in 40 patients.

Because the contaminants in blood products are all biological in nature, they all have mechanisms by which they are metabolized and eliminated. It could be theorized that most individuals have some degree of reserve with which to absorb these products. No understanding exists of when this absorptive capacity is overwhelmed; however, several manufacturers of these devices recommend limiting the volume of reinfused product. The vast majority of postoperative salvage is performed with little quality oversight. This absence may account for limited safety data being published on this topic. The best approach to providing safe and effective postoperative blood recovery is to follow the AABB *Standards for Perioperative Autologous Blood Collection and Administration.*[41] (The components of a quality program are more fully discussed in Chapter 10.) The lack of more serious sequelae reported from the readministration of unwashed blood may be merely a result of lack of observation and auditing.

Postoperative Anemia Management

There are many causes of postoperative anemia (highlighted in Table 14-1). The following discussion highlights some of the areas of postoperative anemia management that warrant the greatest attention.

Table 14-1. Causes of Postoperative Anemia

1. Frequent blood sampling for measurements of various laboratory parameters.
2. Clinically apparent or occult blood loss from the gastrointestinal (GI) tract caused by erosive upper GI mucosal disease or tissue trauma from suction of gastric contents.
3. Blood loss caused by trauma preceding admission to the intensive care unit (ICU).
4. Blood loss at the time of surgical procedures preceding or during an ICU stay.
5. Inappropriately low circulating concentrations of erythropoietin (EPO), the humoral regulator of red cell production.
6. Diminished responsiveness of marrow precursor cells to EPO—for example, because of decreased availability of iron.
7. Iron and other nutritional deficiencies.

Iatrogenic Anemia

During the postoperative period, anemia is most problematic in the ICU. Anemia is a common finding in the ICU, and blood transfusions are commonly used for the treatment. A number of studies[42,43] have documented the prevalence of anemia in the critically ill patient and the high rate of blood transfusions administered in ICUs. The high prevalence of anemia reported in these studies correlates with administration of red cell transfusions in the range of 37% to 44% of patients during their ICU stay.[44] Corwin[44] reports that a total of 23% of all patients admitted to the ICU had a length of stay >1 week. Of these patients, 85% received blood transfusions. Patients were transfused at the rate of 2 to 3 units per week. These transfusions were not entirely the result of acute blood loss. Patients receiving blood transfusions were phlebotomized an average of 61 to 70 mL per day. Within a couple of days, a unit of whole blood is lost. This observation emphasizes the need to minimize the practice of routine blood draws as well as the need to minimize the volume of the draw.

Transfusion Triggers

Many blood transfusions are administered because of an arbitrary "transfusion trigger" rather than a physiologic need for the oxygen-carrying capacity of blood. Current guidelines for transfusion in the critically ill advise that, at a hemoglobin level of 7 g/dL, red cell transfusion is strongly indicated, whereas at hemoglobin values in excess of 10 g/dL, blood transfusion is seldom justified.[45] For patients with hemoglobin values in the 7 to 10 g/dL range, the transfusion trigger should be based on clinical indicators.

Hebert et al, in the Transfusion Requirements in Critical Care (TRICC)[46] multicenter trial, studied 838 critically ill patients to determine whether restrictive and liberal strategies of red cell transfusion produced equivalent results in critically ill patients.

In the restrictive strategy, patients were transfused at a trigger of 7 g/dL; in the liberal strategy, the patients were transfused at the traditional trigger of 10 g/dL. The researchers concluded that a restrictive strategy of red cell transfusion is at least as effective as—and possibly superior to—a liberal transfusion strategy in critically ill patients.

The results of this study may reflect a storage defect of the red cells during storage. This defect may hinder the intended result of the transfusion. Fundamentally, red cell transfusions are advocated to increase oxygen delivery in critically ill patients. From a macrocirculatory perspective, oxygen delivery is enhanced by increasing the hemoglobin concentration. However, the immediate and long-term effectiveness of this mode of therapy in increasing oxygen delivery at the cellular level is questionable because stored red cells have a depressed ability to unload oxygen peripherally, as well as to deform in order to move through the microcirculation. Animal models have suggested that transfusion of stored blood may impair oxygen delivery at the microcirculatory level.[47] No similar evidence is available in humans.

Potential adverse effects related to allogeneic blood transfusion identified in critically ill patients include increased risk of nosocomial infection,[48] altered inflammatory response,[49] pulmonary and systemic vasoconstriction related to the age of blood and nitric oxide binding,[50,51] and immunosuppression.[52] These adverse effects, plus a less-than-well-defined transfusion trigger, suggest that red cell transfusion should take place when a physiologic reason exists.

Optimization of Erythropoiesis

Critical illness is characterized by blunted erythropoietin production and response.[53] This blunted response appears to result from the inhibition of the erythropoietin gene by inflammatory mediators.[54,55] Corwin[44] demonstrated the efficacy of a weekly dosing schedule of recombinant human erythropoietin (erythropoietin) to decrease the occurrence of red cell transfusion in critically ill patients. Patients receiving erythropoietin were less likely to undergo transfusion (60.4% placebo vs 50.5% erythropoietin; p <0.001). There was a 19% reduction in the total units of red cells transfused in the erythropoietin group (1963 units for placebo vs 1590 units for erythropoietin) and a reduction in red cell units transfused per day alive [ratio of transfusion rates = 0.81; 95% confidence interval (CI) = 0.79-0.83; p = 0.04]. Increase in hemoglobin from baseline to study end was greater in the erythropoietin group. Mortality (14% for erythropoietin vs 15% for placebo) and adverse clinical events were not significantly different. The author concluded that in critically ill patients, weekly administration of 40,000 units of erythropoietin reduces allogeneic red cell transfusion and increases hemoglobin.

Anemia Prevention and Management

The greatest defense against anemia in the postoperative period is to be highly vigilant in looking for signs and symptoms of bleeding. Rapid diagnosis and control of hemorrhage with appropriate therapeutic procedures should be anticipated and implemented as early as possible before loss of a patient's physiologic reserves. Surgical interventions should be simple, quick, and well performed. One should consider angiographic embolization as an adjuvant to a multimodality bleeding control strategy.

Uncontrolled bleeding in patients should lead to consideration of restricted fluid resuscitation and toleration of mild to moderate hypotension—ie, blood pressure at the lowest possible level that maintains tissue perfusion (eg, mean arterial pressure of 50-70 mm Hg). Excessive fluid resuscitation may increase bleeding and reduce oxygen delivery by dilution of coagulation factors and promotion of hypothermia.[56]

Pharmacologic enhancement of hemostasis should be considered. Drugs used for this purpose include tranexamic acid, ε-aminocaproic acid, aprotinin, desmopressin, conjugated estrogens, vitamin K, recombinant Factor VIIa, and cryoprecipitate. These pharmacologic hemostatic agents should be used when bleeding is generalized or when the bleeding site is not accessible.

Topical sealants and adhesives such as fibrin sealant or hemostatic agents (collagen-based, gelatin-based, oxidized cellulose, and thrombin hemostat) can be used depending on the site and amount of bleeding.

Hyperbaric Medicine

Hyperbaric oxygen (HBO) therapy is the administration of 100% oxygen under increased atmospheric pressure [usually 2 atmospheres or 10 m (33 ft) under sea]. To fully appreciate the effect of the increased atmospheric pressure, one must understand the variables that determine the oxygen content of blood (CaO_2). The oxygen content of blood is dictated by the following equation:

$$CaO_2 = (Hb \times 1.39 \times SaO_2) + 0.003 \, pO_2$$

where
CaO_2 = oxygen content,
Hb = hemoglobin,
SaO_2 = hemoglobin oxygen saturation, and
pO_2 = partial pressure of oxygen.

The factor 1.39 is the volume of oxygen that combines with a gram of hemoglobin, and 0.003 is the oxygen solubility coefficient. The oxygen content is determined by two components: the oxygen carried by the hemoglobin ($Hb \times 1.39 \times SaO_2$) and the oxygen that is dissolved in the blood ($0.003 \, pO_2$).

Under normal conditions, the partial pressure of oxygen in the alveoli is about 100 mm Hg, the hemoglobin in a normal adult male is around 15 g/dL, and the oxygen saturation is around 98%. With these parameters:

$$CaO_2 = (15 \text{ g/dL of blood} \times 1.39 \text{ mL/g} \times 0.98) +$$
$$(0.003 \text{ mL/dL of blood/mm Hg} \times 100 \text{ mm Hg})$$

or

$$CaO_2 = 20.433 + 0.3 = 20.7 \text{ mL of } O_2/\text{dL of blood}$$

What this formula demonstrates is that the dissolved oxygen makes a very small contribution to total oxygen content under these normal conditions.

Inhalation of 100% oxygen raises the pO_2 seven times to approximately 670 mm Hg. The hemoglobin, normally about 97% to 98% saturated, becomes 100% saturated. In addition, large amounts of oxygen will physically dissolve in the plasma. The following equation reflects those factors:

$$CaO_2 = 20.85 + 2.01 = 22.86 \text{ mL of } O_2/\text{dL of blood}$$

During inhalation of 100% oxygen at 1 atmosphere, the total oxygen content of arterial blood is elevated from 20 volume percent (vol %) to about 22 vol %, or an increase of 2 vol %. If the pressure is raised from 1 to 3 atmospheres absolute (ATA), the alveolar oxygen will increase correspondingly, and the oxygen tension and the content of the arterial blood will also rise. This rise should be approximately 760 mm Hg with each increase in atmospheric pressure. At 3 ATA, the arterial oxygen tension would be >2000 mm Hg. No further gains in the oxygen carried by hemoglobin is achieved; however, the dissolved component goes up so that at 3 ATA the equation is as follows:

$$CaO_2 = 20.85 + 6 = 26.85 \text{ mL of } O_2/\text{dL of blood}$$

An increase of 6 vol % of arterial oxygen is evident.

The resting oxygen needed in a normal person is about 4 to 5 vol %. A severely anemic patient with a hemoglobin level of 1 g/dL who is being given oxygen under 3 ATA would require the following oxygen content equation:

$$CaO_2 = (1 \text{ g/dL of blood} \times 1.39 \text{ mL/g} \times 1.00) +$$
$$(0.003 \text{ mL/dL of blood/mm Hg} \times 2000 \text{ mm Hg})$$

or

$$CaO_2 = 1.39 + 6 = 7.39 \text{ mL of } O_2/\text{dL of blood}$$

Therefore, HBO at 3 ATA can provide enough oxygen for resting metabolism even in the absence of hemoglobin.

HBO Therapy as an Alternative to Blood Transfusion Therapy

HBO is used as an adjuvant therapy for patients with severe anemia, along with erythropoietin, iron, folate, and nandrolone deconate to maximize marrow production. It may be used in a number of different circumstances, such as the following:

1. A patient refuses blood transfusion for religious reasons (Jehovah's Witness).
2. Personal reasons for avoiding transfusion usually stem from a fear of hepatitis or AIDS.
3. In cases of severe hemolysis, as in acute hemolysis, the syndrome is mediated by warm antibodies.
4. A rare blood type is present for which no adequate cross-type can be obtained.
5. A blood shortage exists.

Clinical Parameters to Start HBO

Currently, most centers administer HBO for severe anemia according to the following criteria:

1. Systolic blood pressure below 90 mm Hg or vasopressors required for the patient.
2. Disorientation or coma.
3. Ischemic electrocardiogram (ECG) changes.
4. Ischemic gut.

Unfortunately these criteria have limitations such as difficulty assessing disorientation postoperatively, ECG changes caused by multiple other causes, and ischemic gut being too late a parameter to be useful as a resuscitative measure.

In the authors' opinion, high blood lactate levels or serial lactate blood levels (that show no decreasing trends) are strong indicators of tissue hypoxia and can be used as a parameter to make a decision to initiate HBO therapy.

Also, any condition that leads to tissue hypoxia and that can cause end-organ damage or can be potentially life threatening should be an indication to start HBO therapy to tide the patient over the initial period of hypoxia until such time as the bone marrow can increase the production of red cells.

Delivery Systems

HBO therapy is administered in a pressurized chamber. Three distinct types of chambers are available, namely multiplace chambers, duoplace chambers, and monoplace chambers. Multiplace chambers can accommodate between 2 and 18 patients. The chambers commonly incorporate a minimum pressure capability of 6 ATA. Advantages to a multiplace chamber include constant patient attendance and evaluation, as well as multiple patients treated per session. Disadvantages include high capitalization and staffing costs, large space requirements, and risk of decompression sickness in the attending staff.

In duoplace chambers, the main compartment accommodates one supine patient. An access lock behind the patient's head accommodates one seated attendant. The main disadvantage to this chamber is the high capitalization costs.

A monoplace chamber is a single occupancy chamber with a pressure capability of 3 ATA. The major advantage to this type of chamber is that it is the most cost-efficient delivery method for HBO. The chamber also presents no risk of decompression sickness. The major disadvantage is that the patient is in relative isolation.

Treatment Protocol Guidelines

HBO is repeated as needed, at pressures appropriate to relieve the relative hypoxia, and is discontinued when a hematocrit level of 15% to 22.9% and a hemoglobin level of 5.0% to 7.7% is reached.

Efficacy

The concept of supporting a severely anemic animal model with dissolved oxygen was tested by Boerema et al[57] and Esmond et al[58] where an improved survival was noted, over controls, in animals in hemorrhagic shock treated with HBO. As discussed earlier, the main reason for using HBO is to dissolve enough oxygen in the severely anemic patient to support the basic metabolic needs of the body until sufficient hemoglobin is restored to the circulation to meet the oxygen demand.

In a study by Wright et al,[59] one group of rabbits (n = 12) received no treatment other than Ringer's lactate resuscitation, whereas the other group (n = 12) received five HBO treatments in the 4 days immediately following blood loss. These rabbits were monitored for 14 days after the bleeding episode for hemoglobin levels and reticulocyte counts. The control group was more affected by the blood withdrawal or loss than was the HBO group, reaching a low of 37% hemoglobin loss compared with 29% hemoglobin loss at 48 hours (p <0.001). The animals in the HBO group recovered faster, reaching the baseline level of hemoglobin in 11 days as opposed to 14 days for the control group of animals (p <0.001). Reticulocyte counts were not significantly affected by HBO treatment. Treatment with HBO facilitated recovery from moderate (30%) acute blood loss without any major adverse events, resulting in favorable effects at 48 hours and hastening recovery to baseline hemoglobin levels. These results support the data gained from anecdotal clinical experiences in treating extreme blood loss with HBO.

Successful human use of HBO was first reported by Amonic et al[60] with a patient in chronic hemorrhagic shock. No large trials in humans have been performed to date, although a few case reports regarding effective use in Jehovah's Witness patients with exceptional blood loss have been published.[61,62]

Contraindications

Conditions such as claustrophobia, pneumothorax, history of spontaneous pneumothorax, chronic obstructive pulmonary disease, seizure disorders, pregnancy (except in carbon monoxide poisoning), upper respiratory infection, hyperthermia, malignant tumors, and acidosis, as well as use of certain drugs (such as alcohol, nicotine, and steroids) are some of the contraindications for undergoing HBO therapy.

Safety

Some complications with use of HBO such as barotrauma[63] result in middle ear effusion, and rarely pulmonary or central nervous system oxygen toxicity. HBO therapy is associated with increased peripheral vascular resistance, reducing distal perfusion and compounding difficulty in oxygen delivery associated with severe anemia. Some of the signs and symptoms of oxygen toxicity in the central nervous system and pulmonary system are listed in Table 14-2.

The most common barotrauma is middle ear injury. The gradations of middle ear barotraumas are noted in Table 14-3. Other known barotrauma complications include reversible myopia and pneumothorax. The following may also be affected by barotrauma: the sinuses (congestion or occlusion leading to pain and bloody discharge), the gastrointestinal tract (vomiting, nausea, flatulence, colicky pain), and the teeth (infected or restored teeth may harbor gas leading to tooth pain, tooth implosion, or explosion).

Table 14-2. Signs and Symptoms of Oxygen Toxicity

Central Nervous System	Pulmonary System
Nausea and vomiting	Dry cough
Seizures	Substernal chest pain
Sweating	Bronchitis
Pallor	Shortness of breath
Muscle twitching	Pulmonary edema
Anxiety/respiratory changes	Pulmonary fibrosis
Visual changes	
Tinnitus	
Hallucinations	
Vertigo	
Hiccups	
Decreased level of consciousness	

Table 14-3. Teed Scale of Descent for Middle Ear Barotrauma

Grade	Signs/Symptoms	Treatment
0	Symptoms without signs	Frenzel and Valsalva maneuver
I	Injection of the tympanic membrane, especially along the handle of malleus	Frenzel and Valsalva maneuver
II	Injection plus slight hemorrhage within the substance of the tympanic membrane	Topical decongestants and ear decompression
III	Gross hemorrhage within the substance of the tympanic membrane	Centrally acting decongestant
IV	Free blood in the middle ear as evidenced by blueness and bulging	Otolaryngology evaluation; myringotomy tubes—if significant symptoms persist
V	Perforation of the tympanic membrane	Otolaryngology evaluation; myringotomy tubes—if significant symptoms persist

Treatment Fees and Insurance Coverage

The fees for HBO therapy can range from $150 per hour to almost $1000 per hour. Most of these costs are covered by Medicare, Medicaid, and most commercial insurance, including managed care plans. Prior approval for payment by commercial insurance is required at many hyperbaric centers.

References

1. Stehling LC, Zauder HI, Rodgers W. Intraoperative autotransfusion. Anesthesiology 1975;43:337-45.
2. Martin J, Robitaille D, Perrault LP, et al. Reinfusion of mediastinal blood after heart surgery. Thorac Cardiovasc Surg 2000;120:499-504.
3. Ayers DC, Murray DG, Duerr DM. Blood salvage after total hip arthroplasty. J Bone Joint Surg 1995;77:1347-51.
4. Thurer RL, Lytle BW, Cosgrove DM, Loop FD. Autotransfusion following cardiac operations: A randomized, prospective study. Ann Thorac Surg 1979;27:500-7.
5. Eng J, Kay PH, Murday AJ, et al. Postoperative autologous transfusion in cardiac surgery: A prospective, randomized study. Eur J Cardiothorac Surg 1990;4:595-600.
6. Roberts SR, Early GL, Brown B, et al. Autotransfusion of unwashed mediastinal shed blood fails to decrease banked blood requirements in patients undergoing aortocoronary bypass surgery. Am J Surg 1991;162:477-80.
7. Ritter MA, Keating EM, Faris PM. Closed wound drainage in total hip or total knee replacement: A prospective, randomized study. J Bone Joint Surg Am 1994;76:35-8.
8. Faris PM, Ritter MA, Keating EM, Valeria CR. Unwashed filtered shed blood collected after knee and hip arthroplasties: A source of autologous red blood cells. J Bone Joint Surg Am 1991;73:1169-78.
9. Clements DH, Sculco TP, Burke SW, et al. Salvage and reinfusion of postoperative sanguineous wound drainage: A preliminary report. J Bone Joint Surg Am 1992;74:646-51.
10. Moonen AFCM, Knoors NT, van Os JJ, et al. Retransfusion of filtered shed blood in primary total hip and knee arthroplasty: A prospective randomized clinical trial. Transfusion 2007;47:379-84.
11. Blevins FT, Shaw B, Valeri CR, et al. Reinfusion of shed blood after orthopaedic procedures in children and adolescents. J Bone Joint Surg Am 1993;75:363-71.
12. Munoz M, Garcia-Vallejo JJ, Ruiz MD, et al. Transfusion of post-operative shed blood: Laboratory characteristics and clinical utility. Eur Spine J 2004;13 (Suppl 1):S107-13.

13. Huet C, Salmi LR, Fergusson D, et al. A meta-analysis of the effectiveness of cell salvage to minimize perioperative allogeneic blood transfusion in cardiac and orthopedic surgery. International Study of Perioperative Transfusion (ISPOT) Investigators. Anesth Analg 1999:89:861-9.

14. Society of Thoracic Surgeons Blood Conservation Guideline Task Force, Ferraris VA, Ferraris SP, et al. Perioperative blood transfusion and blood conservation in cardiac surgery: The Society of Thoracic Surgeons and the Society of Cardiovascular Anesthesiologists clinical practice guideline. Ann Thorac Surg 2007;83(Suppl 5):S27-86.

15. Waters JH, Dyga RM. Postoperative blood salvage: Outside the controlled world of the blood bank. Transfusion 2007;47:362-5.

16. Sinardi D, Marino A, Chillemi S, et al. Composition of the blood sampled from surgical drainage after joint arthroplasty: Quality of return. Transfusion 2005; 45:202-7.

17. Dalén T, Bengtsson A, Brorsson B, Engström KG. Inflammatory mediators in autotransfusion drain blood after knee arthroplasty, with and without leucocyte reduction. Vox Sang 2003;85:31-9.

18. Blevins FT, Shaw B, Valeri CR, et al. Reinfusion of shed blood after orthopaedic procedures in children and adolescents. J Bone Joint Surg Am 1993;75: 363-71.

19. Duchow J, Ames M, Hess T, Seyfert U. Activation of plasma coagulation by retransfusion of unwashed drainage blood after hip joint arthroplasty: A prospective study. J Arthroplasty 2001;16:844-9.

20. Krohn CD, Reikeras O, Bjornsen S, Brosstad F. Fibrinolytic activity and postoperative salvaged untreated blood for autologous transfusion in major orthopaedic surgery. Eur J Surg 2001;167:168-72.

21. Andersson I, Tylman M, Bengtson JP, Bengtsson A. Complement split products and proinflammatory cytokines in salvaged blood after hip and knee arthroplasty. Can J Anaesth 2001;48:251-5.

22. Bengtsson A, Avall A, Hyllner M, Bengtson JP. Formation of complement split products and proinflammatory cytokines by reinfusion of shed autologous blood. Toxicol Lett 1998;100-101:129-33.

23. Jensen CM, Pilegaard R, Hviid K, et al. Quality of reinfused drainage blood after total knee arthroplasty. J Arthroplasty 1999;14:312-18.

24. Handel M, Winkler J, Hornlein RF, et al. Increased interleukin-6 in collected drainage blood after total knee arthroplasty: An association with febrile reactions during retransfusion. Acta Orthop Scand 2001;72:270-2.

25. Krohn CD, Reikeras O, Aasen AO. Inflammatory cytokines and their receptors in arterial and mixed venous blood before, during and after infusion of drained untreated blood. Transfus Med 1999;9:125-30.

26. Tylman M, Bengtson JP, Avall A, et al. Release of interleukin-10 by reinfusion of salvaged blood after knee arthroplasty. Intensive Care Med 2001;27:1379-84.

27. Hansen E, Pawlik M. Reasons against the retransfusion of unwashed wound blood. Transfusion 2004;44(Dec Suppl):45S-53S.

28. Arnestad JP, Bengtsson A, Bengtson JP, et al. Release of cytokines, polymorphonuclear elastase, and terminal C5b-9 complement complex by infusion of wound drainage blood. Acta Orthop Scand 1995;66:334-8.

29. Wixson RL, Kwaan HC, Spies SM, Zimmer AM. Reinfusion of postoperative wound drainage in total joint arthroplasty: Red blood cell survival and coagulopathy risk. J Arthroplasty 1994;9:351-8.

30. Faris PM, Ritter MA, Keating EM, Valeri CR. Unwashed filtered shed blood collected after knee and hip arthroplasties: A source of autologous red blood cells. J Bone Joint Surg Am 1991;73:1169-78.

31. Krohn CD, Reikerås O, Mollnes TE. Complement activation and increased systemic and pulmonary vascular resistance indices during infusion of postoperatively drained untreated blood. Br J Anaesth 1999;82:47-51.

32. Carless PA, Henry DA, Moxey AJ, et al. Cell salvage for minimising perioperative allogeneic blood transfusion. Cochrane Injuries Group. Cochrane Database of Syst Rev 2006;3:CD001888. [Available at http://www.cochrane.org/reviews/en/ab001888.html (accessed July 30, 2007).]

33. Howie C, Hughes H, Watts AC. Venous thromboembolism associated with hip and knee replacement over a ten-year period: A population-based study. J Bone Joint Surg Br 2005;87:1675-80.

34. Majkowski RS, Currie IC, Newman JH. Postoperative collection and reinfusion of autologous blood in total knee arthroplasty. Ann R Coll Surg Engl 1991; 73:381-4.

35. Newman JH, Bowers M, Murphy J. The clinical advantages of autologous transfusion: A randomized, controlled study after knee replacement. J Bone Joint Surg Br 1997;79:630-2.

36. Klodell CT, Richardson JD, Bergamini TM, Spain DA. Does cell-saver blood administration and free hemoglobin load cause renal dysfunction? Am Surg 2001;67:44-7.

37. Spain DA. Miller FB, Bergamini TM, et al. Quality assessment of intraoperative blood salvage and autotransfusion. Am Surg 1997;63:1059-63.

38. Yoshida M, Roth RI, Levin J. The effect of cell-free hemoglobin on intravascular clearance and cellular, plasma, and organ distribution of bacterial endotoxin in rabbits. J Lab Clin Med 1995;126:151-60.

39. Thurer RL, Lytle BW, Cosgrove DM, Loop FD. Autotransfusion following cardiac operations: A randomized, prospective study. Ann Thorac Surg 1979;27: 500-7.

40. Hartz RS, Smith JA, Green D. Autotransfusion after cardiac operation. J Thorac Cardiovasc Surg 1988;96:178-82.

41. Ilstrup S, ed. Standards for perioperative autologous blood collection and administration. 3rd ed. Bethesda, MD: AABB, 2007.

42. Corwin H. RBC transfusion in the ICU. Is there a reason? Chest 1995;108: 767-71.

43. Vincent JL, Baron JF, Reinhart K, et al. Anemia and blood transfusion in critically ill patients. JAMA 2002;288:1499-507.

44. Corwin HL. Anemia and blood transfusion in the critically ill patient: role of erythropoietin. Crit Care 2004;8(Suppl 2);S42-4.

45. Practice guidelines for blood component therapy: A report by the American Society of Anesthesiologists Task Force on Blood Component Therapy. Anesthesiology 1996;84:732-47.

46. Hebert PC, Wells G, Blajchman MA, et al. A multicenter, randomized, controlled clinical trial of transfusion requirements in critical care. Transfusion Re-

quirements in Critical Care Investigators, Canadian Critical Care Trials Group. N Engl J Med 1999;340:409-17.

47. Tsai AG, Cabrales P, Intaglietta M. Microvascular perfusion upon exchange transfusion with stored red blood cells in normovolemic anemic conditions. Transfusion 2004;44:1626-34.

48. Taylor R. Impact of allogenic packed red blood cell transfusion on nosocomial infection rates in the critically ill patient. Crit Care Med 2002;30:2249-54.

49. Johnson JL, Moore EE, Gonzalez RJ, et al. Alteration of the postinjury hyperinflammatory response by means of resuscitation with a red cell substitute. J Trauma 2003;54:133-9.

50. Fernandes CJ Jr, Akamine N, De Marco FV, et al. Red blood cell transfusion does not increase oxygen consumption in critically ill septic patients. Crit Care 2001;5:362-7.

51. Reiter CD, Wang X, Tanus-Santos JE, et al. Cell-free hemoglobin limits nitric oxide bioavailability in sickle-cell disease. Nat Med 2002;8:1383-9.

52. Goodnough LT, Brecher ME, Kanter MH, AuBuchon JP. Transfusion medicine: First of two parts—blood transfusion. N Engl J Med 1999;340:438-47.

53. Rodriguez RM, Corwin HL, Gettinger A, et al. Nutritional deficiencies and blunted erythropoietin response as causes of the anemia of critical illness. J Crit Care 2001;16:36-41.

54. Frede S, Fandrey J, Pagel H, et al. Erythropoietin gene expression is suppressed after lipopolysaccharide or interleukin-1 beta injections in rats. Am J Physiol 1997;273(3 Pt 2):R1067-71.

55. Jelkmann W. Proinflammatory cytokines lowering erythropoietin production. J Interferon Cytokine Res 1998;18:555-9.

56. Roberts I, Evans P, Bunn F, et al. Is the normalisation of blood pressure in bleeding trauma patients harmful? Lancet 2001;357:385-7.

57. Boerema I, Meyne NG, Brummelkamp WH, et al. Life without blood. Ned Tijdschr Geneesk 1960;104:949-54.

58. Esmond WG, Attar S, Cowley RA. Hyperbaric oxygenation in experimental hemorrhagic shock: Experimental chamber design and operation. Trans Am Soc Artif Intern Organs 1962;8:384-93.

59. Wright JK, Ehler W, McGlasson DL, Thompson W. Facilitation of recovery from acute blood loss with hyperbaric oxygen. Arch Surg 2002;137:850-3.

60. Amonic RS, Cockett AT, Lorhan PH, Thompson JC. Hyperbaric oxygen therapy in chronic hemorrhagic shock. JAMA 1969;208:2051-4.

61. Greensmith JE. Hyperbaric oxygen reverses organ dysfunction in severe anemia. Anesthesiology 2000;93:1149-52.

62. McLoughlin PL, Cope TM, Harrison JC. Hyperbaric oxygen therapy in the management of severe acute anaemia in a Jehovah's Witness. Anaesthesia 1999;54:891-5.

63. Hamilton-Farrell M, Bhattacharyya A. Barotrauma. Injury 2004;35:359-70.

In: Waters JH, ed.
Blood Management: Options for Better Patient Care
Bethesda, MD: AABB Press, 2008

15

Special Surgical Management: Liver Surgery

VIVEK MAHESHWARI, MD;
T. CLARK GAMBLIN, MD; AND
DAVID A. GELLER, MD

MAINTENANCE OF GOOD HEMOSTASIS, WHICH is an integral part of any surgical procedure, remains a challenge for operative liver surgery.[1] Traditionally, the principal cause of morbidity and mortality in hepatic resection has been directly related to intraoperative bleeding.[2] Many anatomical limitations make liver surgery complex. The liver has a dual blood supply consisting of the hepatic artery and the portal vein, and it receives a significant proportion of the cardiac output. Most high-volume medical centers still report median blood losses of 800 to 1800 mL for major

Vivek Maheshwari, MD, Surgical Oncology Fellow; T. Clark Gamblin, MD, Assistant Professor of Surgery; and David A. Geller, MD, Richard L. Simmons Professor of Surgery and Codirector, UPMC Liver Cancer Center, Department of Surgery, University of Pittsburgh, Pittsburgh, Pennsylvania liver resections.[3] Various authors have reported the use of allogeneic blood transfusion, with a rate varying from 23% to 98%.[1,4] Ability to minimize blood loss during hepatic resection makes the procedure safer, reduces the requirement for blood component transfusion, and eventually improves patient outcome.

The increasing experience and technological advances in surgical techniques, anesthesia refinements, and preoperative radiology imaging, coupled with a better understanding of liver anatomy, make it increasingly possible to perform major liver resections with a minimal blood loss and a declining perioperative morbidity and mortality.[2,5,6] Those advances have led to a widespread acceptance of live donor hepatectomies for liver transplantation.[7] Further recent technological advances have resulted from an explosion in minimally invasive technology. As a corollary, many of these innovative instruments have been applied in open surgical procedures to reduce blood loss. Today, liver surgeons have an array of electrosurgical devices, staplers, and hemostatic agents to choose from for operative hepatic surgery.

Preoperative Evaluation

The preparation for liver resection starts with careful evaluation of the indications and with assessment of the patient's medical condition. The liver is the site for synthesis of several coagulation factors, and some liver disorders are associated with platelet dysfunction. The coagulation and platelet disorders should be corrected preoperatively, along with optimizing the patient's medical condition.

Preoperative planning includes a good radiological assessment of the liver pathology and its relationship with inflow and outflow vessels of the liver. In most circumstances, assessment can be achieved with a good triphasic computed tomography (CT) scan. The CT scan provides an opportunity to identify aberrant anatomical variations in vascular anatomy, thus obviating the need for more invasive angiographic procedures. Improvements in multiplanar imaging and software processing have allowed for preoperative reconstruction of virtual 3-D liver anatomy and will be available for wider clinical use in the future. Other diagnostic imaging techniques such as ultrasound, magnetic resonance imaging, or angiography can be used, depending on the need. Information obtained from diagnostic imaging helps surgeons by providing a road map for liver resection. A careful preoperative assessment of portal and hepatic vein anatomy helps the surgeon avoid catastrophic bleeding events.

Anesthesia for Liver Surgery

During surgery, close cooperation between the surgeon and the anesthesiologist is essential. Various anesthetic techniques minimize blood loss and transfusion requirements. Troublesome bleeding is often encountered during the parenchymal transection phase from the hepatic sinusoids or from injury to the hepatic veins at their junction with the inferior vena cava (IVC).[4,8] The pressure in the sinusoids and the hepatic veins is directly related to the central venous pressure (CVP). The maintenance of low CVP (<5 mm Hg) during the operation precludes vena caval distension and facilitates mobilization of the liver and dissection of the retrohepatic and major hepatic veins. More important, such an approach minimizes hepatic venous bleeding during parenchymal transection, and it facilitates control of inadvertent venous injury, particularly of the intrahepatic course of the middle hepatic vein.[4] However, low CVP increases the risk for air embolism; a 0.4% incidence of clinically significant air embolism without mortality has been reported.[4] Air embolism can be avoided by the immediate oversewing of any holes in the hepatic veins.

Low CVP can be maintained by restricting intravenous fluid infusions to 1 mL/kg/hour and by accepting lower urine outputs of 25 mL/hour. It is acceptable to maintain a systolic blood pressure above 90 mm Hg until the liver resection has been completed and until the patient can be rendered euvolemic after hemostasis is achieved at the cut edge of the liver. Occasionally, intravenous nitroglycerine or the venodilating properties of narcotic agents can be used to lower CVP.[4] Avoiding positive end-expiratory pressure, or PEEP, can help keep hepatic venous pressure low.

Another technique to minimize allogeneic transfusion is intraoperative isovolemic hemodilution (see Chapter 8).

Surgical Techniques

Adequate surgical exposure is requisite for a safe, controlled liver resection. Adequate exposure can usually be accomplished by a right subcostal incision and its extension to midline toward the xiphoid. The incision can be extended to the left subcostal if required. Exposure is facilitated by use of a self-retaining retractor with rib-grip blades. Adequate mobilization of the liver is the next essential step. During that phase, it is important to avoid traction injury to short hepatic veins and the right adrenal gland, which is often adherent to the posterior capsule of the liver. Such injuries are a potential source of significant but avoidable blood loss.

Intraoperative ultrasound is a valuable tool. Not only does it allow identification of unsuspected pathology, but also it is crucial in mapping intrahepatic vascular anatomy and variations. The depth and location of vascular pedicles and hepatic veins can be identified and marked. Furthermore, if inflow occlusion is used, ultrasound performed at the end of the procedure can confirm the adequacy of portal venous inflow and hepatic vein outflow in the liver.

Because most blood loss occurs during the parenchymal transection phase, various methods have been described to minimize blood loss. These approaches can be divided into two major categories: 1) methods to reduce liver blood flow, both antegrade and retrograde (see Table 15-1), and 2) methods to divide liver parenchyma (see Table 15-2).

Table 15-1. Methods to Reduce Blood Flow to the Liver

Control of antegrade blood flow

Pringle maneuver
Extrahepatic pedicle control
Intraparenchymal pedicle control

Control of retrograde blood flow

Low central venous pressure
Extrahepatic hepatic vein division

Control of both antegrade and retrograde blood flow

Total vascular isolation
Selective hepatic vascular exclusion

Techniques to Reduce Liver Blood Flow

Pringle Maneuver

In 1908, J. H. Pringle described a method of temporarily compressing the portal inflow vessels in the hepatoduodenal ligament to reduce liver bleeding.[9] It remains the single most popular method of controlling liver bleeding.

Huguet and colleagues and Bismuth and coworkers demonstrated convincingly that the normally functioning liver can tolerate up to 65 minutes of warm ischemia, but that the functionally compromised liver, including the cirrhotic liver, is less tolerant.[9] To minimize ischemic injury, inflow occlusion can be applied intermittently, with 15 minutes of occlusion alternating with 5 minutes of reperfusion.[10] Other modifications are selective, such as a "half-Pringle" maneuver, whereby inflow is occluded to only that part of the liver to be resected.[11] In addition to causing warm ischemia, the Pringle maneuver has other limitations. In the presence of an aberrant left hepatic artery, inflow occlusion may not be complete. Furthermore, the clamping of

Table 15-2. Methods of Dividing Liver Parenchyma

Method	Manufacturer	Method of Action	Function
Finger fracture/ clamp and crush technique	N/A	Manual disruption of tissue	Tissue separation
Ultrasonic surgical aspirator	CUSA EXcel system (Integra, Plainsboro, NJ)	Two rupturing effects at the tissue interface: 1) forces impacted tissue to vibrate, accelerate, and decelerate with the tip, and 2) tip produces localized pressure waves that cause vapor pockets around cells	Tissue fragmentation leaving intact vessels and portal ducts
Water jet	Multiple manufacturers	High-pressure pump transfers energy to a liquid jet	For jet cutting of parenchymal tissue
Staplers	Multiple manufacturers	Metal staple across tissue surface	Dividing major hepatic veins and portal pedicles

Electrosurgical devices	Multiple manufacturers	Converts standard electrical current with frequency of 60 cycles per second to 300,000 cycles per second with a variety of waveforms that have variable tissue effects	Used to cut, coagulate, or vaporize tissue
Bovie electrocautery	Multiple manufacturers	High-power electrocautery	Used to score tissue and seal off small blood vessels (1-2 mm)
Radiofrequency electro-surgery	TissueLink (TissueLink Medical, Dover, NH)	Radiofrequency electrical energy with a low irrigation of saline to conduct energy	Sealing structures up to 3 to 6 mm
Bipolar vessel sealing device	LigaSure (Tyco Valleylab, Boulder, CO)	High-current, low-voltage output	Seals vessels up to 7 mm
Argon beam coagulator	Birtcher Medical Systems (Irvine, CA)	Conduction of high-frequency current to target tissue via a plasma arc	Limit or stop bleeding from large open surfaces
Ultrasonic shear devices	Ethicon Endo-Surgery (division of Johnson & Johnson, New Brunswick, NJ)	Coaptive coagulation at low temperatures ranging from 50 to 100 C	Seals vessels up to 6 mm

the hepatoduodenal ligament does not control retrograde hepatic venous bleeding. The Pringle maneuver can occasionally induce spasm or other injury to the hepatic artery, although such injuries are uncommon. Fortunately, portal venous or splanchnic venous congestion is usually not a significant clinical problem with this maneuver.

Other techniques that have been described provide selective vascular occlusion by compression of parenchyma.[2] The Longmire liver clamp has been designed for such use. The clamp is difficult to apply, especially with thick liver parenchyma, which is typically the case in hemihepatectomy. The Longmire clamp is most frequently used for left lateral segmentectomy, but its use has recently declined.

Total Vascular Isolation

Total vascular isolation (TVI) is capable of achieving control over both antegrade and retrograde blood flow. That phenomenon was first described by Heaney et al in 1948. They used an abdominothoracic approach, which was modified in 1966 to include occlusion of the infra- and suprahepatic vena cavae, the porta hepatis, and the infradiaphragmatic aorta.[12] The technique, which is recommended for experienced liver surgeons undertaking difficult liver resections,[12] is accomplished by applying inflow occlusion at the hepatoduodenal ligament and occlusion of the infra- and suprahepatic vena cava.[12] Volume loading may be required to minimize hemodynamic consequences of caval occlusion. In patients who do not tolerate reduction in venous return, supraceliac cross-clamping of the aorta may be required, which can also reduce splanchnic congestion. Hemodynamic instability can be circumvented by various techniques that bypass systemic and portal venous circulation, but their use adds complexity to the liver procedure.

The principal advantage of TVI is to prevent profuse hemorrhage and air embolism. The maneuver is technically complex and cannot be applied intermittently. It is associated with warm ischemia to the liver and, in the case of supraceliac aorta occlusion, to other visceral organs, thus resulting in reperfusion injuries. Approximately 14% of patients will not tolerate the hemodynamic consequences.[4] In most reported series, TVI is associated with significant morbidity—but such morbidity may be a reflection of more complex and difficult resections being performed with this technique. Most liver centers reserve TVI for tumors that are located close to the hepatic vein confluence or to the IVC.

Selective Hepatic Vascular Exclusion

For patients who are unable to tolerate the hemodynamic consequences of IVC occlusion, an alternative technique is to selectively occlude the hepatic veins in combination with a Pringle maneuver, leaving the IVC patent. However, this technique, which requires dissection of hepatic veins, can be technically demanding and potentially hazardous.[13]

Pedicle Control

The amount of operative blood loss can be further reduced by ligation of corresponding inflow blood vessels, combined with hepatic vein division or without it, before liver parenchymal transection. The corresponding hepatic artery and portal vein can be divided either extraparenchymally or intraparenchymally. Many surgeons reserve division of the right or left hepatic duct to the parenchymal transection to minimize the chance of injury to the remaining contralateral hepatic duct.

Extraparenchymal pedicle control requires dissection of the appropriate branch of the hepatic artery or the portal vein by hilar dissection. During dissection of the portal vein, it is important not to injure small caudate lobe branches, and such injuries should be controlled before isolation of a main portal vein branch. Any anomalous portal venous anatomy, such as the right anterior portal vein branch emanating from the left portal vein, should be identified by preoperative imaging and intraoperative ultrasound. Care should be taken with the hepatic artery to identify any anomalous arterial supply to the contralateral lobe. Extrahepatic pedicle control may require longer operative time, but it reduces the need for the Pringle maneuver and warm ischemia time. It may also expedite parenchyma transection by inducing a line of demarcation.

An alternative approach to pedicle control is intraparenchymal division as described by Launois and Jamieson.[14] Portal structures carry the Glisson's sheath around them as they enter the liver parenchyma. By making appropriate hepatotomies under inflow control with the Pringle maneuver, a surgeon can isolate and divide a desired pedicle en masse with vascular staples, or the surgeon can divide the pedicle between clamps. While dividing the pedicle, the surgeon should take care not to narrow inflow to the contralateral pedicle. The major advantage of that approach is shorter operative time because the surgeon avoids extrahepatic hilar vascular dissection.[15] Disadvantages to that approach are the requirement for initial inflow control with the Pringle maneuver, blunt dissection to isolate the pedicle, and, rarely, injury to the hepatic duct confluence. The approach should not be used if the tumor is close to the hilum.

Hepatic Vein Division

For formal right hepatic lobectomy, the right hepatic vein is usually divided outside the liver at the junction with the IVC. Before the surgeon attempts dissection of the right hepatic vein, the entire liver should be elevated off the IVC in "piggyback" fashion by individually ligating the short hepatic vein branches. Care should be taken to identify and oversew any dominant inferior accessory right hepatic veins. Once the right hepatic vein is exposed and dissected from above and below the liver, it can safely be divided with an ENDO GIA (Tyco, Princeton, NJ) vascular stapler or between vascular clamps.

For left hepatic lobectomy, the left and middle hepatic veins usually form a common trunk as they insert into the IVC. They can be divided together with a vascular stapler after ensuring adequate identification of the right hepatic vein.

Liver Parenchyma Transection

Most of the blood loss during liver resection is encountered during division of the liver parenchyma. With anatomical resection, blood loss can be minimized with prior control of blood flow, as discussed earlier. Nonanatomical resections and division of diseased liver parenchyma, as in a cirrhotic or fatty liver, are notoriously difficult because of bleeding from the parenchyma. Various methods and techniques have been used to divide the liver parenchyma, but none are ideal. Future improvements in liver surgery will be needed. The desire to minimize blood loss and the ability to control blood vessels and bile ducts encountered during parenchymal division have to be balanced against lateral damage to the remaining tissue and vital structures.

Finger Fracture and the Clamp and Crush Technique

Finger fracture was an early technique to divide liver parenchyma and the controlling blood vessels with suture ligatures or clips. However, finger fracture does not provide the precise control that is needed, and it is associated with significant avulsion injuries to blood vessels. The finger fracture technique was replaced with the clamp-and-crush technique because it allows finer control. The clamp-and-crush technique remains one of the most popular techniques, although problems associated with it include oozing from the transected surface, inadvertent injuries to venous tributaries, slow pace of the transection, and requirements for inflow occlusion.

Ultrasonic Surgical Aspiration

The Cavitron ultrasonic surgical aspirator (CUSA) EXcel system (Integra, Plainsboro, NJ) consists of a console unit and a variety of surgical tip handpieces. The console unit houses the electrosurgery unit and control panel. From the control panel, the amplitude, the irrigation, and the tissue select mode can be changed. Within the water-cooled handpiece, a transducer activates a hollow titanium tip along its longitudinal axis at a frequency of either 23 kHz or 36 kHz. The ultrasonic aspirator has two rupturing effects at the tissue interface. The first is caused by suction that couples tissue to the tip and forces impacted tissue to vibrate, accelerate, and decelerate with the tip, eventually fragmenting away from the nonaffected tissue. The second important effect is cavitation. The rapidly oscillating tip produces localized pressure waves that cause vapor pockets around cells in tissue with high water content, like hepatocytes, and the collapse of these pockets causes the cells to rupture. Tissues with strong intracellular bonds and high content of collagen and elastin are difficult to fragment. The speed of tissue fragmentation depends on the amplitude setting of the system. Thus, hepatocytes can be destroyed. The cell debris is removed by constant irrigation and suction, thereby exposing vascular structures and bile ducts, which subsequently can be controlled by clips or ties. The dissector itself has no hemostatic properties, and the optimal setting for amplitude and frequency varies from patient to patient.

In general, division of a cirrhotic liver requires high-energy settings, although the liver of older patients may require lower settings. High-energy settings may destroy thin-walled structures like veins and can cause significant bleeding. To optimize the use of the ultrasonic aspirator requires keeping the operating hand supple and using gentle forward movements. Because the power is directed forward, side-to-side waving of the handpiece is unproductive.[16] The device's greatest advantages are that it causes minimal lateral damage and that it can be used to dissect around portal triad and hepatic veins. The disadvantages are the slow pace of the liver resection and the cumbersome machine setup.

Water Jet Cutting

Another technique involves a high-pressure pump that transfers energy to a liquid jet. With jet cutting, the loosely connected liver parenchyma is washed away from the more resilient blood vessels and bile ducts by a water beam. Pressures of 10 to 80 bar and nozzles with a diameter of 0.1 to 0.2 mm produce an adequate beam for jet cutting of parenchymal tissue.[17] The device, which requires a certain amount of practice to be used adeptly, has only recently been approved by the Food and Drug Administration for use in liver surgery.

Staplers in Liver Surgery

Besides conventional methods of controlling blood vessels and bile ducts by using clips or sutures, various new devices are available for rapid control of these structures. Use of vascular stapling devices has gained rapid acceptance in hepatic surgery. A slim design makes the ENDO GIA staplers very helpful in liver surgery, where the surgeon has to work in an anatomically limited space. The staples, besides dividing major hepatic veins and portal pedicles, can effectively and rapidly divide liver parenchyma, often without the need for the Pringle maneuver.

In stapling technique, the liver capsule and parenchyma are divided superficially by using any of the methods described earlier. Once a depth of 2 to 3 cm has been reached or whenever major blood vessels are encountered, vascular staplers can be used to crush the parenchyma and divide the vessels—after creating a tunnel over and under the crossing veins with the help of a blunt instrument such as a Kelly clamp. After the surgeon completes the parenchyma transection, a few figure-eight sutures are occasionally required to achieve hemostasis of small, avulsed crossing veins. Cost of the staplers is a consideration; at times, the transected surface of the liver may not be as flat as when other methods are used.

Electrosurgical Devices

Various electrosurgical devices are routinely used in liver surgery. The electrosurgical generator is the source of the electron flow and voltage. The circuit is composed of the generator, an active electrode, the patient, and a patient return electrode. As current passes through tissues, impedance leads to heat production. An electrosurgical generator converts standard electrical current with a frequency of 60 cycles per second to 300,000 cycles per second. At that frequency, electrosurgical energy can pass through the patient with minimal neuromuscular stimulation and no risk of electrocution.

Different variables, such as power and types of waveforms, can affect tissue impact. Electrosurgical generators can produce a variety of waveforms with variable tissue effects. Constant waveforms produce the cutting current, which produces heat very rapidly and can be used to cut or vaporize the tissue. An intermittent waveform produces the coagulating effect by generating less heat so that a coagulum is formed instead of tissue vaporization. Size of the electrode affects current concentration. The smaller the electrode, the higher the current concentration delivered to the tissue. The longer the generator is activated, the more heat is produced and the farther it will spread to adjacent tissue. Thermal spread has the potential to cause lateral damage. Such damage is one of the significant shortcomings of electrosurgical devices and limits their use to the immediate vicinity of vital structures. Manipulation of the electrode—whether sparking or holding the electrode in direct contact—determines coagulation vs vaporization of tissue.

Bovie Electrocautery. In liver surgery, bovie electrocautery can be used to score the liver capsule and to seal off small blood vessels (1-2 mm). The production of effective hemostasis for larger blood vessels in the liver parenchyma requires high power. Such high power results in excessive heat; temperature exceeding 350 C causes significant lateral damage, charring, and eschar formation. Eschar usually sticks to the electrode and has a tendency to separate from liver parenchyma as the electrode is moved. This sticking can be somewhat overcome by keeping a distance between the liver parenchyma and the electrode. Charring makes it difficult to distinguish between parenchymal, vascular, and biliary structures. It is difficult to divide liver parenchyma with conventional bovie electrocautery alone without risking major blood loss. Various modifications have been designed to overcome some of these shortcomings.

Radiofrequency Electrosurgery. The TissueLink device (TissueLink Medical Inc, Dover, NH) combines radiofrequency electrical energy with a low irrigation of saline to conduct energy and to provide a cooling effect to tissue. The device is capable of sealing structures between 3 and 6 mm in diameter without producing either high temperatures or excessive charring and eschar. Structures >6 mm in diameter should be divided in the conventional manner with clips or ties. The device requires constant suction to clear saline used for irrigation, so the pace of the liver resection may be slow. The first-generation TissueLink device used a floating ball tip that "precoagulated" liver tissue, which was then divided with scissors[18] or bovie cautery. Later-generation devices have a blunt or sharp (cone-head) tip that allows dissection and sealing. The newer devices can be used in combination with the CUSA system or hydrojet to shorten parenchymal transection time. When properly used, that approach can significantly reduce blood loss during liver parenchyma transection.[18] Application of a cooled-tip radiofrequency probe to precoagulate liver tissue along the planned transection line has also been used.[19]

Bipolar Vessel-Sealing Device. A bipolar vessel-sealing device such as the LigaSure (Valleylab, division of Tyco Healthcare Group, Boulder, CO) uses a generator that produces a high-current, low-voltage output that corresponds to at least four times the current of a standard electrosurgery generator, with one-fifth to one-twentieth the amount of voltage. That current allows the collagen in the vessel wall to melt and form a seal.

The feedback-control mechanism in the generator allows the generator to adjust the energy level according to tissue type. The device is capable of sealing blood vessels with high collagen content and in diameters up to 7 mm. Thermal spread is limited to 2 mm and minimal charring is produced. The instrument is bulky, and the cross-sectional area of the blade is 4 mm × 3 mm and can cause mechanical injury if the instrument is pushed through parenchyma. Creating a tunnel with the help of a blunt instrument (similar to creating one with a stapler) can minimize such injury. Liver parenchyma should also be crushed by a gentle maneuver of opening and closing the blades several times or cleared by an ultrasonic dissector before applying (twice if necessary). This action prevents sticking of parenchyma to the blades. Because the technique depends on collagen content of the blood vessel, it cannot be relied on for extremely thin-walled veins.[20]

Electrocoagulation. The Argon beam coagulator (ABC) (Birtcher Medical Systems, Irvine, CA) is a monopolar electrocoagulator that can be used to limit or stop bleeding from large open surfaces. The basic mechanism uses conduction of a high-frequency current to target tissue through an argon plasma arc. The argon gas has been partially or completely ionized. The arc may be initiated and maintained at larger electrode-tissue gaps, thereby preventing contact with tissue and sticking of the coagulum to the electrode. The ABC also allows uniform distribution of energy by a multichanneling effect and enables the painting of bleeding surfaces with precision while delivering a superficial eschar. The ABC is very effective in controlling oozing from transected liver parenchyma or surface bleeding that occurs after a liver capsule tear.

Ultrasonic Shearing

Ultrasonic energy can also be used to coagulate and cut blood vessels. Since its introduction in the 1990s, this method has become very popular, especially for laparoscopic procedures. The Harmonic Scalpel (Ethicon Endo-Surgery Inc, Cincinnati, OH), which uses ultrasonic sheer technology, controls bleeding by coaptive coagulation at low temperatures ranging from 50 to 100 C, thereby limiting lateral thermal spread and damage. As described by the manufacturer, "Coagulation occurs by means of collagen denaturation when the blade, vibrating at 55,500 Hz, couples with protein, thereby denaturing it to form a coagulum that seals" vessels up to 6 mm in size.[21]

Cutting speeds and coagulation are inversely related and can be easily controlled and balanced by manipulating four factors: power, blade sharpness, tissue tension, and grip force or pressure. Increasing the power level increases cutting speed and decreases coagulation. Shear mode cuts faster than blunt mode but provides less coagulation. Less tissue tension and a gentle grip force allow for more coagulation. The blade has been designed for an intermittent operation of 15 seconds on and 15 seconds off. During prolonged activation in tissue, the instrument blade may become hot, and unintended contact with tissue should be avoided.

Ultrasonically activated shears have been used to divide liver parenchyma. Ultrasonic shearing has a few shortcomings, however; the most notable is a higher incidence of biliary leakage because it does not effectively seal biliary radicals.[3] The transection blades are of insufficient length to divide large portal vein branches.[22] Because the technology depends on the presence of sufficient collagen, thin-walled structures like hepatic vein branches may be difficult to seal.

Topical Agents

Certain pharmacological hemostatic agents can also be of aid in achieving hemostasis on the transected surface of the liver. Oxidized cellulose such as Surgicel (Johnson & Johnson Gateway, Piscataway, NJ) and microfibrillar collagen have been used as an adjunct to achieve hemostasis. More recently, the use of fibrin sealants has become increasingly popular because the sealants effectively stop oozing from the surface and may also seal minor bile leaks. Fibrin sealants are supplied as two components: human fibrinogen and thrombin. They also have Factor XIII as a fibrin stabilizer and an antifibrinolytic agent. When these two components are mixed, they form a coagulum in a manner similar to the final steps of physiologic coagulation. These products are plasma derived and undergo rigorous screening and inactivation procedures for viruses. So far, there has not been a reported case of viral transmission with use of these products, although there is always a theoretical risk of viral transmission with use of plasma products.

Two commercial products are available in the United States for the purpose of achieving hemostasis during liver surgery. Tisseel (Baxter, Deerfield, IL) and Crosseal (Ethicon Inc, Johnson & Johnson Gateway) differ in the concentration of various components—the most significant difference being in the antifibrinolytic agent. Tisseel contains bovine aprotinin and carries a small risk for hypersensitivity reaction whereas Crosseal contains tranexamic acid, a synthetic product. In clinical trials, mean time to hemostasis for liver surgery with fibrin sealant was 5.3 minutes vs 7.7 minutes[23]—a statistically significant difference. Because these products have been introduced recently, any long-term adverse effects are unknown.

Summary

Over the past several years, new surgical techniques and advances in biomedical devices have resulted in improved safety of hepatic resections. Consequently, most major medical centers have seen a decreased need for blood transfusion, and many cases of liver surgery are now accomplished as "bloodless." Further advances in imaging and hemostatic technology should allow for continued improvements in blood management.

References

1. Mariette D, Smadja C, Naveau S, et al. Preoperative predictors of blood transfusion in liver resection for tumor. Am J Surg 1997;173:275-9.

2. Buell JF, Koffron A, Yoshida A, et al. Is any method of vascular control superior in hepatic resection of metastasis cancers? Arch Surg 2001;136:569-75.

3. Kim J, Ahmad SA, Lowy AM, et al. Increased biliary fistulas after liver resection with the Harmonic Scalpel. Am Surg 2003;69:815-19.

4. Melendez JA, Arslan V, Fischer ME, et al. Perioperative outcomes of major hepatic resections under low central venous pressure anesthesia: Blood loss, blood transfusion, and the risk of postoperative renal dysfunction. J Am Coll Surg 1998;187:620-5.

5. Gozzetti G, Mazziotti A, Grazi GL, et al. Liver resection without blood transfusion. Br J Surg 1995;82:1105-10.

6. Iwatsuki S, Starzl TE. Personal experience with 411 hepatic resections. Ann Surg 1988;208:421-34.

7. Marcos A, Fisher RA, Ham JM, et al. Right lobe living donor liver transplantation. Transplantation 1999;68:798-803.

8. Jones RM, Moulton CE, Hardy KJ. Central venous pressure and its effect on blood loss during liver resection. Br J Surg 1998;85:1058-60.

9. Fortner JG, Blumgart LH. A historic perspective of liver surgery for tumors at the end of the millennium. J Am Coll Surg 2001;193:210-22.

10. Imamura H, Seyama Y, Kokudo N, et al. One thousand fifty-six hepatectomies without mortality in 8 years. Arch Surg 2003;138:1198-206.

11. Horgan PG, Leen E. A simple technique for vascular control during hepatectomy: The half Pringle. Am J Surg 2001;182:265-7.

12. Hansen PD, Isla AM, Habib NA. Liver resection using total vascular exclusion, scalpel division of the liver parenchyma, and a simple compression technique for hemostasis and biliary control. J Gastrointest Surg 1999;3:537-42.

13. Smyrniotis V, Kostopanagiotou G, Theodoraki K, et al. The role of central venous pressure and type of vascular control in blood loss during major liver resections. Am J Surg 2004;187:398-402.

14. Launois B, Jamieson GG. The importance of Glisson's capsule and its sheaths in the intrahepatic approach to resection of the liver. Surg Gynecol Obstet 1992;174:7-10.

15. Figueras J, Lopez-Ben S, Llado L, et al. Hilar dissection versus the "Glissonean" approach and stapling of the pedicle for major hepatectomies: A prospective, randomized trial. Ann Surg 2003;238:111-19.

16. Rees M, Plant G, Wells J, Bygrave S. One hundred and fifty hepatic resections: Evolution of technique towards bloodless surgery. Br J Surg 1996;83:1526-9.

17. Rau HG, Buttler ER, Baretton G, et al. Jet-cutting supported by high-frequency current: New technique for hepatic surgery. World J Surg 1997;21:254-60.

18. Sturgeon C, Helton WS, Lamba A, et al. Early experience employing a linear hepatic parenchyma coagulation device. J Hepatobiliary Pancreat Surg 2003;10:81-6.

19. Zacharoulis D, Asopa V, Navarra G, et al. Hepatectomy using intraoperative ultrasound-guided radiofrequency ablation. Int Surg 2003;88:80-2.

20. Strasberg SM, Drebin JA, Lineban D. Use of a bipolar vessel-sealing device for parenchymal transection during liver surgery. J Gastrointest Surg 2002;6:569-74.

21. Harmonic Scalpel. Piscataway, NJ: Johnson & Johnson Gateway, 2008. [Available at http://www.jnjgateway.com/home.jhtml?loc=USENG&page=viewContent&

contentId=09008b9880a2d37a&parentId=09008b9880a2d37a (accessed January 3, 2008).]

22. Wrightson WR, Edwards MJ, McMasters KM. The role of the ultrasonically activated shears and vascular cutting stapler in hepatic resection. Am Surg 2000; 66:1037-40.

23. Busuttill RW. A comparison of antifibrinolytic agents used in hemostatic fibrin sealants. J Am Coll Surg 2003;197:1021-8.

In: Waters JH, ed.
Blood Management: Options for Better Patient Care
Bethesda, MD: AABB Press, 2008

16

Special Surgical Management: Obstetrics

EGLE BAVRY, MD, AND
JONATHAN H. WATERS, MD

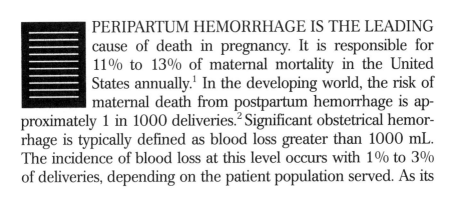 PERIPARTUM HEMORRHAGE IS THE LEADING cause of death in pregnancy. It is responsible for 11% to 13% of maternal mortality in the United States annually.[1] In the developing world, the risk of maternal death from postpartum hemorrhage is approximately 1 in 1000 deliveries.[2] Significant obstetrical hemorrhage is typically defined as blood loss greater than 1000 mL. The incidence of blood loss at this level occurs with 1% to 3% of deliveries, depending on the patient population served. As its

Egle Bavry, MD, Consultant, Pain Management, Cleveland Clinic, Cleveland, Ohio, and Jonathan H. Waters, MD, Chief and Visiting Associate Professor, Department of Anesthesiology, Magee-Womens Hospital, University of Pittsburgh Medical Center, Pittsburgh, Pennsylvania rate of occurrence increases, cesarean section is expected to be associated with increasing rates of hemorrhage.

Physiologic Changes of Pregnancy

Over the course of gestation, one of the most dramatic physiologic changes occurs in the cardiovascular system. At around 30 weeks of gestation, blood volume reaches its peak (up to a 60% increase).[3] The red cell mass expansion is surpassed by a plasma volume expansion so that a physiologic anemia of pregnancy results. This relative anemia decreases viscosity, which is one of the contributors to overall increase in cardiac output. These changes provide significant compensatory reserve should possible acute blood loss occur.

Debate exists regarding the effect on platelet count during gestation.[4-6] It would seem plausible that platelet concentration, like red cell mass, would decrease as a result of a relative greater increase in plasma volume; however, some investigators feel that increased platelet destruction occurs. Along with platelet concentration, most coagulation factors increase during pregnancy. At delivery, this leads to a hypercoagulable state. Of greatest importance is a 50% increase in fibrinogen concentration.[7]

After delivery, the hemoglobin level returns to that of a nonpregnant state. Immediately following delivery, hemoglobin concentration reflects the combined contributions of hemoglobin and iron status during pregnancy and blood loss associated with delivery. The expected fall in hemoglobin within the first 3 days following vaginal delivery ranges from 0.1 to 0.6 g/dL.[8] As the physiologic plasma volume expansion of pregnancy reverses after delivery, diuresis ensues, resulting in a rapid hemoconcentration. As a result, the hemoglobin level rises rapidly from the third postpartum day forward.[9] In uncomplicated patients, the hemoglobin concentration should normalize within 4 to 6 weeks.[10]

Indications for Transfusion

Debate regarding the appropriate trigger for transfusion for all patients is ongoing. The debate has focused on the appropriate transfusion of red cells but is evolving to include plasma and platelet transfusion. For red cells, the Transfusion Requirements in Critical Care Investigators trial[11] suggests that a reasonable threshold for critically ill patients is a hemoglobin below 7 g/dL. Obstetric patients make up a unique population of usually healthy women in their twenties and thirties with pregnancy-induced cardiovascular changes. The optimal hematocrit at which peripartum blood transfusion should be given remains undefined in this patient group. In general, most practitioners allow their asymptomatic patients to drop to hemoglobin levels of 5 to 6 g/dL, a level not generally tolerated in other patient populations. In the days following delivery, hemoconcentration occurs through decreases in plasma volume. With this hemoconcentration, immediate postpartum anemia will be ameliorated without transfusion. Blood transfusion in this population should be performed recognizing that any complication resulting from transfusion will have a greater impact on the quality of life of young and healthy patients and the benefit-to-risk ratio should be weighed carefully.

As with red cells, the optimal platelet and plasma transfusion triggers for the peripartum patient are also poorly defined. Peripartum platelet transfusion should take place when evidence of bleeding is accompanied by platelet counts consistent with surgical triggers—that is, less than 50,000/μL. A rational approach for plasma is to transfuse when international normalized ratio (INR) levels increase beyond 1.6 in association with clinical evidence of bleeding. For the nonpregnant patient, INR levels greater than this are associated with coagulation factor concentrations of less than 30%. Whether this is true for pregnancy has not been elucidated. Because plasma transfusion carries the greatest risk of transfusion-related acute lung injury, serious thought should be given before administration in a young, healthy, peripartum female.

Preoperative Autologous Blood Donation

Several studies[12,13] have shown that autologous blood donation in the third trimester of pregnancy is safe for both mother and fetus. Nonetheless, the need for blood obtained during preoperative autologous donation is unpredictable, and therefore the practice is generally not cost effective.[14] Placenta previa is one obstetric condition for which autologous donation may be appropriate.[15] In patients with placenta previa, the majority of units donated (81%) are eventually used for autologous transfusion.[16] However, 25% of these patients required additional allogeneic blood—a rate similar to the 25% to 30% transfusion rate reported in other series of placenta previa without blood donation.

Although, in general, autologous blood donation is thought to be safe, some potential risks should always be considered: blood donation decreases maternal iron stores and can adversely affect iron delivery to the fetus, and maternal hypovolemia after blood donation can impair uteroplacental perfusion. Women who deliver within 1 week of autologous donation have lower predelivery hematocrit levels and may be more likely to require peripartum transfusion than women who do not donate.

Furthermore, specific limitations of autologous blood donation in obstetric patients include difficulty in timing the donation, increased vasovagal reactions during blood donation, and difficulty in predicting blood loss, which makes patient selection difficult. Most donor centers use a hemoglobin cutoff of 11 g/dL before allowing donation to take place. This is a level that is routinely seen in the antepartum female because of the physiologic anemia of pregnancy; thus many patients are ineligible for autologous donation. In addition, the number of units of blood that can be safely collected over a period of time without any maternal or fetal hemodynamic compromise is uncertain, and there is insufficient information on the effect of preoperative blood donation on the fetus.

Acute Normovolemic Intraoperative Hemodilution

Acute normovolemic hemodilution has been advocated by some practitioners but its effect on fetal safety has been little studied. The concern in pregnancy is that impaired fetal oxygenation might result from maternal blood volume changes. Although no controlled placental flow studies have been performed in human pregnancy during hemodilution, it is known that the oxygen affinity of fetal hemoglobin F is capable of maintaining fetal oxygenation in an environment of decreased blood flow. Additional studies are required to document the safety and benefits of this procedure during pregnancy.

Intraoperative Blood Recovery

The use of blood recovery in obstetrics is classically contraindicated; however, little data are available to substantiate this contraindication. In fact, significant data exist to support its use. The contraindication arises from a concern that shed blood can be contaminated with amniotic fluid, and readministration may lead to an iatrogenic amniotic fluid embolism. The incidence of amniotic fluid embolism is so rare that a study to demonstrate the safety of blood recovery would require 1.7 million patients. Because this sample size is unrealistic, an evaluation of what is known about blood recovery along with an evaluation of the alternative therapy, allogeneic transfusion, is warranted.

Support for the use of blood recovery in obstetric hemorrhage now encompasses 390 reported cases where blood contaminated with amniotic fluid has been washed and readministered without filtration.[17-19] None of these cases were complicated by amniotic fluid embolism. Only one adverse report has been made: a letter to the editor of the *International Journal of Obstetric Anesthesia* described a 22-year-old Jehovah's Witness patient at 30 weeks gestation with preeclampsia and

HELLP (hemolysis, elevated liver enzymes, low platelet count) syndrome.[20] Her presenting laboratory values were a hemoglobin level of 7.1 g/dL, a platelet count of 48,000, aspartate aminotransferase of 194 IU/L, and alanine aminotransferase of 330 IU/L. A Continuous Auto Transfusion System [C.A.T.S (Fresenius, distributed by Terumo, Ann Arbor, MI)] was used to recover 600 mL of blood and amniotic fluid, which was subsequently processed to 200 mL. It is important to note that no leukocyte depletion filter was used. Ten minutes after starting the reinfusion, the patient became dyspneic, hypoxic (O_2 Sat = 85%), and, finally, arrested. A clinical diagnosis of amniotic fluid embolism was followed by a pathologic diagnosis which "did not reveal any other cause."[20]

Whether blood recovery was responsible for the death of the patient in this report is highly suspect. First, the patient was severely ill when presenting to the labor suite and may have succumbed by a number of different mechanisms. Second, the report provides little description of how the blood was processed other than that a C.A.T.S machine was used. This is important because blood recovery can be associated with the "cell salvage syndrome," which is a coagulopathy that results from the readministration of a partially washed product and is typically due to a lack of knowledge of the parameters necessary for a quality wash. Last, it can be questioned whether the volume of reinfused blood was adequate to cause an amniotic fluid embolism. Tio[21] demonstrated a therapeutic effect of amniotic fluid when he infused amniotic fluid into 27 peripartum women with prolonged coagulation times. Volumes ranged from 5 to 500 mL and resulted in resolution of the clotting abnormalities. He then proceeded to administer amniotic fluid to 73 patients of various ages without effect.[22] Thus, it seems unlikely that any remnant amniotic fluid in the 200 mL of recovered blood could be responsible for the demise of the aforementioned patient.

Because of the rarity of amniotic fluid embolus, evaluations of surrogate markers of amniotic fluid have been made. Unfortunately, because the mechanism for amniotic fluid embolism is not clear, any studies demonstrating that recovered blood is clean for one parameter may not extrapolate to the unknown mechanism of amniotic fluid embolism. Tissue factor is thought to be involved in the disseminated intravascular coagulopathy that typically follows the acute embolic event.[23] Bernstein and colleagues[24] evaluated the washout of tissue factor and found that routine washing eliminated all tissue factor activity. Because tissue factor may be only one of many components that lead to the syndrome of amniotic fluid embolism, washing of this tissue factor would not guarantee that amniotic fluid embolism would not occur.[25,26] Nevertheless, several studies evaluating the efficacy of blood recovery washout—including studies on the removal of free hemoglobin, bromocreosol green dye, and heparin—have suggested that if one factor is effectively removed, the other factors are equally removed.[27,28] Therefore, if tissue factor is effectively removed from blood contaminated with amniotic fluid, these previous studies would suggest that the other biochemical components of amniotic fluid would also be similarly removed or reduced significantly in concentration.

In a pig model, clear amniotic fluid (meconium-free) injected into the pig in quantities up to 10 mL/kg caused only minor effects.[29] However, when meconium-stained amniotic fluid was infused at volumes of 3 mL/kg, severe coagulopathy and cardiorespiratory abnormalities ensued. This would suggest that it is important to remove the particulate matter of amniotic fluid. Durand and colleagues[30] showed cell washing alone did not remove fetal squamous cells. Waters et al[31] demonstrated that leukocyte-reduction filters along with cell washing will remove fetal squamous cells to an extent comparable to the concentration of these cells in a maternal blood sample following placental separation. From this study it was concluded that the combination of recovered-blood washing and filtration produces a blood component comparable to circulating maternal blood, with the exception of the fetal hemoglobin contamination. The filters use a small-pore microfiber web and a negative surface charge.[32]

This discussion may become irrelevant because recent articles[33-35] have suggested that amniotic fluid embolus is in fact not an embolic disease but rather an anaphylactic reaction. This suggestion implies that amniotic fluid embolus would occur with or without blood recovery because amniotic fluid is routinely entrained during delivery. Therefore, any debate regarding remnant amniotic fluid in recovered blood may be irrelevant.

Despite what appears to be substantial reassuring data, several precautions should be taken when recovering blood in obstetrics. First, it is advisable to minimize the aspiration of amniotic fluid through a double suction setup. One suction should be connected to the blood recovery reservoir and used for suctioning blood. The other should be connected to the regular wall suction and used only for aspiration of amniotic fluid. In this way, the volume of amniotic fluid contamination is minimized. Second, the use of leukocyte-reduction filters at the completion of processing can reduce the fetal squamous cell contamination to a level comparable to maternal blood contamination. These filters should be used by the anesthesiologist, placing <300 mm Hg pressure on the reinfusion bag. Last, because fetal red cell contamination is present, an Rh incompatibility between mother and infant may suggest that the Rhogam (Ortho-Clinical, Rochester, NY) dose following delivery may need to be modified.

The practice of medicine frequently requires evaluation of risks when applying different treatment strategies. In this area, the purely theoretical risk of blood recovery in obstetrics is compared to the transfusion of allogeneic blood, which has multiple known adverse consequences. Until proven otherwise, the use of recovered blood appears to offer the safer treatment modality for the hemorrhaging obstetric patient.

Pharmacological Treatment

Role of Erythropoietin in Obstetrics

During pregnancy, endogenous erythropoietin levels are normally increased. This accounts for an increased red cell mass, provided that stores of vitamin B_{12}, folate, and iron are adequate. Erythropoietin levels increase with increasing gestational age and peak at 40 weeks with levels at term that are 2 to 4 times higher than those found in nonpregnant nonanemic controls.[36]

Exogenous erythropoietin administered during pregnancy is considered to be a teratogenic risk factor C drug. There are no adequate and well-controlled studies in pregnant women treated with erythropoietin; it should be used only if potential benefits outweigh potential risks to the fetus. Overall, there are few cases in the literature documenting the use of erythropoietin in pregnancy. No maternal or fetal side effects have been described.

Role of Iron Supplementation in Obstetrics

In many surgical environments, the greatest risk factor for transfusion is preoperative anemia. Though not definitively demonstrated in pregnancy, one can assume that anemia would also be a risk factor for transfusion. Inadequate available iron is responsible for the majority of anemia in pregnant women.[37] Therefore, focus on maintaining available iron stores should be paramount. Over the course of gestation, maternal iron stores are severely reduced as a result of the expansion of the mother's red cell mass and the iron needs of the developing fetus.[38] Even with supplemental oral iron, marrow stores during the third trimester show only small traces of remaining iron.[39] Because the prevalence of iron deficiency anemia is so high in pregnant women, the Centers for Disease Control and Prevention recommends universal iron supplementation despite inconclusive evidence of its benefits.[40] Unfortunately, the compliance with oral iron supplementation is typically poor, especially in lower-income populations.[41] Every effort should be made to limit supplemental iron to the oral route, but in some patients, parenteral iron might be needed. Parenteral iron can be given either intravenously or intramuscularly. Two intramuscular injections of iron sorbitol given 6 weeks apart has been demonstrated to be equivalent to daily oral iron in hemoglobin and iron store response.[42]

Uterotonics

Uterotonics are drugs used to stimulate uterine contraction and, in turn, to reduce postpartum hemorrhage. There are three primary agents used in the United States for this purpose: oxytocin, ergots, and prostaglandins.

Oxytocin

Oxytocin has been demonstrated to reduce the risk of significant postpartum hemorrhage by up to 40%.[43] As a result, the American College of Obstetrics and Gynecology (ACOG) recommends routine oxytocin, 10 to 40 U intravenously by continuous infusion following delivery. The British National Formulary recommends 5 U intravenously.[44,45] Little data are available on adequate dosing of oxytocin following delivery; dosing strategies are primarily empiric. Minimum dosing strategies for oxytocin have been more clearly defined for elective cesarean section[46] and for cesarean delivery after labor arrest.[47] In these up-down sequential allocation scheme studies, it appears that the effective dose for 90% of the population is 1 U for elective cesarean section and 3 U for cesarean labor after labor arrest. These doses are significantly lower than the commonly used US recommendations. The primary reason for minimizing the dosing is concern about hypotension,[48] although it is not clear whether the concern is valid. Other adverse reactions that have been described occur in less than 1% of patients: premature ventricular contractions, arrhythmias, hypertension, severe water intoxication with convulsions, coma, and death.[49]

For oxytocin, a receptor mechanism depends on gestational age and increases over the course of gestation. The pattern of uterine contractions after postpartum administration of intravenous oxytocin is described as a short period of hypercontractibility followed by an increased frequency in contractions. Because of its short half-life, the response to a single dose diminishes in as little as 10 minutes.[50]

Ergots

Grains exposed to specific moisture conditions grow ergot fungus. Reports of ergot poisoning date back to the ninth century, when plagues occurred and victims suffered from gangrene. Ultimately the vasoconstrictive properties of these fungi have become recognized as the cause of what was termed "Saint Anthony's fire."[51]

Ergot alkaloids act as partial agonists at alpha receptors and have a direct vasoconstrictive action.[52] Little is known about how ergot alkaloids achieve their oxytocic effects. Care is needed in the administration of this drug. Many cases of myocardial infarction have been reported with dosing of methylergonovine.[53] These cases recommend intramuscular dosing of the drug to avoid peak levels of the drug and its associated coronary vasospasm. When administered intravenously, it should be diluted and given slowly. Typical dosing of methylergonovine is 0.2 mg intramuscularly every 2 to 4 hours.

Ergot alkaloids are contraindicated in the presence of hypertensive disease because severe hypertension may develop secondary to vasoconstriction. In cases of significant postpartum hemorrhage, the risk of hypertension following methylergonovine needs to be balanced with the need for enhancement of uterine tone to prevent ongoing blood loss where hypotension is present.

Prostaglandins

The third most commonly used group of uterotonic agents is prostaglandins. Prostaglandins include natural substances [prostaglandin (PG) 2-alpha and PGE2] and synthetic substances (15-methyl PGF2-alpha and sulprostone). The uterotonic effect of prostaglandins is independent of gestational age. Although the exact mechanism is not fully understood, prostaglandins produce a strong myometrial contraction resulting in increased uterine tone. According to the ACOG education bulletin,[54] 15-methyl PGF2-alpha may be given in a dose of 0.25 mg intramuscularly every 15 to 90 minutes (no more than 8 doses). Refractory uterine atony may respond to 250 mg of intramuscular carboprost [Hemabate (Pharmacia and Upjohn, Kalamazoo, MI), an analog of PGF2-alpha.[55] This agent may also be given by intramyometrial injection at cesarean delivery or transabdominally after vaginal delivery.

Diarrhea (11%), raised blood pressure (7%), and vomiting (7%) are the most common unwanted effects of carboprost (Hemabate), whereas bronchospasm and pulmonary edema are very rare.[56]

Recombinant Factor VIIa

There is growing interest in using recombinant activated factor VII (rFVIIa) for treatment of postpartum hemorrhage.[57] Only case reports with varying dosing regimens of its use have been published. In the largest series[58] (43 cases), 72% of the cases were reported to have stopped bleeding following administration of rFVIIa. (The problem with case series is that significant biasing results from the tendency of investigators to report positive results more frequently than negative ones.) Caution is advised when considering use of this drug because of the very high cost: The 1.2-mg, 2.4-mg, and 4.8-mg vials cost $1200, $2400, and $4800, respectively. Although there is no standard dose for rFVIIa in obstetrics, Franchini et al[59] list the average dose used in a series of case reports as 65 µg/kg with a range of 13 to 120 µg/kg. If an average weight of 70 kg for postpartum females is considered, the average cost per patient would be $4550 per dose. Further work is needed to identify the appropriate dose and indication.

Mechanical Maneuvers

Postpartum hemorrhage for suspected uterine atony should be managed initially by bimanual uterine massage and compression. Bimanual compression is performed by massaging the uterus between one hand on the abdomen and the other hand or fist in the vagina or within the uterus. Uterine cavity packing is another mechanical maneuver that has been successfully used in treatment of postpartum hemorrhage. Historically, it was frequently performed to control postpartum hemorrhage. However, care should be taken to ensure that packing does not conceal significant hemorrhage or prevent the uterus from contracting firmly, as well as to systematically pack the fundus from side to side, avoiding creation of dead space for blood to accumulate. Prophylactic antibiotic therapy should be started at the time of uterine packing, and oxytocin should be continued for 12 to 24 hours after the pack has been removed. The recommendation for the time interval until removal of the pack is controversial, but most authors favor 24 to 36 hours, with removal at the bedside after pretreatment with analgesics.[60]

A variation on uterine cavity packing is based on balloon tamponade. There have been at least 45 cases in the literature describing balloon tamponade of the bleeding uterus. Balloon tamponade has been achieved with a number of different types of balloons, ranging from Foley catheters to condoms. The Sengstaken-Blakemore tube is traditionally used for the control of bleeding from esophageal varices but is the most widely used device for balloon tamponade of the uterus.[61] The Sengstaken-Blakemore tube combines an esophageal balloon with a gastric balloon. When used for uterine bleeding, the gastric balloon is cut off. The advantage of the Sengstaken-Blakemore tube over other types of balloon catheters is that the balloon can accommodate up to 500 mL of solution. The alternative Foley catheter bursts at volumes approaching 150 mL. Additionally, the Sengstaken-Blakemore tube is advocated because its sausage shape better conforms to the postpartum uterus.

The "tamponade test" is commonly described with the use of the Sengstaken-Blakemore tube.[62] This test determines the need for curative hysterectomy. In this test, the Sengstaken-Blakemore tube is placed through the cervix via the vagina. The balloon is inflated until it becomes visible at the cervical canal. Generally, this requires 75 to 300 mL of saline. In order to maintain uterine contraction over the balloon, an oxytocin infusion is run continuously during the test. The balloon is left inflated, with constant monitoring of bleeding either around the balloon or through the lumen of the attached catheter. In addition, hemoglobin levels are checked periodically. If the patient continues to show evidence of ongoing hemorrhage, the patient has failed the "tamponade test" and requires a curative hysterectomy. In most reports of successful tamponade, the balloon is left in place for 12 to 24 hours, after which it is deflated and the patient is observed for further bleeding.

Despite the retrospective nature and small numbers of cases reporting on the use of balloon tamponade, the low cost of these tubes and the noninvasiveness of the technique should make the use of these tubes part of the standard algorithm for managing postpartum hemorrhage. Prospective randomized trials would be attractive in further elucidating the effectiveness of this technique, although the infrequency of postpartum hemorrhage would make this difficult.

Interventional Radiology

Balloon catheterization and occlusion of the aorta or internal iliac vessels can be helpful in treatment and prevention of postpartum hemorrhage. The procedure involves retrograde placement of a balloon catheter through the femoral artery under fluoroscopic guidance. The catheter is then guided into the internal iliac arteries. The balloon may be inflated intermittently throughout the dissection, thus markedly decreasing blood loss and keeping the operative field drier.

Balloon catheterization is often not considered for women with uncontrolled hemorrhage because of 1) the limited number of modern angiography units with a skilled, around-the-clock, on-call team, and 2) the risk of transferring an unstable patient to the angiography table. It takes 1 to 2 hours to gain control of the major bleeding after the initial consultation.[63,64]

In patients at high risk for postpartum hemorrhage the catheters can be placed before labor or cesarean section. Studies
have compared patients undergoing prophylactic catheterization to those under emergent conditions. Patients undergoing
prophylactic angiographic catheter placement were noted to
have significantly reduced blood loss and transfusion requirements.

Surgical Techniques

Bilateral uterine artery ligation is a first-line procedure for controlling uterine bleeding during cesarean section.[65] As described
by O'Leary and O'Leary,[66] it is relatively simple, and in the absence of uterine rupture, or broad ligament hematoma, it is successful in 95% of cases for controlling postpartum hemorrhage.
The complication rate is less than 1% and future fertility is not
affected. Collateral circulation and recanalization occurs within
6 to 8 weeks.

AbdRabbo[65] described a technique of stepwise uterine devascularization to control intractable postpartum hemorrhage. The
technique involves performing one vessel ligation at a time before proceeding to the next step if bleeding is not completely
controlled. B-Lynch et al[67] described a technique in which the
uterus remains in situ and a "brace suture" (B-Lynch suture) is
placed around the uterus, which may lead to satisfactory hemostasis.

When most medical and conservative surgical therapies have
failed, emergency hysterectomy remains an acceptable and potentially life-saving procedure.[68] Uterine atony and placenta ac-
cretia (each make up 28% of all cases) are the most common
indications for peripartum hysterectomy. The mortality of hysterectomy should be less than 1%, even in emergency cases.
Subtotal hysterectomy is an acceptable alternative in an unstable patient to decrease operative time.[69]

References

1. Prochat RW, Koonin LM, Atrask HK, et al, for the Maternal Mortality Collaborative: Maternal mortality in the United States: Report from the Maternal Mortality Collaborative. Obstet Gynecol 1988;72:91-97.
2. Abou Zahr C, Royston E. Global mortality. Global fact-book. Geneva: World Health Organization, 1991.
3. Scott DE. Anemia during pregnancy. Obstet Gynecol Annu 1972;1:219-44.
4. Tygart S, McRoyan D, Spinnato J, et al. Longitudinal study of platelet indices during normal pregnancy. Am J Obstet Gynecol 1986;154:883.
5. Sejeny S, Eastham R, Baker S. Platelet counts during normal pregnancy. J Clin Pathol 1975;28:812.
6. Fay R, Hughes A, Farron N. Platelets in pregnancy: Hyperdestruction in pregnancy. Obstet Gynecol 1983;61:238.
7. Maternal adaptations to pregnancy. In: Cunningham FG, MacDonald PC, Gant NF, et al, eds. Williams obstetrics. 20th ed. Stamford, CT: Appleton & Lange, 1997:205.
8. Prendiville WJ, Harding JE, Elbourne DR, Stirrat GM. The Bristol third stage trial: Active versus physiological management of third stage of labour. BMJ 1988;297:1295-300.
9. Lund CJ. Studies on the iron deficiency anemia of pregnancy; including plasma volume, total hemoglobin, erythrocyte protoporphyrin in treated and untreated normal and anemic patients. Am J Obstet Gynecol 1951;62:947-63.
10. Jansen AJ, van Rhenen DJ, Steegers EA, Duvekot JJ. Postpartum hemorrhage and transfusion of blood and blood components. Obstet Gynecol Surv 2005; 60:663-71.
11. Hebert PC, Wells G, Blajchman MA, et al. A multicenter, randomized, controlled clinical trial of transfusion requirements in critical care. Transfusion Requirements in Critical Care Investigators, Canadian Critical Care Trials Group. N Engl J Med 1999;340:409-17.
12. O'Dwyer G, Mylotte M, Sweeney M, Egan EL. Experience of autologous blood transfusion in an obstetrics and gynaecology department. Br J Obstet Gynaecol 1993;100:571-4.
13. Lindenbaum CR, Schwartz IR, Chibber G, et al. Safety of predeposit autologous blood donation in the third trimester of pregnancy. J Reprod Med 1990; 35.537-40.
14. Combs CA, Murphy EL, Laros RK Jr. Cost-benefit analysis of autologous blood donation in obstetrics. Obstet Gynecol 1992;80:621-5.
15. American College of Obstetrics and Gynecology. Blood component therapy. Technical bulletin #199. Washington, DC: ACOG, 1994.
16. McVay PA, Hoag RW, Hoag MS, Toy PT. Safety and use of autologous blood donation during the third trimester of pregnancy. Am J Obstet Gynecol 1989; 160:1479-86.
17. Rainaldi MP, Tazzari PL, Scagliarini G, et al. Blood salvage during caesarean section. Br J Anaesthesia 1998;80:195-8.
18. Grimes DA. A simplified device for intraoperative autotransfusion. Obstet Gynecol 1988;72:947-50.

19. Jackson SH, Lonser RE. Safety and effectiveness of intracesarean blood salvage (letter). Transfusion 1993;33:181.

20. Oei SG, Wingen CBM, Kerkkamp HEM. Cell salvage: How safe in obstetrics? (letter). Int J Obstet Anesth 2000;9:143.

21. Tio AG. [no title (letter).] Rev Peruana Obstet 1955;3:84.

22. Tio AG. Clinical use of amniotic fluid. JAMA 1956;161:996.

23. Lockwood CJ, Bach R, Guha A, et al. Amniotic fluid contains tissue factor, a potent initiator of coagulation. Am J Obstet Gynecol 1991;165:1335-41.

24. Bernstein HH, Rosenblatt MA, Gettes M, Lockwood C. The ability of the Haemonetics 4 cell saver system to remove tissue factor from blood contaminated with amniotic fluid. Anesth Analg 1997;85:831-3.

25. Halmagyi DFJ, Starzecki B, Shearman RP. Experimental amniotic fluid embolism: mechanism and treatment. Am J Obstet Gynecol 1962;84:251-6.

26. Morgan M. Amniotic fluid embolism. Anaesthesia 1979;34:20-32.

27. Kling D, Börner U, von Bormann B, Hempelmann G. [Heparin elimination and free hemoglobin following cell separation and washing of autologous blood with Cell Saver 4 (article in German).] Anasth Intensivther Notfallmed 1988; 23:88-90.

28. Umlas J, O'Neill TP. Heparin removal in an autotransfusor device. Transfusion 1981;21:70-73.

29. Malek WH, Petroianu GA. Autologous blood transfusion. Br J Anaesth 1999; 82:154.

30. Durand F, Duchesne-Gueguen M, Le Bervet JY, et al. [Rheologic and cytologic study of autologous blood collected with Cell Saver 4 during cesarean (article in French).] Revue Francaise de Transfusion et d' Hemobiologie 1989;32:179-91.

31. Waters JH, Biscotti C, Potter P, Phillipson E. Amniotic fluid removal during cell-salvage in the cesarean section patient. Anesthesiology 2000;92:1531-6.

32. Dzik S. Leukodepletion blood filters: Filter design and mechanisms of leukocyte removal. Transfus Med Rev 1993;7:65-77.

33. Fineschi V, Gambassi R, Gherardi M, Turillazzi E. The diagnosis of amniotic fluid embolism: An immunohistochemical study for the quantification of pulmonary mast cell tryptase. Int J Legal Med 1998;111:238-43.

34. Farrar SC, Gherman RB. Serum tryptase analysis in a woman with amniotic fluid embolism. A case report. J Reprod Med 2001;46:926-8.

35. Ray BK, Vallejo MC, Creinin MD, et al. Amniotic fluid embolism with second trimester pregnancy termination: A case report. Can J Anaesth 2004;51:139-44.

36. Barton DP, Joy MT, Lappin TR, et al. Maternal erythropoietin in singleton pregnancies: A randomized trial on the effect of oral hematinic supplementation. Am J Obstet Gynecol 1994;170:896-901.

37. Routine iron supplementation during pregnancy. Review article. US Preventive Services Task Force. JAMA 1993;270:2848-54.

38. Taylor DJ, Mallen C, McDougall N, Lind T. Effect of iron supplementation on serum ferritin levels during and after pregnancy. Br J Obstet Gynaecol 1982; 89:1011-7.

39. Svanberg B, Arvidsson B, Norrby A, et al. Absorption of supplemental iron during pregnancy: A longitudinal study with repeated bone-marrow studies

and absorption measurements. Acta Obstet Gynecol Scand 1975;48(Suppl): 87-108.

40. Recommendations to prevent and control iron deficiency in the United States. Centers for Disease Control and Prevention. MMWR Recomm Rep 1998; 47(RR-3):1-29.

41. Jasti S, Siega-Riz AM, Cogswell ME, et al. Pill count adherence to prenatal multivitamin/mineral supplement use among low-income women. J Nutr 2005; 135:1093-101.

42. Kumar A, Jain S, Singh NP. Singh T. Oral versus high dose parenteral iron supplementation in pregnancy. Int J Gynaecol Obstet 2005;89:7-13.

43. Prendiville W, Elbourne D, Chalmers I. The effects of routine oxytocic administration in the management of the third stage of labour: An overview of the evidence from controlled trials. Br J Obstet Gynaecol 1988;95:3-16.

44. Obstetrics, gynaecology, and urinary-tract disorders. In: British national formulary. 42nd ed. London (UK): British Medical Association and Royal Pharmaceutical Society of Great Britain, 2001:373-6.

45. Thomas TA, Cooper GM on behalf of the Editorial Board of the Confidential Enquiries into Maternal Deaths in the United Kingdom. Maternal deaths from anaesthesia. An extract from Why Mothers Die 1997–1999, the Confidential Enquiries into Maternal Deaths in the United Kingdom. Br J Anaesth 2002; 89:499-508.

46. Carvalho JC, Balki M, Kingdom J, Windrim R. Oxytocin requirements at elective cesarean delivery: A dose-finding study. Obstet Gynecol 2004;104(5 Pt 1):1005-10.

47. Balki M, Ronayne M, Davies S, et al. Minimum oxytocin dose requirement after cesarean delivery for labor arrest. Obstet Gynecol 2006;107:45-50.

48. Balestrieri PJ. Maternal hemodynamics after oxytocin bolus compared with infusion in the third stage of labor: A randomized controlled trial (letter). Obstet Gynecol 2005;105:1486.

49. Lacy CF, Armstrong LL, Goldman MP, Lance LL. Drug information handbook. Hudson, OH: Lexi-Comp, 1978 to present.

50. Hendricks CH. Uterine contractility changes in the early puerperium. Clinical Obstet Gynecol 1968;11:125-44.

51. Maclean AB. Ergometrine. J Obstet Gynaecol 2005;25:1-2.

52. Muller-Schweinitzer E, Weidemann H. Basic pharmacological properties. In: Berde B, Schild HO, eds. Ergot alkaloids and related compounds. Berlin: Springer-Verlag, 1978:87-196 (handbook of experimental pharmacology, 49).

53. Lin YH, Seow KM, Hwang JL, Chen HH. Myocardial infarction and mortality caused by methylergonovine. Acta Obstet Gynecol Scand 2005;84:1022.

54. American College of Obstetrics and Gynecology. Postpartum hemorrhage. Educational bulletin #243. Int J Gynecol Obstet 2001;61;79-86.

55. Selo-Ojeme DO. Primary postpartum haemorrhage. J Obstet Gynaecol 2002; 22:463-9.

56. The management of postpartum haemorrhage. Drug Ther Bull 1992;30:89-92.

57. Moscardo F, Perez F, de la Rubia J, et al. Successful treatment of severe intra-abdominal bleeding associated with disseminated intravascular coagulation using recombinant activated factor VII. Br J Haematol 2001;114:174-6.

58. Sobieszczyk S, Breborowicz GH, Platicanov V, et al. Recombinant factor VIIa in the management of postpartum bleeds: An audit of clinical use. Acta Obstet Gynecol Scand 2006;85:1239-47.

59. Franchini M, Lippi G, Franchi M. The use of recombinant activated factor VII in obstetric and gynaecological haemorrhage. Br J Obstet Gynaecol 2007;114: 8-15.

60. Maier RC. Control of postpartum hemorrhage with uterine packing. Am J Obstet Gynecol 1993;169:317-21.

61. Seror J, Allouche C, Elhaik S. Use of Sengstaken-Blakemore tube in massive postpartum hemorrhage: A series of 17 cases. Acta Obstet Gynecol Scand 2005;84:660-4.

62. Tamizian O, Arulkumaran S. The surgical management of postpartum haemorrhage. Curr Opin Obstet Gynecol 2001;13:127-31.

63. Vendantham A, Goodwin SC, McLucas B, Mohr G. Uterine artery embolization: An underused method of controlling pelvic hemorrhage. Am J Obstet Gynecol 1997;17:938-48.

64. Alvarez M, Lockwood CJ, Ghidini A, et al. Prophylactic and emergent arterial catheterization for selective embolization in obstetric hemorrhage. Am J Perinatol 1992;9:441-4.

65. AbdRabbo SA. Stepwise uterine devascularization: A novel technique for management of uncontrolled postpartum hemorrhage with preservation of the uterus. Am J Obstet Gynecol 1994;171:694-700.

66. O'Leary JL, O'Leary JA. Uterine artery ligation for control of postcesarean section hemorrhage. Obstet Gynecol 1994;43:849-53.

67. B-Lynch C, Coker A, Lawal AH, et al. The B-Lynch surgical technique for the control of massive postpartum haemorrhage: An alternative to hysterectomy? Five cases reported. Br J Obstet Gynaecol 1997;104:372-5.

68. Smith J, Mousa HA. Peripartum hysterectomy for primary postpartum haemorrhage: Incidence and maternal morbidity. J Obstet Gynaecol 2007;27:44-7.

69. Roberts WE. Emergent obstetric management of postpartum hemorrhage. Obstet Gynecol Clin North Am 1995;22:283-302.

In: Waters JH, ed.
Blood Management: Options for Better Patient Care
Bethesda, MD: AABB Press, 2008

17

Special Surgical Management: Pediatrics

DOREEN E. SOLIMAN, MD, AND ANTONIO CASSARA, MD

ALLOGENEIC BLOOD TRANSFUSIONS IN INFANTS and children carry numerous risks and consequences, including potential transmission of infectious diseases, metabolic derangements, and immunologic reactions. Blood transfusion, especially in the pediatric population, can carry lifelong effects.[1] The risk of transmitting viral infections, such as the hepatitis A, B, and C viruses as well as human immunodeficiency virus, is one of the main concerns of parents[2]—despite the fact that the risk of infection from blood transfusion has decreased tremendously over the past 20 years, especially in the United States.[3]

Doreen E. Soliman, MD, Assistant Professor of Anesthesiology, and Antonio Cassara, MD, Pediatric Anesthesia Fellow, Children's Hospital of Pittsburgh, Department of Anesthesiology and Critical Care Medicine, University of Pittsburgh Medical Center, Pittsburgh, Pennsylvania

Transfusion guidelines and triggers in neonates and children are dictated by the physiologic and hematologic differences between adults and children.[4] The decision to transfuse children should not be guided solely by the patient's hemoglobin concentration. Several factors should be taken into account, including the patient's physiological condition, lactate concentration in the serum, mixed venous oxygenation, and the propensity to bleed after certain surgical procedures.[2]

In the context of various situations and surgical procedures, this chapter addresses conditions that are unique to the pediatric population. It presents the special strategies that have been developed to minimize the use of blood components in the treatment of acute anemia and blood loss sustained during these procedures.

Pediatric Care and the Jehovah's Witness Perspective

Jehovah's Witnesses accept up-to-date, standard-of-care medicine and surgery, but they believe blood transfusion is forbidden, according to their interpretation of the Bible (see Genesis 9:4, Leviticus 17:11, and Acts 15:20,29). The prohibition is based on the belief that blood must not be ingested and that, in transfusion, blood acts as a nutrient that is ingested.[5] Moreover, they believe that the punishment for accepting blood components or products is loss of eternal life and excommunication on earth.[5] Their religious beliefs do not, however, prohibit the use of all blood products; that is, products such as albumin, immunoglobulins, and blood clotting factors may be used at the discretion of each individual.

Because blood removed from the body must be discarded according to their beliefs, preoperative autologous donation (PAD) is not an option.[6] Moreover, intraoperative blood collection and hemodilution that involves blood storage separated from the body is not acceptable,[7] although dialysis circuits, cardiopulmonary bypass (CPB) equipment, and intraoperative blood recovery equipment can be used if the extracorporeal circulation is uninterrupted from the body.[7] Because of the complexity and individual variability of the issues surrounding transfusion and blood management strategies, it is imperative that the physician consult with Jehovah's Witness patients regarding their preferences.

For the pediatric patient the situation is even more complex. In life-threatening situations that involve severe anemia or bleeding, the physician is obligated to follow federal laws and state guidelines for the care of minors.[8-10] State guidelines can vary. In essence, every effort should be made to avoid blood transfusion for children of Jehovah's Witnesses, but children and teenagers under the age of 18 cannot be denied blood transfusion when it is considered a life-saving therapy.[8,10]

Principles of Bloodless Medicine

A series of interventions, created from attempts to avoid transfusion for populations such as the Jehovah's Witnesses, have evolved into the practice of bloodless medicine.[11,12] This practice is being applied to an increasing number of fields from organ transplantation and open-heart surgery to the trauma patient.[12-15]

The practice of bloodless medicine has two goals:

1. Blood augmentation through the use of recombinant human erythropoietin (rHuEPO), iron, vitamin B_{12}, and folic acid.[11,16,17]

2. Reduction of blood loss through blood conservation practices such as the following[11,15,18]:
   - Deliberate hypotension.
   - Acute normovolemic hemodilution (ANH).
   - Intraoperative blood recovery.
   - Drugs to minimize perioperative blood loss.

Although not included in the scope of this chapter, modifications in surgical techniques such as rigorous maintenance of hemostasis, the argon beam coagulator, and topical coagulants have also been used to reduce the amount of blood lost on the surgical field.

Recombinant Human Erythropoietin

rHuEPO has been used for various elective surgeries to increase preoperative red cell mass.[11,15-18] rHuEPO is commercially available as epoetin alfa, epoetin beta, and darbepoetin. Some formulations are suspended in albumin, whereas others are albumin free. Most Jehovah's Witnesses prefer albumin-free formulations, although erythropoietin containing albumin has been accepted.

rHuEPO is usually started 3 weeks before surgery. Doses can vary from 300 U/kg/week to 900 U/kg/week according to the rise of hematocrit and hemoglobin.[12,16,17,19] Iron sulfate, vitamin B_{12}, and folic acid are used as adjuncts during this period to facilitate the rise of the red cell mass.[11,19]

Deliberate Hypotension

Deliberate hypotension is the practice of decreasing arterial blood pressure to hypotensive levels during surgery. The decrease in blood pressure can be achieved with inhaled anesthetics or by a variety of intravenous drugs such as propofal, nitroglycerin, nitroprusside, clonidine, and esmolol. The systolic blood pressure in normotensive patients is decreased to 80 to 90 mm Hg, and the mean arterial pressure (MAP) is decreased to 50 to 65 mm Hg or decreased by 30% of baseline MAP.[11]

The purpose is to decrease blood loss during surgery and improve visibility in the surgical field. There are some concerns over the effects that low perfusion pressures can have on the central nervous system and end organs such as the heart, kidneys, and eyes, but current literature seems to indicate that normotensive patients can tolerate a MAP of 50 to 55 mm Hg without damage to these organs.[20,21]

Acute Normovolemic Hemodilution

ANH involves the exchange of whole blood for crystalloid or colloid solutions. Whole blood is rich in platelets and coagulation factors, which are not present in washed or preoperatively donated blood. A maximum of 30% of the estimated blood volume is removed through a central line and drained by gravity into a citrate-phosphate-dextrose-adenine bag, while colloids or crystalloids are administered to maintain blood volume. The blood is kept in continuous contact with the body through the central line. In other words, the column of blood is uninterrupted.[16,22]

The whole blood is stored at room temperature and returned to the patient when needed. The technique decreases the absolute loss of red cells during surgery and preserves clotting factors and platelets that can be returned when needed.[16,23] International Study of Perioperative Transfusion reviewers concluded that ANH could be useful in the reduction of perioperative blood transfusion.[23] More recent studies support the use of ANH in procedures with potential for high blood loss.[24,25]

The limitations of this technique are related to the patient's age and weight. The red cell volume available to be diluted on a per kilogram basis is small. Furthermore, infants less than 4 months of age are not good candidates for ANH because the neonatal myocardial function may not be able to compensate for the anemic state, even though normovolemia is maintained.[26]

The combination of rHuEPO and ANH increases the amount of blood available for hemodilution and was found to be effective in reducing the requirement of blood transfusion in infants. Meara et al[27] found that the combination of rHuEPO, ANH, and controlled hypotension reduced the transfusion requirement noticeably with respect to the control group. They concluded that the addition of rHuEPO significantly increased the efficacy of blood management strategies.

Blood Recovery Techniques

Blood from blood recovery techniques is accepted by most Jehovah's Witnesses if continuity with the body is maintained. Acceptance is on an individual basis. The blood is suctioned from the surgical field and collected in a reservoir. From there, the blood enters a bell-shaped canister that is a centrifuge where the red cells are washed and concentrated.[13] (It could be argued that during the centrifugal phase the red cells are separated from the system and the body.) After this process, the red cells are stored in a collection bag. The collection bag must also be in connection with the body through venous access. Therefore, it is important that this section of the circuit be primed so that no air is admitted into the circuit. There are no platelets or clotting factors in a recovered blood product. A meta-analysis review on blood recovery showed that this technique is useful in decreasing the need for intraoperative transfusion.[22]

Drugs to Minimize Perioperative Blood Loss

Minimizing perioperative blood loss by using pharmacologic agents is a useful adjunct, especially in the treatment of the Jehovah's Witness patient. Antifibrinolytic agents such as tranexamic acid, aminocaproic acid, and aprotinin have long been used to decrease blood loss during surgeries.[28] A meta-analysis of randomized trials evaluating the efficacy of aprotinin, desmopressin, tranexamic acid, and aminocaproic acid in decreasing the number of transfusions showed that aprotinin, tranexamic acid, and, to a lesser extent, aminocaproic acid significantly reduced blood loss, whereas desmopressin was not effective in reducing blood loss.[28] A recent observational study, however, found that the use of aprotinin to control bleeding during cardiac surgery caused significant end-organ damage, namely myocardial infarction and renal failure.[27] More recently, the off-label use of recombinant Factor VIIa (rFVIIa) for uncontrolled intra-operative bleeding has shown noticeable efficacy in the reduction of bleeding, thus reducing the need for transfusion.[11,16,18,29,30]

The Premature Infant

Term infants develop a physiologic anemia the first few months after birth. This anemia results from changes in endogenous erythropoietin concentration. During fetal development low arterial oxygen saturation in utero stimulates erythropoietin production. Erythropoietin stimulates the marrow, as well as the liver and kidney, to vigorously produce red cells. After birth, the arterial oxygen saturation increases, causing suppression of erythropoietin production and, in turn, red cell mass decreases until erythropoietin production resumes at a hemoglobin level of 10 to 11 g/dL. Fetal hemoglobin has a higher affinity for oxygen and a shorter life span. It declines by 6 to 12 weeks and is replaced by adult hemoglobin, which shifts the oxygen-hemoglobin dissociation curve to the right.

Preterm infants experience a greater drop in hemoglobin levels known as the anemia of prematurity. It is considered an exaggeration of the physiologic anemia of infancy and it lasts longer. It is a normocytic normochromic anemia associated with a low erythropoietin concentration.[31] Hemoglobin concentration decreases to 7 to 8 g/dL in infants <32 weeks gestation.[32] The neonatal myocardium adapts to anemia by increasing contractility.[33] This includes increases in stroke volume and left ventricular output, which can be reversed by transfusion of Red Blood Cells (RBCs).

Transfusion Triggers

The decision to transfuse preterm infants is based on the presence of underlying cardiopulmonary disease. In infants with severe bronchopulmonary dysplasia, hemodynamic compensatory responses are normalized after transfusion. This is reflected in decreases in heart rate, cardiac output, stroke volume, shortening fraction, and plasma lactate.[34]

The tendency of preterm infants to frequently require blood transfusions because of the anemia of prematurity, frequent phlebotomies, and associated comorbidities has led investigators to seek methods for minimizing transfusions in this patient population. Transfusion practices for preterm infants in neonatal intensive care units have been scrutinized, and more rigorous guidelines have been instituted. Factors that have been identified to indicate the need for transfusion include the use of mechanical ventilation, chronic lung disease, sepsis, lower birth hematocrit, and increased phlebotomy losses.

Recombinant Human Erythropoietin

The association of the anemia of prematurity with low serum erythropoitin levels has led to the evaluation, in several trials, of rHuEPO for use in minimizing blood transfusion in preterm infants. The results of these clinical trials have been somewhat contradictory regarding the efficacy of rHuEPO in treating preterm infants. The European Multicenter Erythropoietin Study Group[35] evaluated the effect of rHuEPO on the need for transfusion. Infants <34 weeks gestation and weighing 750 to 1499 g were enrolled in the study. The dose of rHuEPO used was 250 U subcutaneously, three times a week for 42 days. A total of 13 doses was administered. In addition, the infants received oral supplemental iron (2 mg/kg/day). Patients were randomized to receive rHuEPO or a placebo. Success was defined as maintaining hematocrit above 32% without transfusion. The treatment group received fewer transfusions, and the success rate of weaning infants off ventilators by day of life 6 was 44%, vs 28% in the placebo group.

In a multicenter, randomized, double-blind, and placebo-controlled study,[36] 172 infants weighing <1000 g and 118 infants weighing 1001 to 1250 g were treated with rHuEPO and placebo. The treatment dose was 400 U/kg intravenously or subcutaneously, three times weekly. All infants received supplemental enteral and parenteral iron. This study could not demonstrate the effect of rHuEPO use and iron supplementation on transfusion requirements.

The adverse side effects of rHuEPO reported in adult studies have not been reported in infants—ie, hypertension, pain, rash, and seizures.[37] Although transient neutropenia was reported in early studies, this finding has not been validated in recent randomized clinical trials.[38]

Craniofacial Surgery

Craniosynostosis is premature closure of skull sutures in infants. The incidence is 0.6 per 1000 births.[26,39] The normal newborn skull accommodates the rapid growth of the brain with the presence of unfused sutures and open fontanelles.[29,40] Craniosynostosis causes dysmorphic features and, rarely, increased intracranial pressure.

Cranial vault remodeling (CVR) procedures, which are commonly performed in infants, can correspond with the occurrence of the physiologic anemia of the newborn. These procedures typically involve significant blood loss ranging from 42% to 126% of the blood volume.[26,30,41,42] Allogeneic blood transfusion occurs in 96.3% of patients undergoing craniosynostosis repair.[40,43] Estimation of blood loss is challenging and frequently underestimated by the anesthesiologist. The blood loss varies with the type of suture repaired but is about 24% of estimated blood volume for sagittal suture repair, 21% for unicoronal, 65% for bicoronal, and 42% for metopic suture repair.[30,41]

Surgical techniques to repair craniosynostosis range from strip craniectomy to extensive CVR, and the approach chosen influences the degree of blood loss that will occur. CVR involves extensive osteotomies with bone repositioning.[30,41] Endoscopic techniques first described by Jimenez and Barone in 1998 are gaining widespread acceptance.[44] The endoscopic techniques result in advantages such as reduced blood loss, shorter operative time, and decreased cost and length of stay.[42,45] Several strategies have been proposed for reducing allogeneic blood use during the perioperative care of the pediatric patient.

Preoperative Strategies

The preoperative use of rHuEPO has been studied in infants and children undergoing CVR. Fearon and Weinthal,[46] in a randomized, controlled, and blinded study, used 600 U/kg per week subcutaneously for 3 weeks in the study group.[43,46] Iron supplementation (4 mg/kg per day) was administered to both the study and control groups, and 93% of the control group required transfusion, whereas 57% of the erythropoietin group were transfused. Three of the patients in the erythropoietin group were under 12 months of age. The preoperative hemoglobin level increased from 12.1 to 13.1 g/dL in the rHuEPO group.

The disadvantages of this technique are the multiple needle sticks, the subcutaneous rHuEPO injection, and repeated blood samples for hemoglobin measurement, which are distressing to the children. Cost has become an issue, as the average cost of rHuEPO is $109 per 10,000 U. In a 10-kg child, 6000 U administered per week preoperatively for 4 weeks would cost $262. The preparation and storage of a donor-directed unit of RBCs is $180.[27,44] With the risks of allogeneic blood transfusion, which include immunosuppression, hemolytic reactions, and transfusion-related acute lung injury, an argument can be made for the preoperative use of rHuEPO.[45] A careful discussion with parents on a case by case basis is recommended.

ANH, another option, has been described in children.[46,47] A combination of ANH with preoperative administration of erythropoietin and iron supplementation has been effective in reducing the transfusion requirement in infants and children. Increased red cell mass preoperatively allows for the performance of this technique. In a retrospective study, Meneghini et al[48] demonstrated the use of autologous blood in 11 of 16 patients who received erythropoietin. ANH alone as a method of blood conservation during CVR surgery has not been shown to be beneficial.[46,47]

The challenges with PAD in the pediatric population undergoing craniosynostosis repair are that the blood volume in infants and children less than 3 years of age is small and needle phobia is likely to render these children less cooperative and make vascular access more difficult. Therefore, PAD can be achieved only under deep sedation or general anesthesia. A prospective study examined the role of PAD in children undergoing simple cardiac procedures. Children from 3 to 9 years old and weighing less than 20 kg donated 5 to 10 mL/kg per donation about six times before surgery. The study group was slightly anemic preoperatively but did not require any allogeneic transfusion, whereas 80% of the control group was transfused.[47,49]

Intraoperative Strategies

Advances in the blood recovery equipment available for pediatric use have contributed to the successful use of intraoperative blood recovery during CVR.[48-52] With the introduction of small-volume centrifugation bowls such as the Fresenius Continuous Auto Transfusion System (C.A.T.S, Fresenius, distributed by Terumo, Ann Arbor, MI), it is feasible to recover blood in young children intraoperatively. The C.A.T.S has a chamber in the shape of a double spiral with a capacity of 30 mL that processes shed blood continuously.

Fearon[50] reported a prospective nonrandomized study involving 60 children who underwent major CVR. All surgeries were performed with the use of a blood recovery machine equipped with a 55-mL pediatric bowl. The average age of the patients was 4 years, and half the patients were less than 18 months of age. Of 60 patients, 58 received recycled autologous blood. On average, about 110 mL was returned for transfusion. The hematocrit level for the recycled blood varied between 50% and 70%. The blood was available for transfusion about 130 minutes after the start of the procedure. Transfusion of allogeneic blood occurred in 18 of 60 patients (30%). Only two patients did not receive recycled blood, because of an insufficient amount in one case and a purulent sinus infection in the other. It should be noted that Deva et al[53] could not demonstrate a significant benefit in autologous transfusion of recovered blood.

Postoperative retrieval of blood in infants weighing less than 10 kg has been described with the use of the CBCII ConstaVac system (Stryker Instruments, Kalamazoo, MI). A retrospective study that compared the efficacy of intraoperative blood recovery using the CATS with the postoperative blood salvaging system CBCII ConstaVac in 204 patients showed that the latter is also effective in decreasing blood transfusion.[54]

In addition to the changes in equipment, surgeons have also modified their techniques, which involve technologies such as microneedle electrocautery. Craniotomies are performed with an air-driven craniotome, and dural bleeding is stopped with bipolar cautery and oxidized cellulose sheets.[53,54] Dissecting scalp flaps in the subgaleal plane instead of the subperiosteal plane causes less bleeding.

The use of antifibrinolytic agents during craniosynostosis repair has been reported.[55,56] Tranexamic acid can potentially decrease blood loss. The average blood loss in a study group of patients who received tranexamic acid was 190 mL, compared to 290 mL in the control group. The dose of tranexamic acid used was 15 mg/kg before incision, repeated every 4 hours during surgery, followed by administration of the drug every 8 hours for 48 hours.

In summary, the care of infants and children undergoing CVR should be carried out by a team of experienced surgeons, anesthesiologists, nurses, and perfusionists. Communication between these various groups is critical for the accurate assessment of blood loss and for making appropriate transfusion decisions.

Pediatric Cardiac Surgery

Over the past 60 years, tremendous advances in the repair of congenital heart defects in infants and children have been made. These advances include improvements in surgical techniques, CPB equipment, and anesthesia care. The concept of early repair of congenital cardiac defects has led to performance of certain procedures during the newborn period and infancy.[54,57] Procedures requiring CPB involve autologous blood transfusions. Many factors influence the use of blood components during pediatric cardiac surgery, including hemodilution, effects of the pump prime, fibrinolysis, repeat surgery, and coagulation abnormalities associated with severe cyanotic cardiac disease.[56-59] In neonates and infants, the effects of hemodilution led to the use of blood components in the pump prime.

Pediatric patients and, in particular, neonates and infants who have cardiac surgery with CPB are at higher risk for postoperative bleeding than adult patients because of physiologic differences. In particular, hemodilution is more pronounced in pediatric patients because the smaller blood volume and immaturity of the coagulation system create less capacity for compensation. Furthermore, clearance of heparin is impaired because of hepatic and renal immaturity. When Platelets, FFP, and Cryoprecipitated AHF are not able to control the bleeding, re-exploration is the next step.

Many strategies have been developed for minimizing the use of blood components during pediatric cardiac surgery. These strategies include ANH, miniaturizing the bypass circuit, the use of antifibrinolytic agents, and techniques such as modified ultrafiltration to decrease blood loss and offset the deleterious effects of CPB.[58,60]

Acute Normovolemic Hemodilution

Performing cardiac surgery on pediatric patients is challenging, especially in neonates because of the limited blood volume. Boettcher et al[13] reported the use of CPB during open heart surgery in three infants weighing 4.5 kg, 3.5 kg, and 3.1 kg, respectively, without the use of allogeneic blood components. A small CPB circuit with a priming volume of 200 mL of crystalloid solution was used to decrease the hemodilution. Average hemoglobin levels decreased from 10.5 to 5.5 g/dL during CPB. All of the patients tolerated the procedure, and no blood or additional blood components were necessary during the procedure and hospital stay. This case report confirms that pediatric patients are capable of tolerating more extreme levels of hemodilution than previously considered.

Equipment and Technique Modifications

The equipment used for CPB has evolved over the past 10 years. High priming volumes and rates of transfusion enhance inflammatory response to CPB and increase myocardial and pulmonary dysfunction. The use of low-priming-volume CPB systems has been successful in decreasing transfusion requirements. As a result of the introduction of vacuum-assisted CPB circuits to reduce priming volume for pediatric patients, the percentage of transfusion-free neonatal CPB operations has increased.[60,61] However, the recent modifications introduced by several manufacturers to the various components of the extracorporeal circuit carry the risk of introducing gaseous microemboli into the arterial system.[62]

Modifications in the bypass circuit involving the size of the oxygenators (neonatal arterial oxygenator size is 45-60 mL), shorter arterial and venous cannulae, and placement of centrifugal pump close to the patient's head have reduced the size of the pump prime to as low as 160 mL.[61-64]

The systemic inflammatory response and capillary leak syndrome effects of extracorporeal circulation have deleterious effects on vital organ functions in the postoperative period. The use of modified ultrafiltration during and after the cessation of bypass has been studied by many investigators. The effects of modified ultrafiltration include an increase in hematocrit and decreases in platelet levels, chest tube drainage, and transfused blood components, as well as decreased mechanical ventilation support. Greater hemodynamic stability and decreased length of stay were shown in the intensive care unit.[63-66]

Antifibrinolytics

The use of antifibrinolytic agents has been successful in decreasing bleeding during neonatal surgery and reoperations in congenital cardiac surgery. Aprotinin is a potent antifibrinolytic agent that has demonstrated efficacy in diminishing bleeding, and it exerts anti-inflammatory effects that improve postoperative function.[65,67] Recently, two large observational studies addressed the effects of aprotinin on renal function in adults.[39,66-68] The results of the studies led to caution in the use of aprotinin in neonates and children undergoing CPB. A recent prospective study[69] investigated the safety of aprotinin use in pediatric cardiac surgery. The authors concluded that despite the higher incidence of renal dysfunction and failure in the aprotinin group (incidence of dialysis = 9.6% vs 4.1%; renal dysfunction = 26.3% vs 16.1%), an independent effect of the drug to produce renal failure could not be demonstrated.[68,69]

Tranexamic acid has been effective in decreasing blood loss in pediatric patients undergoing repeat sternotomy for repair of congenital heart defects. Reid et al[70] prospectively studied the use of tranexamic acid in 41 children. After induction of anesthesia and before skin incision, patients received a bolus of 100 mg/kg of tranexamic acid, followed by an infusion of 10 mg/kg/hr. An additional bolus of 100 mg/kg was given at the onset of CPB. The blood loss in the tranexamic acid group was 24% less than the placebo group. Additionally, the transfusion requirements and the cost for transfusion components were less for the treated group.

Although the use of rFVIIa in pediatric cardiac surgery is limited, there are several reports of successful use of the drug to control excessive postoperative bleeding. Tobias et al[71] evaluated the efficacy of rFVIIa in nine postsurgical cardiac patients with chest tube drainage exceeding 4 mL/kg/hr. The chest tube output was 5.8 mL/kg/hr for the initial three hours after surgery and decreased to 2.0 mL/kg/hr after the administration of rFVIIa.

In a retrospective chart review by Egan et al,[72] four of the children who received rFVIIa had severe postoperative bleeding, and two had severe uncontrolled intraoperative bleeding. Patients received prior conventional therapy with FFP, Platelets, and Cryoprecipitated AHF. The median age was 32 months. Patients received a bolus dose of 180 µg/kg of rFVIIa. This dose was repeated 2 hours later in all patients except for one, in whom bleeding stopped after the first dose. There was a significant decrease in the bleeding volume after the second dose, accompanied by normalization of prothrombin time (PT), international normalized ratio, and activated partial thromboplastin time. All patients survived and no thromboembolic events were noted.

In another retrospective chart review, Reiter et al[73] report the use of rFVIIa in 46 pediatric patients for postoperative and intraoperative bleeding complications. This represents the largest case review on the use of rFVIIa to date. In the study, 11 patients had post-CPB bleeding. The dose of 160 µg/kg and a repeat dose were administered, although timing was not documented. All patients survived, coagulation parameters normalized, and no thromboembolic events were observed.

Veldman et al[74] describe the use of rFVIIa in pediatric patients on extracorporeal membrane oxygenation (ECMO) following surgery for congenital heart disease. Patients requiring ECMO frequently are subject to severe bleeding. The use of rFVIIa in ECMO patients is limited by the increased risk of thrombotic events, especially in the ECMO circuit. In this retrospective study, 7 patients on ECMO with severe intractable bleeding were treated with rFVIIa at a dose of 90 µg/kg. Three patients died. The rates of occlusion in the ECMO system and mortality did not differ from the historic controls. There was statistical significance neither in the reduction of bleeding volume nor in the reduction of transfusion requirements. Pychynska-Pokorska et al[75] describe the use of rFVIIa in post-CPB bleeding in 7 patients ranging in age from 5 days to 4 years. A first dose of 30 µg/kg or 60 µg/kg was administered, and a second dose was given if bleeding did not show signs of decreasing after 15 minutes. All patients received conventional therapy before rFVIIa was started. Bleeding was controlled in all patients, with significant reduction in blood loss in the first hour. Hemostasis was achieved within 3 hours of the first dose. The use of rFVIIa prevented re-exploration in all 7 patients with no thromboembolic complications.

A retrospective and unmatched case-control study evaluated the efficacy and safety of rFVIIa therapy in postsurgical pediatric patients.[76] It compared patients with severe bleeding who received rFVIIa with patients treated with blood components only. In the group of 46 patients studied, 23 of 24 patients receiving the drug responded. There was significant reduction in chest tube drainage from 52.3 to 18.8 mL/kg/hr. Twelve of the study patients were on ECMO. The study reported a 25% incidence of thrombotic complications in the study group. Consequently, this drug should be considered for use with caution in situations of excessive intractable bleeding after cardiac surgery in pediatric patients.

Scoliosis Surgery

The etiology of spinal deformities in children and adolescents may be congenital, neuropathic, or idiopathic. Surgery for scoliosis correction is commonly associated with major blood loss.[77] The surgery involves decortication of the transverse processes and lateral laminae with facetectomy, followed by segmental spinal instrumentation.[77,78] The most commonly used segmental fixation technique is sublaminar wire fixation. More recently, a combination of sublaminar wires, hooks, and pedicle screws has been used in spinal fusion.[79] Blood loss related to surgical technique is caused by disruption of internal vertebral veins and decortication of large areas of bone.[78,80]

There are many factors that influence the degree of blood loss in scoliosis surgery, including the number of vertebrae fused, the complexity of the curvature, the duration of surgery, and the underlying cause of scoliosis (idiopathic or neuromuscular). In a prospective observational study, Kannan et al[80] demonstrated that children with neuromuscular scoliosis had significantly greater blood loss than those with idiopathic scoliosis (median blood loss of the former group was 78% of total blood volume, compared to 20% for the latter).

Patients with neuromuscular disorders that are strongly associated with spinal deformities such as Duchenne muscular dystrophy or cerebral palsy are more likely to receive allogeneic transfusions. These patients are more likely to have nutritional deficiencies, such as vitamin K deficiency, leading to increased PT.[81] In Duchenne muscular dystrophy, lack of dystrophin in the vascular smooth muscle causes lack of vasoconstriction, leading to increased bleeding. In addition, paraspinal muscles are dystrophic and fibrotic, rendering the subperiosteal stripping more difficult.[80,81]

Chronic anticonvulsant therapy in patients with cerebral palsy may contribute to increased blood loss during scoliosis repair. Anticonvulsants such as valproic acid have been associated with thrombocytopenia. The mechanism is poorly understood, but causes have been postulated to include hepatotoxicity, immune thrombocytopenia, or marrow suppression.[81-83]

Several techniques are described below for reducing blood loss during scoliosis repair in children. Generally, a combination of these techniques is successful in reducing the requirements for allogeneic transfusion.

Preoperative Autologous Donation

PAD in children is an attractive method of avoiding allogeneic transfusion.[84] PAD has many advantages, including a minimizing of the effect of blood shortages in blood banks. It offers hemodynamic stability during the processing of recovered blood as well as a reduction in the use of platelets and clotting factors. It is also well accepted by parents who are anxious about their children receiving allogeneic banked blood. The logistics of collection of PAD in pediatric patients can be challenging. PAD should occur in centers where transfusion professionals are familiar with dealing with children and are able to handle adverse reactions to blood donation such as nausea, dizziness, and hemodynamic instability.

Several complications have been attributed to PAD, including bacterial contamination, wastage of collected units, and iatrogenic anemia before surgery. The latter can be offset by the use of erythropoietin and iron supplementation preoperatively. The cost of PAD and the expense of the service may outweigh the benefit for the pediatric patient. However, several studies have reported reduction in perioperative blood transfusions with the use of PAD before spinal fusion surgery.

Acute Normovolemic Hemodilution

Fontana et al[85] demonstrated that in extreme normovolemic anemia, cardiac output and oxygen transport are not impaired in the pediatric population. In this study, eight pediatric patients undergoing scoliosis surgery were treated with ANH. Intravascular volume was maintained with 5% albumin and the impact of hemodilution was evaluated by mixed venous oxygen saturation (SVO_2). An SVO_2 level >60% was considered capable of providing adequate oxygen carrying capacity. If SVO_2 levels decreased below 60% during surgery, then transfusion was deemed necessary. Hemoglobin levels decreased from 10.0 ±1.6 g/dL to 3.0 ±0.8 g/dL. On 100% oxygen, SVO_2 levels decreased from 90.8% ±5.4% to 72.3% ±7.8%, and oxygen extraction increased from 17.3% ±6.2% to 44.4% ±5.9%. This evidence suggests that more extreme levels of normovolemic hemodilution than previously reported may be clinically acceptable in young, healthy patients.

Antifibrinolytic Agents

Various drugs have been used successfully to reduce bleeding in patients undergoing spinal fusion. A lysine antifibrinolytic agent, ε-aminocaproic acid, binds the lysine site on plasminogen and plasmin, preventing plasmin from binding to fibrin. The efficacy and safety of ε-aminocaproic acid in decreasing intraoperative bleeding has been shown in several studies.[86,87] The pediatric dose used is similar to the adult dose: a loading dose of 100 mg/kg/hr intravenously over 15 minutes, followed by an infusion of 10 mg/kg/hr until the end of the procedure. It is an inexpensive drug, compared to other antifibrinolytic agents such as aprotinin.

Tranexamic acid, a synthetic agent similar to ε-aminocaproic acid, has been effective in reducing blood loss and transfusions in spinal fusions for Duchenne muscular dystrophy scoliosis. Shapiro et al[88] demonstrated that blood loss in a study group that received tranexamic acid was reduced by 42%. The tranexamic acid dose used was 100 mg/kg over 15 minutes before incision, followed by 10 mg/kg/hr until the end of surgery.

Similarly, the efficacy of aprotinin was studied in a prospective, randomized, blinded, and controlled study in children undergoing spinal fusions of seven segments or greater.[89] High-dose aprotinin was administered as a 240-mg/m^2 loading dose over 30 minutes before incision. The load was followed by a continuous infusion of 56 mg/m^2 throughout the case and for 4 hours after surgery. The blood loss in the aprotinin group was significantly lower than the placebo group (545 ±312 mL vs 930 ±772 mL). This decrease in blood loss resulted in fewer blood transfusions in the aprotinin group and eliminated the need for component therapy such as Platelets and Fresh Frozen Plasma.

Desmopressin is an analog of vasopressin. It causes the endothelial cells to release von Willebrand factor and promotes platelet adhesiveness. There are conflicting results on the efficacy of this drug. Kobrinsky[90] reported a reduction of intraoperative bleeding by 30% in patients undergoing spinal fusion surgery with a normotensive anesthesia technique. Other investigators could not demonstrate any reduction in blood loss with the use of desmopressin.[91]

Deliberate Hypotension

Many drugs are used to achieve an ideal MAP. The remainder of the chapter addresses only the agents that are of practical clinical use, in the authors' opinion.

Nicardipine is a dihydroxypiridine derivative that dilates systemic, cerebral, and coronary vessels. It decreases MAP through its effects on systemic vascular resistance while maintaining cardiac contractility, stroke volume, and cardiac filling pressures. Rebound hypotension does not commonly occur because of its negative chronotropic effects. Tobias et al[92] studied the use of nicardipine in 24 children undergoing anteroposterior spinal fusion as well as posterior spinal fusion. The dose of nicardipine was 5 or 10 μg/kg/min until the desired MAP (55-65 mm Hg) was achieved. The infusion was decreased and titrated to maintain a MAP of 55 to 65 mm Hg.[92,93] Following the discontinuation of the infusion, MAP returned to baseline within 8 to 60 minutes. This prolonged hypotension seems to be a disadvantage of the use of nicardipine as a hypotensive agent. However, no adverse effects were noted. Nicardipine was compared with sodium nitroprusside in 20 adolescents during posterior spinal fusion for idiopathic scoliosis. Decreased blood loss was noted with the nicardipine group as compared to the sodium nitroprusside group (761 vs 1297 mL).[92,94]

Vasodilators cause increased cerebral blood volume and intracranial pressure. Reflex tachycardia occurs more commonly with the use of sodium nitroprusside than with nicardipine. The α2-adrenoceptor agonists clonidine and dexmedetomidine are being used perioperatively. Through their effects on the central and peripheral receptors, they cause sedation, opioid-sparing effects, and a dose-dependent decrease in blood pressure and heart rate. Dexmedetomidine has a differential specificity for the α2:α1 receptors of 1620:1, compared with 200:1 for clonidine.[95] These agents decrease the central sympathetic output with the absence of reflex tachycardia and rebound hypertension, which is common with direct vasodilators.

Tobias and Berkenbosch et al[96] reported the use of dexmedetomidine for controlled hypotension in a 14-year-old adolescent during anterior spinal fusion for idiopathic scoliosis repair. Controlled hypotension was initiated with an infusion of 0.2 µg/kg/hr and increased to 0.5 to 0.7 µg/kg/hr. The MAP decreased from a range of 70 to 80 mm Hg to a range of 55 to 60 mm Hg. The heart rate decreased from a range of 90 to 100 bpm to a range of 70 to 80 bpm. The heart rate increased 7 minutes after the discontinuation of the infusion to 102 bpm, and the MAP increased to 76 mm Hg.

There is a paucity of data addressing the use of dexmedetomidine for controlled hypotension. However, there is abundant information regarding the sympatholytic effects caused by stimulation of the presynaptic α2 receptors, decreasing the sympathetic tone while increasing the parasympathetic tone.[87,93] Reported side effects of bradycardia (5.3%), hypotension (22.8%), and hypertension (16%) can be avoided by eliminating the initial loading dose or limiting it to 0.5 µg/kg.[96,97]

Conclusion

Advancements in surgical techniques and technologies for blood management, together with drugs that are now available to minimize blood loss, have made possible the surgical treatment of the pediatric patient without the need for allogeneic blood. This includes viable solutions for children of the Jehovah's Witness population. Of course, in such cases it is necessary to consult with the patient's parents, unless the patient is an adolescent. The adolescent Jehovah's Witness patient needs to decide what his or her own preferences are regarding allogeneic transfusion and blood management techniques.

References

1. Tynell E, Norda R, Shanwell A, et al. Long-term survival in transfusion recipients in Sweden. Transfusion 2001;41:251-5.

2. Woloszczuk-Gebicka B. How to limit allogenic blood transfusion in children. Paediatr Anaesth 2005;15:913-24.

3. Luban NL. An update on transfusion-transmitted viruses. Curr Opin Pediatr 1998;10:53-9.

4. Barcelona A, Thompson SL, Alexis A, Cote CJ. Intraoperative pediatric blood transfusion therapy: A review of common issues. I: Hematologic and physiologic differences from adults. Metabolic and infectious risks. Paediatr Anaesth 2005;15:716-26.

5. Woolley S. Ethics: Children of Jehovah's Witnesses and adolescent Jehovah's Witnesses: What are their rights? Arch Dis Child 2005;90:715-19.

6. Questions from Readers. The Watchtower 1951(July 1):415.

7. Mann MC, Votto J, Kambe J, McNamee MJ. Management of the severely anemic patient who refuses transfusion: Lessons learned during the care of a Jehovah's Witness. Ann Intern Med 1992;117:1042-8.

8. Prince v. Massachusetts, 321 US 158 at 170 (1944).

9. People ex rel. Wallace et al v. Labrenz et al, 104 N.E.2d 769 (IL 1952).

10. In the matter of baby girl Newton. WL 54916 (Del.Ch.) (1990).

11. Maness CP, Russell SM, Altonji P, Allmendinger P. Bloodless medicine and surgery. AORN 1998;67:144-52.

12. Bodnaruk ZM, Wong CJ, Thomas MJ. Meeting the clinical challenge of care for Jehovah's Witnesses. Transfus Med Rev 2004;18:105-16.

13. Boettcher W, Merkle F, Heubler M, et al. Transfusion-free cardiopulmonary by-pass in Jehovah's Witness patients weighing less than 5 kg. J Extra Corpor Technol 2005;37:282-5.

14. Pasic M, Ruisz W, Koster A, Hetzer R. Bloodless surgery of acute type A aortic dissection in a Jehovah's Witness patient. Ann Thorac Surg 2005;80:1507-10.

15. Remmers PA, Spencer AJ. Clinical strategies in the medical care of Jehovah's Witnesses. Am J Med 2006;119:1013-18.

16. Jabbour N, Gagandeep S, Thomas D, et al. Transfusion-free techniques in pediatric live donor liver transplantation. J Pediatr Gastroenterol Nutr 2005;40:521-3.

17. Snook NJ, O'Beirne HA, Enright S, et al. Use of recombinant human erythropoietin to facilitate liver transplantation in a Jehovah's Witness. Br J Anaesth 1996;76:740-3.

18. Jabbour N, Nicolas MD, Gagandeep S, et al. Live donor liver transplantation without blood products: Strategies developed for Jehovah's Witnesses offer broad application. Ann Surg 2004;240:350-7.

19. Feagan BG, Wong CJ, Kirkley A, et al. Erythropoietin with iron supplementation to prevent allogenic blood transfusion in total hip joint arthroplasty. A randomized controlled trial. Ann Intern Med 2000;133:845-54.

20. Boonmak S, Boonmak P, Laopaiboon M. Deliberate hypotension with propofol under anesthesia for functional endoscopic sinus surgery (FESS). Cochrane Database Syst Rev 2007;3:CD006623. DOI:10.1002/14651858.CD006623.

21. Andel D, Andel H, Horaufk K, et al. The influence of deliberate hypotension on splanchnic perfusion balance with use of either isofluorine or esmolol and nitroglycerin. Anesth Analg 2001;93:1116-20.

22. Huet C, Salmi LR, Fergusson D, et al. A meta-analysis of the effectiveness of cell salvage to minimize peri-operative allogenic blood transfusion in cardiac

and orthopedic surgery: International Study of Peri-operative Transfusion (ISPOT) investigators. Anesth Analg 1999;89:861-9.

23. Bryson GL, Laupacis A, Wells GA. Does acute normovolemic hemodilution reduce peri-operative allogenic transfusion? A meta-analysis. The International Study of Peri-operative Transfusion. Anesth Analg 1998;86:9-15.

24. Matot I, Scheinin O, Jurim O, et al. Effectiveness of acute normovolemic hemodilution to minimize allogenic blood transfusion in major liver resections. Anesthesiology 2002;97:794-800.

25. Sanders G, Coker A, Mellor N, et al. Acute normovolemic hemodilution in colorectal surgery. Eur J Surg Oncol 2002;28:520-2.

26. Shuper A, Merlob P, Grunebaum M, Reisner SH. The incidence of isolated craniosynostosis in the newborn infant. Am J Dis Child 1985;139:85-6.

27. Meara JG, Smith EM, Harshbarger RJ, et al. Blood-conservation techniques in craniofacial surgery. Ann Plast Surg 2005;54:525-9.

28. Laupacis A, Fergusson D. MHA for the International Study of Peri-operative Transfusion (ISPOT) investigators. Drugs to minimize peri-operative blood loss in cardiac surgery: Meta-analysis using peri-operative blood transfusion as outcome. Anesth Analg 1997;85:1258-67.

29. Martinowitz U, Michealson M, Israeli Multidisciplinary rFVIIa Task Force. Guidelines for the use of recombinant activated Factor VII in uncontrolled bleeding: Report by the Israeli Multidisciplinary rFVIIa Task Force. J Thromb Haemost 2005;3:638-9.

30. Tanaka KA, Waly AA, Cooper WA, et al. Treatment of excessive bleeding in a Jehovah's witness patient after cardiac surgery with recombinant factor VIIa. Anesthesiology 2003;98:1513-15.

31. Kling PJ, Schmidt RL, Roberts RA, et al. Serum erythropoietin levels and erythropoiesis. J Pediatr 1996;128:791-6.

32. Stockman JA, Oski FA. Red blood cell values in low-birth-weight infants during the first seven weeks of life. Am J Dis Child 1980;134:945-6.

33. Cambonie G, Matecki S, Milési C, et al. Myocardial adaptation to anemia and red blood cell transfusion in premature infants requiring ventilation support in the 1st postnatal week. Neonatology 2007;92:174-81.

34. Bard A, Fouron JC, Chessex P, Widness JA. Erythropoietic and metabolic adaptations to anemia of prematurity in infants with bronchopulmonary dysplasia. J Pediatr 1998;132:630-4.

35. Maier MP, Obladen M, Scigalla P, et al. The effect of epoetin beta (recombinant human erythropoietin) on the need for transfusion in very low birth weight preterm infants. N Engl J Med 1994;330:1173-8.

36. Ohls RK, Ehrenkranz RA, Wright LL, et al. Effects of early erythropoietin therapy on the transfusion requirements of preterm infants below 1250 grams birth weight: A multicenter, randomized controlled trial. Pediatrics 2001;108: 934-42.

37. Halperin DS, Wacker P, Lacourt G, et al. Effects of recombinant human erythropoietin in infants with anemia of prematurity: A pilot study. J Pediatr 1990; 116:779-86.

38. Meister B, Aurer H, Simma B, et al. The effect of recombinant human erythropoietin in circulating hematopoietic progenitor cells in anemic premature infants. Stem Cells 1997;15:359-63.

39. Mangano DT, Miao Y, Vuylsteke A, et al. Investigators of the Multicenter Foundation. Mortality associated with aprotinin during 5 years following coronary artery bypass graft surgery. JAMA 2007;297:471-9.

40. Koh J, Gries H. Perioperative management of pediatric patients with craniosynostosis. Anesthesiol Clin 2007;25:465-81.

41. Kearney RA, Rosales JK, Howes WJ. Craniosynostosis: An assessment of blood loss and transfusion practices. Can J Anaesth 1989;36:473-7.

42. Meyer P. Blood loss during repair of craniosynostosis. Br J Anaesth 1993;71: 854-7.

43. Faberowski LW, Black S, Mickle JP. Blood loss and transfusion practice in the perioperative management of craniosynostosis repair. J Neurosurg Anesthesiol 1999;3:167-72.

44. Jimenez DE, Barone CM. Endoscopic craniectomy for early surgical correction of sagittal craniosynostosis. J Neurosurg 1998;88:77-81.

45. Clayman MA, Murad GJ, Steele MH, et al. History of craniosynostosis surgery and the evolution of minimally invasive endoscopic techniques: The University of Florida experience. Ann Plast Surg 2007;58:285-7.

46. Fearon JA, Weinthal J. The use of recombinant erythropoietin in the reduction of blood transfusion rates in craniosynostosis repair in infants and children. Plast Reconstr Surg 2002;109:2190-6.

47. Hans P, Collin V, Bonhomme V, et al. Evaluation of acute normovolemic hemodilution for surgical repair of craniosynostosis. J Neurosurg Anesthesiol 2000;12:33-6.

48. Meneghini L, Zadra N, Aneloni V. Erythropoietin therapy and acute preoperative normovolaemic haemodilution in infants undergoing craniosynostosis surgery. Paediatr Anaesth 2003;3:392-6.

49. Weldon BC. Blood conservation in pediatric anesthesia. Anesthesiol Clin North America 2005;23:347-61.

50. Fearon JA. Reducing allogenic blood transfusions during pediatric cranial vault surgical procedures: A prospective analysis of blood recycling. Plast Reconstr Surg 2004;113:1126-30.

51. Dahami S, Orliaguet GA, Meyer PG, et al. Perioperative blood salvage during surgical correction of craniosynostosis in infants. Br J Anaesth 2000;85:550-5.

52. Jimenez DF, Barone CM. Intraoperative autologous blood transfusion in the surgical correction of craniosynostosis. Neurosurgery 1995;37:1075-9.

53. Deva AK, Hopper RA, Landecker A, et al. The use of intraoperative autotransfusion during cranial vault remodeling for craniosynostosis. Plast Reconstr Surg 2001;109:58-63.

54. Orliaguet GA, Bruyere M, Meyer PG, et al. Comparison of perioperative blood salvage and postoperative reinfusion of drained blood during surgical correction of craniosynostosis in infants. Paediatr Anesth 2003;63:797-804.

55. Tunçbilek G, Vargel I, Erdem A, et al. Blood loss and transfusion rates during repair of craniofacial deformities. J Craniofac Surg 2005;16:59-62.

56. Durán de la Fuente P, García-Fernández J, Pérez-López C, et al. Usefulness of tranexamic acid in cranial remodeling surgery. Rev Esp Anestesiol Reanim 2003;50:388-94.

57. Laussen PC. Neonates with congenital heart disease. Curr Opin Pediatr 2001; 13:220-6.

58. Odegard KC, Zurakowski D, Hornykewycz S, et al. Evaluation of the coagulation system in children with two-ventricle congenital heart disease. Ann Thorac Surg 2007;83:1797-803.
59. Odegard KC, McGowan FX Jr, Zurakowski D, et al. Coagulation factor abnormalities in patients with single-ventricle physiology immediately prior to the Fontan procedure. Ann Thorac Surg 2002;73:1770-7.
60. Ungerleider RM, Shen I. Optimizing response of the neonate and infant to cardiopulmonary bypass: Semin Thorac Cardiovasc Surg Pediatr Card Surg Annu 2003;6:140-6.
61. Hayashi Y, Kagisaki K, Yamaguchi T, et al. Clinical application of vacuum-assisted cardiopulmonary bypass with a pressure relief valve. Eur J Cardiothorac Surg 2001;20:621-6.
62. Norman NJ, Sistino JJ, Acsell JR. The effectiveness of low-prime cardiopulmonary bypass circuits at removing gaseous emboli. J Extra Corpor Technol 2004;36:336-42.
63. Golab HD, Takkenberg JM, Gerner-Weelink GL, et al. Effects of cardiopulmonary bypass circuit reduction and residual volume salvage on allogeneic transfusion requirements in infants undergoing cardiac surgery. Interact Cardiovasc Thorac Surg 2007;6:335-9.
64. Hickey E, Karamlou T, You J, Ungerleider RM. Effects of circuit miniaturization in reducing inflammatory response to infant cardiopulmonary bypass by elimination of allogeneic blood products. Ann Thorac Surg 2006;81:S2367-72.
65. Sever K, Tansel T, Basaran M, et al. The benefits of continuous ultrafiltration in pediatric cardiac surgery. Scand Cardiovasc J 2004;38:307-11.
66. Gaynor JW. The effect of modified ultrafiltration on the postoperative course in patients with congenital heart disease. Semin Thorac Cardiovasc Surg Pediatr Card Surg Annu 2003;6:128-39.
67. Mossinger H, Dietrich W, Braun SL, et al. High-dose aprotinin reduces activation of hemostasis, allogeneic blood requirement, and duration of postoperative ventilation in pediatric cardiac surgery. Ann Thorac Surg 2003;75:2:430-7.
68. Aronsib S, Fontes ML, Miao Y, et al. Risk index for perioperative renal dysfunction/failure: Critical dependence on pulse pressure hypertension. Circulation 2007;13:115:733-42.
69. Szekely A, Sapi E, Breuer T, et al. Aprotinin and renal dysfunction after pediatric cardiac surgery. Paediatr Anaesth 2008;18:151-9.
70. Reid RW, Zimmerman AA, Laussen PC, et al. The efficacy of tranexamic acid versus placebo in decreasing blood loss in pediatric patients undergoing repeat cardiac surgery. Anesth Analg 1997;84:990-6.
71. Tobias JD, Simsic JM, Weinstein S, et al. Recombinant factor VIIa to control excessive bleeding following surgery for congenital heart diseases in pediatric patients. Intensive Care Med 2004;19:270-3.
72. Egan JR, Lammi A, Schell DN, et al. Recombinant activated Factor VII in pediatric cardiac surgery. Intensive Care Med 2004;30:682-5.
73. Reiter PD, Valuck RJ, Taylor RS. Evaluation of off-label recombinant activated Factor VII for multiple indication in children. Clin Appl Thromb Haemost 2007;13:233-40.

74. Veldman A, Neuhaeuser C, Akintuerk H, et al. RFVIIa in the treatment of persistent hemorrhage in pediatric patients on ECMO following surgery for congenital heart disease. Pediatr Anesth 2007;17:1176-81.

75. Pychynska-Pokorska M, Mool JJ, Krajewski W, Jarosik P. Use of recombinant coagulation factor VIIa in uncontrolled postoperative bleeding in children undergoing cardiac surgery with cardiopulmonary bypass. Pediatr Crit Care Med 2004;5:246-50.

76. Agarwal HS, Bennett JE, Churchwell KB, et al. Recombinant factor seven therapy for postoperative bleeding in neonatal and pediatric cardiac surgery. Ann Thorac Surg 2007;84:161-8.

77. Shapiro F, Sethna N. Blood loss in pediatric spine surgery. Eur Spine J 2004;13(Suppl 1):6-17.

78. Kim YJ, Lenke LG, Kim J, et al. Comparative analysis of pedicle screw versus hybrid instrumentation in posterior spinal fusion of adolescent idiopathic scoliosis. Spine 2006;31:291-8.

79. Luque ER. Segmental spinal instrumentation for correction of scoliosis. Clin Orthop 1982;163:192-8.

80. Kannan S, Meert K, Mooney J, et al. Bleeding and coagulation changes during spinal fusion surgery: A comparison of neuromuscular and idiopathic scoliosis patients. Pediatr Crit Care Med 2002;3:364-9.

81. Karol L. Scoliosis in patients with Duchenne muscular dystrophy. J Bone Joint Surg 2007;89A:155-62.

82. Chambers H, Weinstein C, Mubarak S, et al. The effect of valproic acid on blood loss in patients with cerebral palsy. J Pediatr Orthop 1999;19:792.

83. Gerstner T, Teich M, Bell N, et al. Valproate-associated coagulopathies are frequent and variable in children. Epilepsia 2007;48:205-6.

84. Lauder GR. Pre-operative predeposit autologous donation in children presenting for elective surgery: A review. Transfus Med 2007;17:75-82.

85. Fontana JL, Welbron L, Mongan PD, et al. Oxygen consumption and cardiovascular functions in children during profound intraoperative normovolemic hemodilution. Anesth Analg 1995;80:219-25.

86. Florentino-Pineda I, Thompson GH, Poe-Kochert C, et al. The effect of ε-aminocaproic acid on perioperative blood loss in idiopathic scoliosis. Spine 2004; 29:23-38.

87. Thompson GH, Florentino-Pineda J, Poe-Kochert C. The role of ε-aminocaproic acid in decreasing perioperative blood loss in idiopathic scoliosis. Spine 2005;30(Suppl):S94-9.

88. Shapiro F, Zurakowski D, Sethna NF. Tranexamic acid diminishes intraoperative blood loss and transfusion in spinal fusions for duchenne muscular dystrophy scoliosis. Spine 2007;32:2278-83.

89. Cole J, Murray D, Snider R, Bassett G, et al. Aprotinin reduces blood loss during spinal surgery in children. Spine 2001;25:2482-5.

90. Kobrinsky NL, Letts RM, Patel LR, et al. 1-Desamino-8-D-arginine (desmopressin) decreases operative blood loss in patients having Harrington rod spinal fusion surgery. A randomized, double-blinded, controlled trial. Ann Intern Med 1987;107:446-50.

91. Guay J, Reinberg C, Poitras B, et al. A trial of desmopressin to reduce blood loss in patients undergoing spinal fusion for idiopathic scoliosis. Anesth Analg 1992;75:405-10.
92. Tobias J, Hersey S, Mencio G, Green N. Nicardipine for controlled hypotension during spinal surgery. J Pediatr Orthop 1996;16:370-3.
93. Tobias JD. Controlled hypotension in children. Pediatr Drugs 2002;4:439-53.
94. Hersey SL, O'Dell NE, Lowe S, et al. Nicardipine versus nitroprusside for controlled hypotension during spinal surgery in adolescents. Anesth Analg 1997; 84:1239-44.
95. Bloor BC, Ward DS, Belleville JP, Maze M. Effects of intravenous dexmedetomidine in humans. II. Hemodynamic changes. Anesthesiology 1992;77:1134-42.
96. Tobias JD, Berkenbosch JW. Initial experience with dexmedetomidine in paediatric-aged patients. Paediatr Anaesth 2002;12:171-5.
97. Riker RR, Frazer G. Adverse events associated with sedatives, analgesics, and other drugs that provide patient comfort in the intensive care unit (review). Pharmacotherapy 2005;25(5 Pt 2):8S-18S.

In: Waters JH, ed.
Blood Management: Options for Better Patient Care
Bethesda, MD: AABB Press, 2008

18

Special Surgical Management: Cardiac Surgery

DAVY H. CHENG, MD, MSc, FRCP(C);
ANN CRAIG, MBChB; AND
FIONA E. RALLEY, BSc, MBChB, FRCA

MORE THAN 1 MILLION CARDIAC SURGERIES are performed worldwide each year. The patient population undergoing cardiac surgery is changing; patients are increasingly older and have more co-morbidities. High-risk cardiac procedures (repeat and combined operations) are becoming more common, accounting for >25% of total cardiac surgeries. Cardiac surgery consumes approximately 16% of the total hospital blood supply. Large institutional variabilities still exist in transfusion practice in cardiac surgery despite the publication of national consensus guidelines.[1,2]

Davy H. Cheng, MD, MSc, FRCP(C), Professor and Chair/Chief; Ann Craig, MBChB, Clinical Fellow; and Fiona E. Ralley, BSc, MBChB, FRCA, Professor and Director, Perioperative Blood Conservation Program, Department of Anesthesia and Perioperative Medicine, University of Western Ontario, London, Ontario, Canada

Strategies for blood management in cardiac surgery may be considered in pre-, intra-, and postoperative categories, as listed in Table 18-1.

Table 18-1. Perioperative Blood Management Modalities in Cardiac Surgery

Phase	Modality
Preoperative	• Treatment of anemia (erythropoietin, iron, folate) • Restriction of iatrogenic blood loss (reducing amount of blood drawn, avoiding hematoma at heart catheterization site) • Discontinuation of antiplatelet agents (aspirin, clopidogrel, ticlopidine, abciximab, tirofiban, and eptifibatide)
Intraoperative	• Pharmacological agents (tranexamic acid, aminocaproic acid, aprotinin, desmopressin, recombinant Factor VIIa, fibrin sealants) • Mechanical devices (enhanced coagulation monitoring, ANH with or without plasmapheresis, blood recovery, Harmonic Scalpel*) • Cardiopulmonary techniques (heparin-bonded circuits, OPCAB, minimized extracorporeal circuits, retrograde autologous priming, ultrafiltration/modified ultrafiltration) • Transfusion threshold (meticulous surgical hemostasis, avoidance of transfusion trigger numbers, oxygen extraction ratio)
Postoperative	• Transfusion threshold • Coagulation monitoring (appropriate and early surgical reexploration) • Transfusion algorithms

*Ethicon Endo-Surgery Inc, Cincinnati, OH.
ANH = acute normovolemic hemodilution; OPCAB = off-pump coronary artery bypass.

Preoperative Management

Preoperative red cell mass and patient age are the principal determinants for blood transfusion during cardiac surgery.[3] Other preoperative predictors of perioperative blood transfusion are emergency or urgent operations, cardiogenic shock, catheterization-induced coronary occlusion, low-body-mass index, left ventricular ejection fraction <30%, female gender, peripheral vascular disease, insulin-dependent diabetes, creatinine level >1.8 mg/dL, albumin value <4 g/dL, and reoperations.[4,5]

Preoperative Anemia

The volume of blood loss that can be tolerated in any surgical setting is directly related to the initial total blood volume [65-75 mL × weight (kg) for males; 55-65 mL × weight (kg) for females]. Preoperative anemia is potentially preventable in most patients, especially those with hospital-acquired anemia (37.3%) and those with iron deficiency (29.3%).[6] Creating a hematocrit to compensate for expected blood loss can be achieved with the use of recombinant human erythropoietin (rHuEPO) in addition to either oral or intravenous iron supplementation. Treatment with erythropoietin (<70 kg = 20,000 IU/week; >70 kg = 40,000 IU/week), iron (ferrous sulphate, 300 mg by mouth three times a day), and folate has been used before surgery to increase hemoglobin levels.[7,8] This induces reticulocytosis within 3 days after the initial injection, provided adequate iron stores are available to support this increased hemoglobin production, with the production of the equivalent of 1 unit of blood by day 7. Alghamdi et al[9] performed a meta-analysis of the preoperative use of rHuEPO in cardiac surgical patients and demonstrated that the administration of erythropoietin before cardiac surgery is associated with a significant reduction in the risk of exposure to allogeneic blood transfusion with or without the use of preoperative autologous donation (PAD). PAD has been performed in at-risk patients but has not been shown to be cost-effective.[10,11]

Antiplatelet Drugs

Patients undergoing cardiac surgery are often on antiplatelet agents (aspirin, clopidogrel, ticlopidine, abciximab, tirofiban, and eptifibatide) before surgery to reduce their risk of atherosclerotic events and stroke. The recommended acute dose of clopidogrel is 300 to 600 mg before cardiac catheterization and possible percutaneous intervention. The recommended maintenance dose is 75 mg per day. After discontinuation of the dosage, platelet aggregation and bleeding time gradually return to normal in about 5 days. Ticlopidine has been associated with serious hematologic abnormalities (neutropenia in 2.4% of patients).[12] Delaying elective operations for 4 to 5 days is recommended for patients on aspirin and clopidogrel. Delaying operations for 12 to 24 hours is advisable for patients on abciximab. Operations should be delayed for 2 to 3 hours, if possible, for patients on tirofiban and eptifibatide.[13] However, emergency surgery should not be delayed when it is otherwise indicated. Use of aprotinin may reduce blood loss and transfusion in such settings.[14]

Intraoperative Management

Strategies to reduce intraoperative anemia should be directed at increasing oxygen delivery to tissues, controlling hemostasis, and limiting unnecessary hemodilution. Techniques for intraoperative blood management can be divided into the following classifications:

1. Pharmacological, including the use of drugs that affect the hematopoietic system: antifibrinolytics, desmopressin, recombinant Factor VIIa, and fibrin sealants.

2. Mechanical: enhanced coagulation monitoring, acute normovolemic hemodilution (ANH) with or without plasmapheresis, blood recovery, and Harmonic Scalpel (Ethicon Endo-Surgery Inc, Cincinnati, OH).
3. Cardiopulmonary bypass techniques: heparin-coated circuits, off-pump coronary artery bypass (OPCAB) surgery, minimal extracorporeal circulation, retrograde autologous prime during cardiopulmonary bypass (CPB), use of microcardioplegia systems, and ultrafiltration.
4. Miscellaneous: meticulous maintenance of surgical hemostasis and establishment of transfusion triggers.

Pharmacological Strategies

Antifibrinolytics

Aprotinin [2.0 million kallikrein inhibitory units (KIU) loading, 2.0 million KIU during CPB, and 0.5 million KIU/hour] is a kallikrein inhibitor that also inhibits soluble proteases involved in inflammation, including trypsin, plasmin, elastase, and thrombin. Lysine analogs such as tranexamic acid (50-100 mg/kg) or aminocaproic acid (10-15 g) administered after anesthesia induction are indicated to enhance hemostasis when fibrinolysis contributes to bleeding. Both lysine analogs attenuate fibrinolysis by inhibiting lysis of plasminogen to plasmin and, to a lesser degree, by directly inhibiting plasmin activity. Desmopressin, a synthetic analog of the natural pituitary hormone 8-D-arginine vasopressin, increases the release of von Willebrand factor into the blood and increases levels of antihemophilic Factor VIII activity in the plasma. The role of desmopressin (16-20 μg) in reducing blood loss in cardiac surgery is limited to postoperative use in patients with bleeding who are on preoperative acetylsalicylic acid or in patients with uremia.

Recently, Mangano et al,[15] in a nonrandomized, observational study of 4374 patients undergoing revascularization procedures, found an association between aprotinin and serious end-organ damage. The authors recommended using tranexamic acid and aminocaproic acid as safer and less expensive alternatives in reducing blood loss in cardiac surgery. Their findings of postoperative renal dysfunction associated with the use of aprotinin were supported by another single-center observational study on high-risk cardiac surgery patients.[16] In addition, the safety issue of aprotinin has been further questioned by a follow-up publication by Mangano et al[17] (on the same study population of 4374 patients) suggesting an increased 5-year mortality in patients who received aprotinin. These concerns are currently being addressed by various regulatory agencies in North America and Europe. Meanwhile, the Canadian prospective, randomized, controlled, multi-center trial of antifibrinolytics (Blood Conservation Using Antifibrinolytics: a Randomized Trial in a Cardiac Surgery Population, or BART) was prematurely terminated because of a trend toward increased mortality seen in patients who received aprotinin. Consequently, the US Food and Drug Administration requested that the manufacturer of aprotinin voluntarily suspend global marketing of the drug until the final analysis of this study is complete.[18]

Therefore, although the efficacy of aprotinin in reducing blood transfusion requirements in patients undergoing cardiac surgery has been well documented, it may be prudent to use other antifibrinolytic alternatives until concerns over its safety have been properly addressed. Tranexamic acid may be used for patients at high risk for bleeding (100 mg/kg) and for patients undergoing routine, first-time coronary artery bypass graft (CABG) (50 mg/kg). Also, aminocaproic acid may be given (5-9 g intravenously before skin incision, followed by 1 g/hour infusion for 6 hours).[19]

Recombinant Factor VIIa

Recombinant activated human coagulation Factor VIIa (rFVIIa) is a vitamin K-dependent glycoprotein that is structurally similar to human-plasma-derived Factor VIIa. At sites of vascular and microvascular injury, rFVIIa is believed to cause local thrombin generation and platelet recruitment.[20] Several reports of beneficial use in cardiac surgery patients with refractory bleeding have been published.[21] The off-label use of rFVIIa (35-70 µg/kg) may be considered in patients with excessive blood loss (>2 L or having received transfusion of >5 units of red cells), with ongoing blood loss (more than 200 cc/hour or inability to close the sternum), and with no surgical bleeding (further exploration or reexploration should be performed) and optimal coagulation—that is, international normalized ratio (INR), partial thromboplastin time (PTT), and fibrinogen should be corrected to at least 50% of normal.[19] Potential complications include myocardial infarction, deep vein thrombosis, pulmonary embolism, and anastomotic or vascular occlusion.[22,23]

Fibrin Sealants

In cardiac surgery, fibrin glues have been used to improve hemostasis, decrease blood transfusions, improve tissue handling, and pretreat vascular grafts. They generally contain two main components: fibrinogen (with or without Factor XIII) and thrombin (plus calcium with or without antifibrinolytic drugs), which can be applied to the bleeding area using a single- or dual-syringe system either in liquid or aerosol format. They mimic the final stage of the clotting cascade through the activation of fibrinogen to thrombin. A meta-analysis by Carless et al demonstrated that fibrin sealants are efficacious in reducing both postoperative blood loss and perioperative exposure to allogeneic red cell transfusion.[24] However, because of the lack of blinding, transfusion practices may have been influenced by knowledge of the patient's treatment status.

Mechanical Strategies

Enhanced Coagulation Monitoring

Monitoring heparin anticoagulation and protamine reversal has been traditionally performed by the use of activated clotting times (ACTs). However, ACT does not correlate well with anti-Xa measures of heparin activity or with heparin concentration, especially with hypothermia and hemodilution during CPB.[25] Other limitations of the celite-activated ACT include its prolongation in the presence of aprotinin and drugs that inhibit platelet glycoproteins IIb and IIIa and its tendency to decrease with surgical stress. The most common point-of-care laboratory technique to measure whole blood heparin concentration is a protamine titration assay called Hepcon (Medtronic, Parker, CO). Thromboelastography assesses clot strength over time; clot strength is a factor of platelet number or function, fibrinogen, and Factor XIII cross-linking. Excess protamine will inhibit clot formation, although insufficient protamine will not fully antagonize heparin. Therefore, the channel with the fastest clot formation will represent the protamine concentration that optimally neutralizes the existing heparin.[25] Such point-of-care testing helps identify patients who could benefit from pharmacologic interventions and those who have a surgical source of bleeding, where coagulation tests are relatively normal despite excessive bleeding.

Acute Normovolemic Hemodilution

The use of intraoperative ANH has been shown to be effective and cheaper than PAD for decreasing perioperative allogeneic transfusion requirements.[2,26] Hemodilution lowers the red cell mass of blood shed during surgery. Whole blood contains clotting factors that would normally be lost with surgical bleeding. Hemodilution should be performed before the onset of surgical bleeding and CPB. During hemodilution, the platelets in blood are protected from the harmful effects of CPB. A study by Van der Linden et al shows that the use of hydroxyethyl starch or modified fluid gelatin for volume expansion did not differ in measured blood loss and transfusion needs.[27] Nonetheless, the efficacy of ANH is controversial.

Segal et al[28] showed that ANH was only moderately effective, reducing transfusions by 10% or 1 to 2 units less than the comparator group. However, an important development may suggest that the role of ANH be revisited: the ability to separate blood collected in the operating room into individual components, such as red cells, platelet-rich plasma, and platelet-poor plasma. This separation allows components to be returned individually, as indicated—preferably after CPB. Furthermore, Licker et al demonstrated that, in addition to conventional myocardial preservation techniques, prebypass ANH achieved further cardiac protection in patients undergoing on-pump myocardial revascularization.[29] Compared with conventional management, prebypass ANH was associated with lower postoperative release of biomarkers of myocardial damage, reduced requirements for inotropic support, and fewer arrhythmias or conduction abnormalities. Increased serum erythropoietin levels triggered by prebypass ANH may be responsible for these findings and represent an alternative mechanism for immediate and delayed cardioprotection.

Blood Recovery

Nitescu et al estimated that more than 75% of the blood lost during cardiac surgery can be recovered and returned to the patient.[30] At the termination of CPB, a significant volume of blood remains in the extracorporeal circuit. This blood can be recovered for retransfusion to the patient using either direct retransfusion of the heparinized, diluted blood or retransfusion after the blood has been washed and concentrated using a cell-saver device.

Transfusion of unprocessed blood has been associated with increases in blood loss and inflammatory mediators.[31] Use of a cell-saver device not only significantly reduces the volume of blood retransfused but also increases the hematocrit to 55% to 60%, which is also free of unbound heparin. Unfortunately, this is achieved with the concurrent removal of all clotting factors. Although it has been shown that there is no significant difference in postoperative hematocrit when either method of retransfusion of the post-CPB circuit volume is used, patients who received the unprocessed blood had significantly greater post-operative blood loss in the intensive care unit (ICU) and received significantly more allogeneic red cell transfusions.[32]

Ultrafiltration and modified ultrafiltration have been demonstrated to reduce blood transfusions following cardiac surgery.[33,34] Advantages of ultrafiltration are that the blood 1) can be processed after CPB and returned to the patient, 2) is volume reduced with a high hematocrit, and 3) retains clotting factors. Its main disadvantage is that the blood still contains a significant amount of heparin. However, Eichert et al found no difference in postoperative blood loss when they compared ultrafiltration with either direct infusion of CPB circuit volume or blood that had been washed before retransfusion.[34] The Hemobag (Global Blood Resources, Somers, CT), specifically designed for ultrafiltration circuit recovery following CPB, effectively produces a product that includes a high concentration of red cells and plasma proteins, including clotting factors and fibrinogen.[35] It has been successfully used in the management of a Jehovah's Witness patient undergoing cardiac surgery.[36]

Postoperative autotransfusion of shed mediastinal blood has mixed results in decreasing blood use. Washing of mediastinal blood that has high hemolytic red cell alterations and high fibrinolytic activity is an alternative to direct reinfusion. Murphy et al[37] compared patients who received either washed intraoperative recovered fluid and postoperative shed mediastinal fluid or allogeneic blood transfusion. Patients in the autotransfused groups not only had a significant reduction in allogeneic blood exposure but also showed no greater derangement of their clotting profiles compared to patients who received allogeneic transfusion.[37]

Intraoperative and postoperative blood recovery has had widespread success in cardiac surgery by significantly reducing the need for autologous transfusion. Its use is limited to the time before heparinization and after protamine administration.[10] Blood recovery is most beneficial when the blood loss is >1 L and when >750 cc of recovered blood is infused.[2]

Harmonic Scalpel

The Harmonic Scalpel was designed to reduce tissue trauma, facilitate dissection, and improve surgical hemostasis. It uses ultrasonic energy to achieve both cutting and coagulation simultaneously, with minimal lateral thermal damage. Although initially used mainly for harvesting of arterial conduits (internal mammary artery[38] and radial artery[39]), it has recently been shown to be associated with better in-hospital outcomes and reduced perioperative blood loss in patients undergoing redo cardiac surgical procedures.[40] Luciani et al showed that by reducing microvascular hemorrhage, the Harmonic Scalpel contributed to decreased blood loss and reduced length of the initial dissection and post-CPB hemostasis phases in redo operations.[40] These results were, in turn, associated with reduced postoperative blood loss and returns to the operating room for bleeding.

An additional advantage is that the Harmonic Scalpel can be used safely in patients with an implanted pacemaker.[41] Future studies are required to address its possible use in patients with a preoperative coagulation disorder. Its main disadvantage is that the device is expensive, but benefits related to lower morbidity and improved postoperative course with reduced length of stay in ICU may outweigh any initial cost of the equipment, especially for redo procedures.

Cardiopulmonary Bypass Strategies

Minimally Invasive Surgical Technique

CBP increases the risk of bleeding by several mechanisms. It causes coagulation factor reduction and dilution, platelet dysfunction, and fibrinolysis. Residual heparinization is also a factor. Therefore, avoiding CPB by performing OPCAB surgery has been promoted to reduce such complications as hemodilution and coagulation deficits and their effect on transfusion requirements. In a meta-analysis of all randomized, controlled trials that compared conventional CPB with OPCAB, Cheng et al reported that OPCAB showed a significant reduction in transfusion rates.[42] Despite this improvement, approximately 25% of OPCAB patients still require allogeneic blood transfusion.[43]

The use of additional blood management strategies with OPCAB has been shown to significantly reduce the need for allogeneic transfusion. Goel et al[44] demonstrated that the use of a blood recovery device during OPCAB reduced the requirement for blood transfusion. In addition, the postoperative hemoglobin concentration was significantly higher in the treated group. The mean volume of blood retransfused was 714 mL. Furthermore, autotransfusion of the washed red cells was not associated with excessive bleeding in the postoperative period.[44] Other blood management strategies that have been used during OPCAB surgery include the use of tranexamic acid[45] and moderate ANH.[46] When combining the use of moderate ANH, tranexamic acid, and the intraoperative retransfusion of washed and processed red cells, Casati et al reduced their transfusion rate in patients undergoing OPCAB from 20% to 4%.[46]

Cardiopulmonary Bypass Circuit

Strategies that are safe and that can decrease transfusion requirements include the use of centrifugal pumps, membrane oxygenators, less traumatic aortic clamping, individualized anticoagulation protocols, improved cardioplegic techniques, and heparin-bonded circuits, plus the elimination of cardiotomy suction and the use of minimal prime volumes with autologous priming.[47] Heparin-coated circuits combined with low systemic heparinization have shown encouraging but inconclusive results in the reduction of postoperative bleeding and blood transfusions. Low systemic heparinization is mostly recommended for first-time CABG patients.[48]

Recently, a mini-extracorporeal circulation [MECC (Jostra AG, Hirrlingen, Germany)] has been introduced to minimize the hemodiluting effect of the conventional extracorporeal circuit.[49]

MECC consists of a minimal priming volume (reduced to 500 mL in place of the 1600 to 2000 mL of the conventional CPB circuit), a heparin-coated closed circuit, a centrifugal pump, an active drainage system, and a blood recovery device. Blood loss and blood requirements for red cell transfusion have been shown to be significantly reduced by using this mini-circuit compared to both OPCAB and conventional CABG techniques.[49] A similar system, PRECiSe (priming reduced extracorporeal circulation setup), has also been associated with a significantly reduced (10% vs 34%) requirement for blood transfusion.[50]

In addition, large volumes of cardioplegia can lead to a significant reduction in the hematocrit during CPB, especially in patients with a small red cell volume. A microplegia system [Quest MPS (Microplegia System), Quest Medical Inc, Allen, TX] has recently been introduced into the CPB circuit at the authors' institution (microplegia is blood cardioplegia without the crystalloid), where it has reduced the mean cardioplegia volume from 700 mL to 140 mL. It also offers tighter potassium and glucose control during CPB.

Retrograde Autologous Priming

Retrograde autologous priming (RAP) of the CPB circuit was developed to minimize hemodilution and, in turn, decrease allogeneic red cell transfusion. After placement of the arterial and venous cannulae, approximately 800 to 1000 mL of the crystalloid prime is displaced with the patient's own circulating blood volume immediately before CPB.

RAP can potentially improve postoperative outcomes by maintaining a higher hematocrit during CPB, thereby reducing intraoperative and postoperative red cell transfusions, and by attenuating the fall in colloid osmotic pressure on initiation of CPB.[51] Although its effectiveness in reducing allogeneic blood transfusion rates is controversial, it has been shown not to produce any increase in perioperative adverse events.[52]

Transfusion Threshold

Meticulous surgical technique plays a vital role in minimizing intraoperative blood loss. In addition, adhering to a transfusion threshold, when appropriate, represents the most cost-effective means of safely decreasing allogeneic exposure. The decision to transfuse a patient should not be based on an arbitrary hemoglobin or hematocrit level (the so-called transfusion trigger) but instead on the patient's clinical condition and comorbidities. Maintenance of normovolemia with colloid infusions to promote tissue oxygenation is essential if the patient is to tolerate a significant degree of anemia. Limited knowledge regarding tolerance of anemia in patients undergoing cardiac surgery has limited advancement in this area. Bracey et al demonstrated the safety of a hemoglobin level of 80 g/L or more in cardiac patients.[53] However, there is an independent, direct association between the degree of hemodilution during CPB and the risk of perioperative stroke[54] and acute renal failure (when hematocrit = 0.21-0.25).[55] One possible effective strategy for reducing transfusion rates would be to avoid transfusion until a critical level for oxygen delivery has been reached. Sehgal et al monitored the oxygen extraction ratio (O_2ER) in patients undergoing CABG surgery and showed that only 15% to 36% of their patients in the transfused group would have been transfused if the O_2ER cutoff had been used.[56]

Postoperative Management

Postoperative bleeding may be caused by platelet dysfunction, coagulation factor depletion or dilution, hypofibrinogenemia, thrombocytopenia, residual heparinization, and fibrinolysis. It is essential to ensure that the patient is normothermic. Fluid warmers and warming blankets should be used. Coagulopathies should be monitored and corrected as dictated by the INR, PTT, and fibrinogen levels. Excessive bleeding in the presence of normal coagulation levels suggests the possibility of surgical bleeding, and reexploration should be considered. Anemia should be treated according to the appropriate transfusion trigger. The use of algorithms to direct blood transfusion strategies in patients after cardiac surgery has been shown to reduce unnecessary exposure to blood components.[57]

Conclusion

Cardiac surgery is being performed with more complex procedures on patients who are older and more critically ill than before. With the dwindling blood supply, the high economic costs of blood transfusion, and the ongoing transfusion risks to the patient despite optimal blood screening, it is vital to maintain as a goal a multidisciplinary team approach that reduces or eliminates perioperative blood transfusions in cardiac surgical patients.

References

1. Stover EP, Siegel LC, Parks R, et al. Variability in transfusion practice for coronary artery bypass surgery persists despite national consensus guidelines: A 24-institution study. Institutions of the Multicenter Study of Perioperative Ischemia Research Group. Anesthesiology 1998;88:327-33.
2. Goodnough LT, Johnston MF, Toy PT. The variability of transfusion practice in coronary artery bypass surgery. Transfusion Medicine Academic Award Group. JAMA 1991;265:86-90.
3. Cosgrove DM, Loop FD, Lytle BW, et al. Determinants of blood utilization during myocardial revascularization. Ann Thorac Surg 1985;40:380-4.
4. Magovern JA, Sakert T, Benckart DH, et al. A model for predicting transfusion after coronary artery bypass grafting. Ann Thorac Surg 1996;61:27-32.
5. Moskowitz DM, Klein JJ, Shander A, et al. Predictors of transfusion requirements for cardiac surgical procedures at a blood conservation center. Ann Thorac Surg 2004;77:626-34.
6. Karksi JM, Mathieu M, Cheng D, et al. Etiology of preoperative anemia in patients undergoing scheduled cardiac surgery. Can J Anaesth 1999;46:979-82.
7. Helm RE, Gold JP, Rosengart TK, et al. Erythropoietin in cardiac surgery. J Card Surg 1993;8:579-606.

8. Laupacis A, Fergusson D. Erythropoietin to minimize perioperative blood transfusion: A systematic review of randomized trials. The International Study of Peri-operative Transfusion (ISPOT) Investigators. Transfus Med 1998;8: 309-17.

9. Alghamdi AA, Albanna MJ, Guru V, et al. Does the use of erythropoietin reduce the risk of exposure to allogeneic blood transfusion in cardiac surgery? A systematic review and meta-analysis. J Card Surg 2006;21:320-6.

10. Etchason J, Petz L, Keeler E, et al. The cost effectiveness of preoperative autologous blood donations. N Engl J Med 1995;332:740-2.

11. Shander A, Rijhwani TS. Clinical outcomes in cardiac surgery: Conventional surgery versus bloodless surgery. Anesthesiol Clin North Am 2005;23: 327-45.

12. Richardson G, Curzen NP, Preston MA, et al. Failure to monitor ticlopidine: The case for clopidogrel. Int J Cardiovasc Intervent 2000;3:29-33.

13. Cheng DKF, Jackevicius CA. Safety of glycoprotein IIb/IIIa inhibitors in urgent or emergency coronary artery bypass graft surgery. Can J Cardiol 2004;20: 223-8.

14. Akowuah E, Shrivastava V, Jamnadas B, et al. Comparison of two strategies for the management of antiplatelet therapy during urgent surgery. Ann Thorac Surg 2005;80:149-52.

15. Mangano DT, Tudor IC, Dietzel C, et al. The risk associated with aprotinin in cardiac surgery. N Engl J Med 2006;354:353-65.

16. Karkouti K, Beattie WS, Dattilo KM, et al. A propensity score case-control comparison of aprotinin and tranexamic acid in high-transfusion-risk cardiac surgery. Transfusion 2006;46:327-38.

17. Mangano DT, Miao Y, Vuylsteke A, et al. Mortality associated with aprotinin during 5 years following coronary artery bypass graft surgery. JAMA 2007; 297:471-9.

18. Food and Drug Administration. Early communication about an ongoing safety review: Aprotinin injection (marketed as Trasylol). (October 25, 2007) Rockville, MD: Center for Drug Evaluation and Research, 2007. [Available at http://www.fda.gov/cder/drug/early_comm/aprotinin.htm (accessed January 10, 2008).]

19. Karksi JM, Karkouti K. Antifibrinolytics and coagulation management. In: Cheng DCH, David TE, eds. Perioperative care in cardiac anesthesia and surgery. Philadelphia: Lippincott Williams & Wilkins, 2006:165-71.

20. Levy JH. Overview of clinical efficacy and safety of pharmacologic strategies for blood conservation. Am J Health Syst Pharm 2005;62:S15-S19.

21. Tanaka KA, Waly AA, Cooper WA, Levy JH. Treatment of excessive bleeding in Jehovah's Witness patients after cardiac surgery with recombinant Factor VIIa (NovoSeven). Anesthesiology 2003;98:1513-5.

22. Rosenfeld SB, Watkinson KK, Thompson BH, et al. Pulmonary embolism after sequential use of recombinant factor VIIa and activated prothrombin complex concentrate in a factor VIII inhibitor patient. Thromb Haemost 2002;87:925-6.

23. Brown JL, Varma S, Morgan Hughes NJ, Rocco G. Thrombosis related to emergency Factor VIIa treatment. Anaesthesia 2003;58:1245.

24. Carless PA, Anthony DM, Henry DA. Systematic review of the use of fibrin sealant to minimize perioperative allogeneic blood transfusion. Br J Surg 2002;89:695-703.

25. Shore-Lesserson L. Evidence-based coagulation monitors: Heparin monitoring, thromboelastography, and platelet function. Semin Cardiothorac Vasc Anesth 2005;9:41-52.

26. Roberts WA, Kirkley SA, Newby M. A cost comparison of allogeneic and pre-operatively or intraoperatively donated autologous blood. Anesth Analg 1996;83:129-33.

27. Van der Linden PJ, De Hert SC, Deraedt D, et al. Hydroxyethyl starch 130/0.4 versus modified fluid gelatin for volume expansion in cardiac surgery patients: The effects on perioperative bleeding and transfusion needs. Anesth Analg 2005;101:629-34.

28. Segal JB, Blasco-Colmenares E, Norris EJ, et al. Preoperative acute normovolemic hemodilution: A meta-analysis. Transfusion 2004;44:632-44.

29. Licker M, Ellenberger C, Sierra J, et al. Cardioprotective effects of acute normovolemic hemodilution in patients undergoing coronary artery bypass surgery. Chest 2005;128:838-47.

30. Nitescu N, Bengtsson A, Bengtson JP, et al. Blood salvage with a continuous autotransfusion system compared with a haemofiltration system. Perfusion 2002;17:357-62.

31. Daane CR, Golab HD, Meeder JHJ, et al. Processing and transfusion of residual cardiopulmonary bypass volume: Effects on hemostasis, complement activation, postoperative blood loss and transfusion volume. Perfusion 2003;18:115-21.

32. Walporth BH, Eggensperger N, Hauser SP, et al. Effects of unprocessed and processed cardiopulmonary bypass blood retransfused into patients after cardiac surgery. Int J Artif Organs 1999;22:210-16.

33. Boodhwani M, Williams K, Babaev A, et al. Ultrafiltration reduces blood transfusions following cardiac surgery: A meta-analysis. Eur J Cardiothorac Surg 2006;30:892-7.

34. Eichert I, Isgrof F, Kiessling AH, et al. Cell saver, ultrafiltration and direct transfusion. Comparative study of three blood processing techniques. J Thorac Cardiovasc Surg 2001;49:149-52.

35. Roeder B, Graham S, Searles B. Evaluation of the Hemobag. A novel ultrafiltration system for circuit salvage. J Extra Corpor Technol 2004;36:162-5.

36. Moskowitz DM, Klein JJ, Shander A, et al. Use of the Hemobag for modified ultrafiltration in a Jehovah's Witness patient undergoing cardiac surgery. J Extra Corpor Technol 2006; 38:265-70.

37. Murphy GJ, Allen SM, Unsworth-White J, et al. Safety and efficacy of perioperative cell salvage and autotransfusion after coronary artery bypass grafting: A randomized trial. Ann Thorac Surg 2004;77:1553-9.

38. Lamm P, Juchem G, Weyrich P, et al. The Harmonic Scalpel: Optimizing the quality of mammary artery bypass grafts. Ann Thorac Surg 2000;69:1833-5.

39. Ronan JW, Perry LA, Barner HB, et al. Radial artery harvest: Comparison of ultrasonic dissection with standard technique. Ann Thorac Surg 2000;69:113-14.

40. Luciani N, Anselmi A, Gaudino M, et al. Harmonic Scalpel reduces bleeding postoperative complications in redo cardiac surgery. Ann Thorac Surg 2005; 80:934-8.

41. Qzeren M, Dogan OV, Duzgun C, et al. Use of an ultrasonic scalpel in the open-heart reoperation of a patient with pacemaker. Eur J Cardiothorac Surg 2002; 21:761-2.

42. Cheng DC, Bainbridge D, Martin JE, et al. Does off-pump coronary artery bypass reduce mortality, morbidity, and resource utilization when compared with conventional coronary artery bypass? A meta-analysis of randomized trials. Anesthesiology 2005;102:188-203.

43. Ascione R, Williams S, Lloyd CT, et al. Reduced postoperative blood loss and transfusion requirement after beating heart coronary operations: A prospective randomized study. J Thorac Cardiovasc Surg 2001;121:689-96.

44. Goel P, Pannu H, Mohan D, et al. Efficacy of cell saver in reducing homologous blood transfusion during OPCAB surgery: A prospective randomized trial. Transfus Med 2007;17:285-9.

45. Murphy GJ, Mango E, Lucchetti V, et al. A randomized trial of tranexamic acid in combination with cell salvage plus a meta-analysis of randomized trials evaluating tranexamic acid in off-pump coronary artery bypass grafting. J Thorac Cardiovasc Surg 2006;132:475-80.

46. Casati V, Benussi S, Sandrelli L, et al. Intraoperative moderate acute normo-volemic hemodilution associated with a comprehensive blood-sparing protocol in off-pump coronary surgery. Anesth Analg 2004;98:1217-23.

47. Borowiec JW, Bozdayi M, Jaramillo A, et al. Influence of two blood conservation techniques (cardiotomy reservoir versus cell-saver) on biocompatibility of the heparin coated cardiopulmonary bypass circuit during coronary revascularization surgery. J Card Surg 1997;12:190-7.

48. Ovrum E, Tangen G, Oystese R, et al. Comparison of two heparin-coated extracorporeal circuits with reduced systemic anticoagulation in routine coronary artery bypass operations. J Thorac Cardiovasc Surg 2001;121:324-30.

49. Gerritsen WB, van Boven WJ, Wesselink RM, et al. Significant reduction in blood loss in patients undergoing minimal extracorporeal circulation. Transfus Med 2006;16:329-34.

50. Beholz S, Zheng L, Kessler M, et al. A new PRECiSe (priming reduced extracorporeal circulation setup) minimizes the need for blood transfusions: First clinical results in coronary bypass grafting. Heart Surg Forum 2005;8:E132-5.

51. Rosengart TK, DeBois W, O'Hara M, et al. Retrograde autologous priming for cardiopulmonary bypass: A safe and effective means of decreasing hemodilution and transfusion requirements. J Thorac Cardiovasc Surg 1998;115:426-39.

52. Murphy GS, Szokol JW, Nitsun M, et al. Retrograde autologous priming of the cardiopulmonary bypass circuit: Safety and impact on postoperative outcomes. J Cardiothorac Vasc Anesth 2006; 20:156-161.

53. Bracey AW, Radovancevic R, Riggs SA, et al. Lowering the hemoglobin threshold for transfusion in coronary artery bypass procedures: Effect on patient outcome. Transfusion 1999;39:1070-7.

54. Karkouti K, Djaiani G, Borger MA, et al. Low hematocrit during cardiopulmonary bypass is associated with increased risk of perioperative stroke in cardiac surgery. Ann Thorac Surg 2005;80:1381-7.
55. Karkouti K, Beattie WS, Wijeysundera DN, et al. Hemodilution during cardiopulmonary bypass is an independent risk factor for acute renal failure in adult cardiac surgery. J Thorac Cardiovasc Surg 2005;129:391-400.
56. Sehgal LR, Zebala LP, Takagi I, et al. Evaluation of oxygen extraction ratio as a physiologic transfusion trigger in coronary artery bypass graft surgery patients. Transfusion 2001;41:591-5.
57. Avidan MS, Alcock EL, DaFonseca J, et al. Comparison of structured use of routine laboratory tests or near-patient assessment with clinical judgement in the management of bleeding after cardiac surgery. Br J Anaesth 2004;92:178-86.

Index